Your Blood Never Lies

HOW TO READ A BLOOD TEST FOR A LONGER, HEALTHIER LIFE

James B. LaValle, RPh, CCN

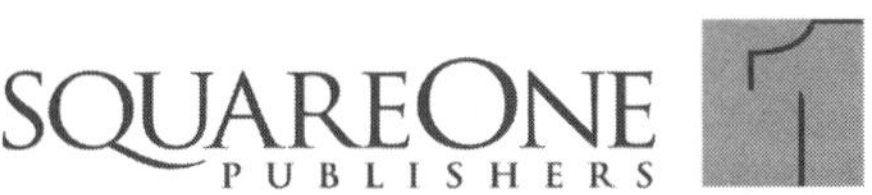

EDITOR: Colleen Day
COVER DESIGNER: Jeannie Tudor
TYPESETTER: Gary A. Rosenberg

The information and advice contained in this book are based upon the research and the personal and professional experiences of the author. They are not intended as a substitute for consulting with a health care professional. The publisher and author are not responsible for any adverse effects or consequences resulting from the use of any of the suggestions, preparations, or procedures discussed in this book. All matters pertaining to your physical health should be supervised by a health care professional. It is a sign of wisdom, not cowardice, to seek a second or third opinion.

Square One Publishers
115 Herricks Road
Garden City Park, NY 11040
(516) 535-2010 • (877) 900-BOOK
www.squareonepublishers.com

Library of Congress Cataloging-in-Publication Data

LaValle, James B.
Your blood never lies : how to read a blood test for a longer, healthier life / James B. LaValle, RPH, CCN, ND.
pages cm
Includes bibliographical references and index.
ISBN 978-0-7570-0350-9 — ISBN 0-7570-0350-8
1. Blood—Analysis—Popular works. I. Title.
RB45.L38 2013
616.07'561--dc23
2013002400

Printed in the United States of America

10 9 8 7 6 5 4 3 2 1

Contents

Part 4 Complete Blood Count

Part 5 Hormones

Part 6 Optional Tests

I dedicate this book to my mother, Freda LaValle,
a witty and caring woman who dedicated her life to the service of others
and made me the person I am today;
to my good friend and colleague, Ernie Hawkins,
who has worked by my side writing
and educating for almost twenty years;
and finally, to my wife and colleague, Laura,
a woman with endless patience who has always been my safe harbor.

Acknowledgments

Several people were involved in putting this book together and bringing it (finally) to fruition. First, I must thank Rudy Shur, the publisher, for his unwavering persistence. I am also grateful for the hard work of Colleen Day, Michael Weatherhead, Ernie Hawkins, Laura LaValle, Rich Mintzer, Marcy Peyser Friedman, Cheryl Kimball, and many others.

Foreword

The world has become a very uncertain place. Rising healthcare costs, political unrest, market downturns, and environmental concerns have created a sense of unpredictability. It is not unreasonable to ask, "What could have been done differently?" For example, were there early warning signs in the mortgage loan crisis that, if detected and acted upon, could have prevented thousands from losing their homes and a $1 billion government bailout?

Our bodies are no different. When physical or psychological symptoms reach crisis, our medical system intervenes swiftly through the use of medications or surgery. But just as the real estate crisis did not miraculously occur overnight, a person does not suddenly wake up one day with diabetes. All major chronic illnesses develop over years, sometimes decades, with minor imbalances evolving into serious abnormalities. But we do not have to wait for a diagnosis to know where our health is headed. Science has learned a tremendous amount about "trends" in physiologic markers that signal impending illness. *Your Blood Never Lies* is a comprehensive manual and guide designed to help people recognize and understand these markers in blood tests, as well as the meanings behind them. In other words, this book places the knowledge—and even the responsibility—in the public domain.

As a physician who has practiced integrative medicine for over twenty years, I have learned to listen to my patients. After all, they are the ones who live in their bodies, so they know what feels normal, and they can often detect subtle shifts in their health long before standard laboratory values become abnormal. Still, normal is not always optimal. And when objective data is viewed through the lens of optimal health and functioning, biological markers can assume a whole new set of meaning and value for both patients and physicians. In this sense, what a person feels as "sub-normal" can actually be detected in laboratory data as "sub-optimal." The power of this book is that it links subjective symptoms to objective data and validates what the patient often already knows—that their health is trending in the wrong direction.

The process of teaching patients about how their bodies work, as well as what is considered normal and abnormal—and more importantly optimal—is key in leveling the playing field between doctors and patients. *Your Blood Never Lies* puts power back in the hands of the patient, facilitates his or her understanding of major issues related to health and illness, and provides a reliable, valid framework for treatment decisions.

I have known Jim LaValle for a number of years now. He is a brilliant clinician and thought-leader who has helped mainstream the notion that health matters as much as illness; that nutrition, lifestyle, and natural products have a rightful place alongside conventional treatments like drugs and surgery; and that there are only two forms of medicine—good and bad. This book reflects his vision for a more humane, interactive, and collegial medical system, and one that is not afraid to place important information in the hands of the public about how the human body works, and what patients can do independently or in collaboration with their doctors. This is an important and timely work that not only makes sense of often confusing and unpredictable symptoms for patients, but also serves as a comprehensive guide to better health.

Andrew Heyman, MD, MHSA
Aldie, VA

Preface

Today, more and more people are taking an interest in their health and becoming active participants in guiding their healthcare. Our present health, as well as its future, relies in large part on self-directed care. After all, who is more invested in your health than you? In fact, personalized medicine in the United States is predicted to exceed $300 billion over the next five years. But while an ever-growing number of people are taking up exercises like yoga, Zumba, and CrossFit, as well as incorporating healthier foods into their diet, many individuals still do not understand some core aspects of health—like the blood.

A blood test is one of the best methods of self care available today. Routine blood testing can provide an accurate picture of not only your current health, but also your future. Even if you eat right, exercise, and eliminate bad habits, you may have an underlying medical condition, nutritional deficiency, or hormone imbalance that only a blood test can detect. As the title of this book asserts, your blood never lies.

Unfortunately, many patients ignore the blood test results they receive in the mail after their annual physical, particularly if their doctor informs them that everything is "normal." The fact of the matter is that "normal" is not always healthy, and certainly not optimal. Historically, blood test results were rarely discussed and recommendations were not made until particular blood values crossed the threshold into the "abnormal," or "out of range," category. In other words, patients have traditionally been told to change their ways only after a disease, disorder, or some other condition has already developed in their bodies.

This book is designed to help change that. *Your Blood Never Lies* will teach you how to interpret your blood test results, and in some cases, patterns that may indicate whether you are at risk for certain conditions in the future. I believe that lab values should be viewed in a similar way to stock market trends. The model used in the business world is predictive. When asked to report on the financial health of a company, an analyst usually points to no fewer than five or six factors indicative of the direction in which the business is headed. By contrast, even though it's common knowledge that chronic conditions like heart disease, diabetes, and cancer develop over many years, the medical field has mainly focused on identifying disease rather than predicting a patient's risk of developing it. Furthermore, incorporating lifestyle and general wellness as part of medicine's continuum of care is still in its infancy.

Thankfully, there is now a growing awareness of the importance of blood tests in preventive care as well as overall health. This change is due in large part to groundbreaking studies like the Kaiser Permanente Study, which revealed that prediabetic conditions can be present even when an individual's blood test is technically normal. Disturbing findings such as these have led more doctors and healthcare professionals to use blood tests as preventive tools and closely evaluate the results, including those in the "normal range." Patients, too, are learning the importance of certain blood markers like cholesterol and triglycerides in assessing cardiovascular health, for example. At the same time, however, most people have never even heard of lab values like homocysteine and blood urea nitrogen (BUN), let alone understood their implications for health.

The good news is that this can change. Recently, my company, Integrative Health Resources, teamed up with Life Time Fitness and Health Check USA to help their members understand the central role that blood tests play in preventing disease as well as optimizing health. Trained healthcare professionals educate clients on positive changes in diet, behavior, and stress response, as well as enhance their knowledge of nutrition and the proper use of dietary supplements, guiding them to understand lab values and trends. This is a truly groundbreaking program, as Life Time Fitness has some 1.2 million members. In fact, it may be the first organized effort of its kind to change the lifestyles of over a million people. I commend Braham Acrotti, the CEO of Life Time Fitness, for broadening the company's focus to include not only physical fitness, but also a wide range of other factors that contribute to a healthy lifestyle, transforming them into the "Healthy Way of Life Company."

In a world with rising rates of chronic disease, it's more important than ever for health-focused institutions to adopt prevention and wellness models. But of equal importance is the need for individuals to be proactive when it comes to matters of health. This begins with having a blood test and, more importantly, understanding the results. By making sense of the various numbers printed on your lab report, you will be able to take the steps necessary to improve your health and, hopefully, steer clear of a future medical condition. When it comes to well-being, your blood is the key to a wealth of information—and it never lies.

INTRODUCTION

A New View of You

If you're like most people, a blood test is an event that comes once a year along with your annual physical. Ideally, within a week, your doctor calls with the results, assuring you that they are normal. You may even receive a copy of the test in the mail, complete with columns of numbers supposedly confirming your health, but to you are probably meaningless and confusing. So you put the results aside, file them away with your other personal records, and carry on with your life free of concern. After all, the doctor says you are in the "normal range," so why worry? While this may be the case, blood tests still raise important questions that even the healthiest of patients should be asking: Does "normal" necessarily mean "healthy"? What can the lab values of a blood test tell you about the current state of your health? And, perhaps more importantly, what can these lab values tell you about your health in the future?

The fact is, blood testing generally has one purpose, and that is to check for disorders, dysfunction, and disease. When blood test results point to a certain condition, measures are taken to bring the appropriate number—the abnormal lab value—into the "normal" range. However, when test results are normal, only rarely is a patient told how to stay in this range or, better yet, how to achieve an optimal, or target, level. It becomes a matter of waiting for the other shoe to drop, leading up to the day when you walk into the doctor's office or pick up the phone and are told, "You are diabetic" or "You have a thyroid disorder." But it does not have to be this way.

A blood test is essentially a blueprint of your health and a glimpse of its future. It tells you so much about what is going on inside your body, and it can speak volumes about what *may* go on inside of it somewhere down the line. The information obtained from lab results can push you to take the needed steps to put (or keep) your health on the right track. A blood test can motivate you to change your dietary habits, start a fitness regimen, or alter certain aspects of your lifestyle, such as your stress level and sleep patterns. A blood test can also be precautionary, helping you to monitor conditions that may be a running concern in your family or personal medical history. If you are already being treated for a particular condition, a blood test is one of the best ways to ensure that your medication is doing its job. In sum, a blood test is a quantitative way of measuring your health so that you can manage it more effectively and easily. But before you can begin to interpret your test results, you should know a thing or two about the blood testing procedure, as well as certain factors that may influence the outcome.

THE BASICS OF BLOOD TESTING

A *blood test* is a common medical procedure in which a small amount of blood is drawn from the body using a needle, which is usually inserted into a vein in the arm. The blood sample is then analyzed by a lab technician to check for any sign or risk of disease, organ dysfunction, nutritional deficiency, or other problem. The technician may examine whole blood or separate the blood cells from the fluid in which they are contained, which is known as the *serum* or *plasma*. The plasma is used to measure levels of various substances in the blood and determine whether or not they fall into the *normal range*. This range is based on the *average* values reported in 95 percent of healthy people of a certain group and, therefore, may vary according to factors such as age, sex, and ethnicity. The reference ranges for normal, high, and low lab values may vary among laboratories depending on the methodology used by the blood analysts. The ranges used in this book reflect the guidelines set by LabCorp, a company that provides testing services to nearly 90 percent of doctors' offices, hospitals, and other medical institutions. (See "A Guide to Reference Ranges" on page 323 for a listing of LabCorp reference ranges.) However, some labs may use slightly different ranges, so you should take this into account when reviewing your blood test results.

Standard blood tests are not always completely accurate. There are a number of factors that may artificially cause your blood levels to fall outside the normal range, resulting in an abnormal reading or false-positive result. Certain foods, physical activity, alcohol and caffeine consumption, and some medications affect metabolism and overall body function, and thus may influence blood test results. Failing to follow pretesting instructions, such as fasting, can also produce abnormal results. By the same token, standard blood tests can indicate normal blood levels when a disease or other condition is actually present, or a false-negative result. The bottom line is that abnormal results may, but do not always, indicate a health problem. If your results show an abnormality, do not panic. Your physician will probably recommend more specific blood tests, which have a higher rate of accuracy.

In general, a blood test is quick and requires little preparation. If you are unfamiliar with the procedure or if it has been a long time since your last blood test, here is a rundown of what you can expect before, during, and after the test.

Before the Blood Test

One of the most common questions people have about blood tests is whether or not they can eat beforehand. Most healthcare professionals recommend fasting for approximately eight hours prior to a blood test. To "fast" generally means to abstain from food and beverages, especially coffee, tea, and alcohol. These liquids in particular should not be in your system for ten to twelve hours before the test, as they can skew readings. However, fasting does not include water, which you should continue to drink not only to prevent dehydration, but also the lightheaded and dizzy feeling that may accompany the loss of even a small amount of blood. If your doctor or health practitioner does not mention fasting, it is best to ask, as it may be advisable to fast for more than eight hours to ensure the accuracy of certain tests.

Pretest preparations may also be tailored to a specific health concern, such as triglycerides or blood sugar. If you are worried that your triglycerides level is high, you may want to avoid fatty foods the day before the test, as these can artificially raise the fat content of your blood and cause a high reading. Even a seemingly harmless food such as salad dressing (unless it is fat-free) can inflate your triglycerides level. If you are concerned about high blood sugar, refrain from eating foods rich in carbohydrates the day before the test, since they remain in your system longer than other foods.

Still, many of your blood levels will not change significantly in the short term, especially if your body is functioning normally. Fasting has the greatest impact on blood sugar, insulin, and triglycerides, so stay away from foods and liquids that can temporarily raise these levels. Keep in mind, though, that there are many blood tests that may require special preparation, so always inquire ahead of time about pretesting instructions. Finally, be sure to tell your doctor or health practitioner if you are taking blood thinners, such as heparin and warfarin (Coumadin), or any other medication, whether prescribed or over-the-counter (OTC). Since medications may interfere with test results, your doctor should be aware of this information before the blood test is administered.

During the Blood Test

Although self-testing kits are now available from online retailers, you should have your blood tested at a doctor's office, lab, or hospital. Drawing blood is not a foolproof procedure and, therefore, should be done by a *phlebotomist*—a specialist trained in drawing blood samples for medical analysis. A skilled phlebotomist should be able to find a vein and draw the blood in a single attempt without causing a patient to feel significant pain or discomfort. Most people feel only a brief pinch when having their blood drawn. Of course, not all phlebotomists are equally skilled at finding veins or inserting needles, so if a vein cannot be found after two tries, you should ask that another technician take your blood instead.

While blood tests are generally neither complicated nor painful, there are a couple things you can do immediately before the test to ensure the procedure is as comfortable and stress-free as possible. First, increase your water intake about an hour before the test, since water helps to fill up the veins, making them plumper and more easily accessible. Second, place a warm towel or heating pad on your arm as you sit in the waiting room. Like water, warmth makes veins less constricted so that the technician taking your blood can easily locate a vein and insert the needle, thereby minimizing discomfort.

You will probably be sitting in a chair or on an examining table for the blood test. Once you are comfortable, the phlebotomist will apply a tourniquet and touch your arm with one or two fingers, feeling for a vein. You may be asked to make a fist to make the veins in your arm more prominent. When the vein is located, the area will be cleaned by applying rubbing alcohol with a cotton swab. Then, it is finally time to draw the blood.

To reduce your anxiety, look away from the needle and focus on another object in the room, or simply close your eyes. Try to relax your arm and make sure you keep it still. Once the needle is in, the hardest part is over—the test will be done in a matter of minutes.

After the Blood Test

Once the needle has been withdrawn from your arm, you will probably be asked to bend your arm and apply pressure to the area while the phlebotomist gets a bandage. Let her know if you are sensitive or allergic to adhesive; you can instead be given a Co-Flex, which is gauze with a rubbery coating. Bandages, which can usually be removed within twenty-four hours, help to minimize bruising, though some people will bruise regardless. This is typically not a concern, but you should speak to your doctor or health practitioner if the bruise lasts for several days. In addition, remember to eat shortly after a blood test to replenish your system and energy. Many people bring a snack, such as a piece of fruit or beverage. At the very least, you should have water or even a glass of juice immediately after your blood is drawn.

It usually does not take long to receive blood test results, especially if the test is administered at a lab. If it is performed at a doctor's office, you may have to wait three to five days for the results, since the blood sample has to be sent out to a lab for analysis. If your doctor or health practitioner does not contact you within a week, you should call and inquire about your results. Keep in mind, though, that most doctors will call right away if a problem is detected, so no news is often a good sign. Even so, it is very important that you are informed of the results and that a copy is mailed to you. This is usually done at the request of the patient, so be sure to ask.

Upon receiving your blood test results, you should carefully review them. The importance of this cannot be stressed enough. Since "your blood never lies," you should be able to understand what it is telling you. This book will be your interpreter and guide.

How to Use This Book

Your Blood Never Lies is designed to be a comprehensive health guide that will enable you to not only understand your blood test results, but also how to improve them. But first you should know how the book is organized, as well as be familiar with some of the information it contains.

Understanding the Format

Your Blood Never Lies is divided into six parts. The first five parts concentrate on specific groups of blood tests, including four traditional blood panels—the lipid panel, the basic metabolic panel, the hepatic function panel, and the complete blood count—as well as commonly administered hormone tests for both men and women. The last part of the book covers tests that, though optional, provide a more complete picture of health. In case you are unfamiliar with blood tests, here is a brief explanation of the labs discussed in this book:

- **Part One—The Lipid Panel.** Used to evaluate heart health, this panel comprises of four biological markers representing the four types of fat found in the blood—triglycerides, total cholesterol, high-density lipoprotein (HDL), and low-density lipoprotein (LDL). Two additional measures of cardiovascular health, homocysteine and c-reactive protein (CRP), may also be measured as part of a more comprehensive profile. These two labs are discussed in Part Six, "Optional Tests" (see page 8).

- **Part Two—The Basic Metabolic Panel.** The labs used to evaluate metabolism measure blood sugar regulation, electrolyte and fluid balance, and kidney function. Biomarkers included in this panel are glucose, calcium, sodium, potassium, blood urea nitrogen (BUN), and creatinine.

- **Part Three—The Hepatic Function Panel.** This panel determines how well your liver is functioning by measuring levels of different proteins produced and processed by the liver, like albumin and globulin, as well as liver enzymes.

- **Part Four—The Complete Blood Count (CBC) Panel.** The lab values measured in the complete blood count (CBC) panel include red blood cells, white blood cells, platelets, and hemoglobin. Maintaining healthy levels of these biomarkers affect your vitality and energy, immune system, and cardiovascular health.

- **Part Five—Hormones.** Although they are not always included in a routine blood test, hormones should be periodically tested, especially in aging adults. Hormones such as estrogen, testosterone, progesterone, DHEA, and prostate specific antigen (PSA) play an integral role in reproductive wellness and affect other aspects of health. Maintaining balanced levels can slow down the aging process, for instance. Hormones involved in metabolism, like the thyroid hormones and the stress hormone cortisol, are also discussed in this section.

- **Part Six—Optional Tests.** This final part of the book highlights four tests—homocysteine, c-reactive protein (CRP), vitamin D, and magnesium—that are not typically measured unless requested, or if a standard blood test shows an abnormality that requires a more in-depth analysis. These tests can provide a more complete picture of heart health, immunity, calcium absorption, blood sugar regulation, and a number of other vital processes.

The chapters in each part cover the various labs included in the panel or test group. Along with reference ranges for the lab value, there is a *target*, or optimal range. While the optimal range may vary slightly for some individuals, this is the general range to which most people should strive. You will also find descriptions of the causes and symptoms of high and low levels, as well as the medical problems that may result from untreated abnormalities.

Additionally, each chapter contains a comprehensive treatment section outlining the various pharmaceutical and natural approaches to correcting abnormal lab values and achieving optimal levels. Treatment options may include medications, doctor-administered therapies, dietary changes, lifestyle adjustments such as exercise and stress reduction, and nutritional supplements. Although lists of drugs are presented in several chapters, it's critical that you follow your doctor's advice when it comes to pharmaceuticals. As supplements do not require a prescription, it's of the utmost importance that you know how to choose and use supplements wisely. The next section covers this topic in more detail.

Choosing and Using Supplements

It's important to point out that in some chapters, the same supplement is recommended to treat both high and low levels of a given lab value. There are two main reasons for this. First, some supplements have normalizing effects, which means they can be used to balance levels that are either elevated or reduced. A substance like magnesium, for example, supports *homeostasis*, or internal balance of the body's chemical system, particularly when it comes to calcium utilization. Therefore, magnesium supplements can be taken to increase the body's absorption of calcium (thereby raising levels), as well as prevent the mineral from accumulating in the kidneys, arteries, and joint cartilage (thereby helping to reduce high levels). The second reason why the same supplement can be used to treat opposing problems has to do with the cause of the abnormal level rather than the chemical properties of the supplement itself. For example, both high and low levels of carbon dioxide (see page 115) can be caused by an adrenal disorder, which is often due to high stress. Thus, "calming" supplements like B vitamins, magnesium, and calcium may be effective against both high and low CO_2.

While supplements do not require a prescription, you should not begin a regimen without first speaking to your doctor, as many medical conditions contraindicate the use of certain substances. Furthermore, choosing quality supplements on your own can be an overwhelming task, especially since the touted advice is often conflicting and filled with misinformation. Even though you are urged to have a discussion with your doctor about this subject, below are some general guidelines for buying supplements to help ensure you purchase the best products.

- **Supplements should be GMP-certified.** With the passage of the Dietary Supplement Health and Education Act (DSHEA) of 1994, dietary supplements were placed under Food and Drug Administration (FDA) regulation, and manufacturers were required to follow good manufacturing practices (GMPs). In order to be considered a GMP-certified manufacturer, a company must be regularly inspected by two third-party organizations, such as the Natural Products Association and NSF International.

- **Do not be fooled by the term "pharmaceutical-grade."** It's commonly believed that supplements labeled pharmaceutical-grade are of higher quality than other products. Although manufacturers may opt to follow drug-level GMPs—which are stricter than supplement GMPs—there is no official pharmaceutical-grade designation. There is, however, a USP designation available for supplement manufacturers. USP, or United States Pharmacopeial Convention, is a voluntary program that involves random inspections of manufacturing plants, as well as testing of products for purity, solubility, and potency. It's important to keep in mind, though, that certifications do not necessarily guarantee the quality of a product. Product quality also depends on factors such as the form of nutrients used, the consistency of ingredients from one batch to another, the types of additives and fillers contained in the product, and the various methods employed to ensure proper absorption of the ingredients. As a consumer, it's important that you research supplement manufacturers to find out how they make their products, rather than simply buy products according to certifications or misleading labels like "pharmaceutical-grade."

- **Food-based supplements are not necessarily superior to other supplements.** While the thought of obtaining nutrients from a food base is appealing, there are a large number of studies showing the effectiveness of non-food-based supplements. More evidence of the superiority of food-based supplements is needed before this assumption can be considered a fact.

- **Look for multivitamins that contain all essential nutrients in optimal amounts.** When choosing a multivitamin or mineral formula, it's important to look for products that contain most or all of the nutrients your body requires. A list of essential daily nutrients and corresponding ranges for optimal intake for men and women is provided on page 11. Keep in mind that you can also purchase lower-strength multivitamins and mineral supplements and follow the Recommended Daily Intake (RDI); however, this dosage will only prevent nutritional deficiency and will not necessarily boost your health.

The bottom line is that you should do your research before purchasing any supplement, and know how well certain products are absorbed and the raw material they contain. Most importantly, though, you should ask your doctor about safe, reliable supplements that will enable you to achieve your health goals.

ESSENTIAL DAILY NUTRIENTS			
Nutrient	**Recommended Daily Dosage for Adult Men**	**Recommended Daily Dosage for Adult Women (Menstruating)**	**Recommended Daily Dosage for Adult Women (Menopausal)**
Boron	1 to 3 mg	1 to 3 mg	1 to 3 mg
Calcium	800 to 1,200 mg	1,200 to 1,500 mg	1,200 to 1,500 mg
Chromium	600 to 1,500 mcg	600 to 1,500 mcg	600 to 1,500 mcg
Coenzyme Q_{10} (CoQ_{10})	50 to 300 mg	50 to 300 mg	50 to 300 mg
Copper	1 to 2 mg	1 to 2 mg	1 to 2 mg
Iron		15 to 30 mg (menstruation increases the body's need for iron)	
Magnesium	400 to 1,000 mg	400 to 800 mg	400 to 800 mg
Manganese	3 to 6 mg	3 to 6 mg	3 to 6 mg
Molybdenum	100 to 150 mcg	100 to 150 mcg	100 to 150 mcg
Selenium	100 to 200 mcg	100 to 200 mcg	100 to 200 mcg
Vanadium	100 to 500 mcg	100 to 500 mcg	100 to 500 mcg
Vitamin A	2,500 to 5,000 IU	2,500 IU	2,500 to 5,000 IU
Natural mixed carotenoids (form of vitamin A)	5,000 to 10,000 IU	5,000 to 10,000 IU	5,000 to 10,000 IU
Vitamin B_1 (thiamine HCl)	10 to 50 mg	10 to 50 mg	10 to 50 mg
Vitamin B_2 (riboflavin-5′-phosphate, riboflavin HCl)	10 to 25 mg	10 to 25 mg	10 to 25 mg
Vitamin B_3 (niacin or niacinimide)	25 to 50 mg	25 to 50 mg	25 to 50 mg
Vitamin B_5 (pantothenic acid)	100 to 500 mg	100 to 500 mg	100 to 500 mg

Nutrient	Recommended Daily Dosage for Adult Men	Recommended Daily Dosage for Adult Women (Menstruating)	Recommended Daily Dosage for Adult Women (Menopausal)
Vitamin B_6 (pyridoxine-5'-phosphate, pyridoxine HCl)	5 to 25 mg	5 to 25 mg	25 to 50 mg
Vitamin B_9 (folic acid, folinic acid, methyltetrahydrofolate)	200 to 1,000 mcg;	800 to 1,000 mcg	200 to 800 mcg
Vitamin B_{12} (methylcobalamin, adenosylcobalamin)	100 to 1,000 mcg	; 100 to 1,000 mcg	100 to 1,000 mcg
Vitamin C (ascorbate)	500 to 1,000 mg	500 to 1,000 mg	500 to 1,000 mg
Vitamin D_3	2,000 to 5,000 IU	2,000 to 5,000 IU	2,000 to 5,000 IU
Vitamin E (mixed tocopherols)	200 to 400 IU	200 to 400 IU	200 to 400 IU
Vitamin K_1	75 to 100 mcg	75 to 100 mg	75 to 100 mcg
Vitamin K_2	90 mcg	90 mcg	90 mcg
Zinc	15 to 50 mg	15 to 30 mg	15 to 30 mg

Reading and Planning Your Blood Test

In addition to the information contained in the chapters, the book offers a number of helpful resources. First, on page 14, you will find a sample blood test to use as a reference when reading your test results. This sample reflects the standard test format used by LabCorp and most laboratories, but not all labs present the information in same order and format. You should compare your personal blood test with the sample to ensure you read it correctly.

The lab values represented on the sample test, which are listed below the appropriate panel heading, are each labeled with a number that corresponds to their chapter number in the book. To the right of the list of tests are a series of columns. On actual tests, lab values are listed in the first column labeled "Result." If a value is out of range, the word "High" or "Low" appears in the column labeled "Flag." The "Units" column lists the standard unit of measurement for each lab value, and the final column, "Reference Interval," provides the generally accepted normal ranges for each blood value so that you can easily compare and understand your results. Keep in mind, though, that a *normal* lab is not necessarily an optimal one. As noted above, while it's important to fall into the "normal" category, it's even more important to achieve the "target" range.

Let's use sodium as an example. The normal range for adults is 134 to 143 millimoles per liter (mmol/L). Therefore, if your sodium level is 133, you are considered out of range. In this case, you will work with your health practitioner to raise this number in a healthy way. But let's say instead that your sodium level is 136, a number at the lower end of the normal range. While such numbers may technically fall into the "normal" category, they warrant a discussion with your doctor or health practitioner. Depending on the test, as well as your medical history and genetics, numbers that are on the low or high end of the normal range may be completely typical for you—and completely healthy. Nevertheless, it may be worthwhile to talk to a healthcare professional about how to prevent that number from creeping into the "low normal" or "high normal" ends of the normal range, or worse, from falling outside the normal range altogether.

Finally, the book provides helpful supplementary material in the appendix (see page 321), including a full reference guide to LabCorp lab value ranges, a list of testing laboratories and their areas of specialization, and a chart for recording the results of your blood test. This book is designed to be a guide, offering advice based on the results of your blood test. It is important that you look for trends in your lab values and take the necessary steps to correct or prevent health problems. At the same time, this book is not intended to replace the professional guidance of a health practitioner, whom you should consult before trying to alter your blood chemistry. Dietary modifications and supplement regimens are significant changes that you should certainly discuss with a healthcare professional, such as a licensed nutritionist, before implementing. Moreover, the information presented in *Your Blood Never Lies* is for educational purposes only, and not meant to diagnose or treat medical conditions.

CONCLUSION

A crucial step towards better health is becoming proactive, and having your blood tested regularly is one of the easiest and most practical ways to do this. Periodic blood tests keep you and your doctor "in the know" about the inner workings of your body so that major health problems can be avoided or curtailed. Having a blood test can be likened to watching the needle on your car's gas gauge—you want to be sure the car has enough fuel to operate properly in order to prevent the warning light from coming on and being stranded on the side of a highway. Blood tests are essentially gauges, and keeping a watchful eye on your blood levels is a way to take control of your health. Unlike a car, however, neither the body nor blood tests come with a manual—but this book can fulfill that role. The pages that follow will give you the insight and practical knowledge you need to become not only an informed patient, but also a responsible and self-advocating individual. Your blood never lies, so it's time to understand what it's saying.

SAMPLE BLOOD TEST

Following is a sample lab report for a blood test, which has been set up to reflect the format used by most testing laboratories. The labs listed each begin with a boldface number that corresponds to their chapter number in the book, so that you can turn to the appropriate page to learn more about a certain blood value. (For instance, "Triglycerides" are explained in Chapter 1.) On an actual blood test, results are printed in the "Results" column, and if the number is abnormal, the word "High" or "Low" appears in the column labeled "Flag." The standard unit of measurement for each lab value is noted in the "Units" column. The reference ranges provided in the last column are the same ranges used in this book, but keep in mind that not all labs use the same values. Compare your blood test to the sample to ensure that you read it correctly, and consult your physician if you have questions or concerns. Finally, keep in mind that under "Reference Interval," you will sometimes find the following symbols used: < means "less than"; > means "greater than."

Specimen #:

Patient ID Number	Patient Phone Number	Patient SSN	
Patient Name	Patient Address	Sex	Date of Birth

Tests Requested: Lipid Panel; Basic Metabolic Panel; Hepatic Function Panel; Complete Blood Count (CBC); Hormones; Homocysteine, C-reactive protein (CRP), Vitamin D, Magnesium

Test	Result	Flag	Units	Reference Interval
Lipid Panel				
1. Triglycerides			mg/dL	< 150
2. Total Cholesterol			mg/dL	< 200
3. LDL Cholesterol			mg/dL	< 100
4. HDL Cholesterol			mg/dL	Men: 40–50 Women: 50–60
Basic Metabolic Panel				
5. Glucose			mg/dL	65–99
6. Calcium			mg/dL	8.6–10.2
7. Potassium			mEq/L	3.5–5.4
8. Sodium			mmol/L	134–143
9. Chloride			mmol/L	97–108
10. Carbon Dioxide			mmol/L	21–33
11. Blood Urea Nitrogen (BUN)			mg/dL	6–20
12. Creatinine			mg/dL	0.5–1.1
13. BUN/Creatinine Ratio				10:1–20:1
14. Glomerular Filtration Rate (GFR)			mL/min	90–120
Hepatic Function Panel				
15. Total Protein			g/dL	6.5–8.0
16. Albumin			g/dL	3.7–5.0
17. Globulin			g/dL	2.0–3.5
18. Albumin/Globulin (A/G) Ratio				1.1–2.4
19. Bilirubin			mg/dL	Total: 0.2–1.4 Direct: 0.0–0.4
20. Alanine Aminotransferase (ALT)			IU/L	0–40
21. Alkaline Phosphatase (ALP)			IU/L	25–150
22. Aspartate Aminotransferase (AST)			IU/L	5–40
23. Gamma-Glutamyl Transferase (GGT)			IU/L	0–45

Test	Result	Flag	Units	Reference Interval			
Complete Blood Count							
24. Red Blood Cells (RBCs)			cells/mcL	Men: 4.7–6.1 million Women: 4.2 million–5.4 million Children (under 18 years old): 4.0–5.5 million Infants: 4.8–7.1 million			
25. Hemoglobin			g/dL	Men: 14–18 Women: 12–16 Children (under 18 years old): 11–13			
26. Hematocrit			%	Men: 36–50 Women: 34–44 Children (under 18 years old): 29–40			
27. Mean Corpuscular Volume (MCV)			fL	80–100			
28. Mean Corpuscular Hemoglobin (MCH)			pg/cell	26–43			
29. Mean Corpuscular Hemoglobin Concentration (MCHC)			g/dL	31–37			
30. Platelets			mm^3	150,000–400,000			
31. White Blood Cells (WBCs)			mcg/L				
Total				4,500–11,000			
Neutrophils				1,800–7,800			
Lymphocytes				1,000–4,800			
Monocytes				0–800			
Eosinophils				0–450			
Basophils				0–200			
Hormones							
32. Dehydroepi-androsterone (DHEA)		mcg/dL		**Men**		**Women**	
				18–19 years old	108–441	18–19 years old	145–395
				20–29	280–640	20–29	65–380
				30–39	120–150	30–39	45–270

Test	Result	Flag	Units	Reference Interval			
DHEA *(continued)*			mcg/dL	**Men**		**Women**	
				40–49	95–530	40–49	32–240
				50–59	70–310	50–59	26–200
				60–69	42–290	60–69	13–130
				69 and over	28–175	69 and over	17–90
33. Cortisol			mcg/dL	6.2–19.4 (AM) 2.3–11.9 (PM)			
34. Estrogen (Total)			pg/mL	**Men**		**Women**	
				Prepubertal	12–55	Prepubertal	12–57
				Adults	40–115	Follicular	61–394
						Ovulation	122–437
						Luteal	156–350
						Postmeno-pausal	20–40
35. Thyroid Hormones							
TSH			mcIU/mL	0.45–4.5			
T_3, *Free*			pg/dL	200–440			
T_3, *Total*			ng/dL	71–180			
T_4, *Free*			ng/dL	0.82–1.77			
T_4, *Total*			mcg/dL	4.5–12.0			
TPO			IU/mL	0–34			
36. Progesterone			ng/mL	**Men**		**Women**	
				0.2–1.4		Pre-ovulation	< 1.0
						Mid-menstrual cycle	5.0–20.0
						Pregnant, 1st trimester	11.2–90.0
						Pregnant, 2nd trimester	25.6–89.4
						Pregnant, 3rd trimester	42.5–48.4
						Postmeno-pausal	< 1.0

Test	Result	Flag	Units	Reference Interval			
37. Testosterone			pg/mL	**Total**		**Free**	
				Men, 13–17 years old	28–1,110	Men, 20–29 years old	9.3–26.5
				Men, 18 and older	280–800	Men, 30–39	8.7–25.1
						Men, 40–49	7.2–24.0
						Men, 50–59	6.8–21.5
						Men, over 59	6.6–18.1
				Women, under 18	6–82	Women, 20–59	0–2.2
						Women, over 59	0–1.8
38. Prostate-Specific Antigen (PSA)			ng/mL	0–4.0			
			Other				
39. Homocysteine			µmol/L	< 11			
40. C-Reactive Protein (CRP)			mg/L	< 1.0 (Low risk)			
41. Vitamin D			ng/mL	25–85			
42. Magnesium, Serum			mEq/L	Adults: 1.8–2.6 Children (2 to 18 years old): 1.7–2.1 Infants: 1.5–2.2			

Key to Measurement Abbreviations

cells/mcL = cells per microliter
fL = femtoliters
g/dL = grams per deciliter
IU/dL = international units per deciliter
IU/mL = international units per milliliter
IU/L = international units per liter
mcg/dL = micrograms per deciliter
mcg/L = micrograms per liter
mcIU/mL = microinternational units per milliliter
mEq/L = milliequivalents per liter
mg/dL = milligrams per deciliter
mg/L = milligrams per liter
mL/min = milliliters per minute
mm^3 = millimeters cubed
mmol/L = millimoles per liter
ng/dL = nanograms per deciliter
lng/mL = nanograms per milliliter
pg/cell = picograms per cel
pg/dL = picograms per deciliter
pg/mL = picograms per milliliter
µmol/L = micromoles per liter

PART 1

The Lipid Panel

According to the American Heart Association, *heart disease*—a term often used interchangeably with *cardiovascular disease*—is the leading cause of mortality in the United States, responsible for one out of every four deaths. It's estimated that 70 million people in the United States alone suffer from heart-related problems, which may include blood clots, clogged arteries, heart attack, and stroke. Risk factors for these conditions include high cholesterol and triglycerides, as well as elevated levels of certain proteins and amino acids found in the blood. The "biomarkers" of heart disease make up the *lipid panel,* also called the *cholesterol test* or *lipid profile,* on a standard blood test. Thus, regular blood testing is essential when it comes to treating and, more importantly, preventing heart disease.

Lipids, a group that includes triglycerides and cholesterol, are fatty substances found in the blood. *Triglycerides* can originate in dietary fats, but they are also produced by the liver when there is excessive intake of sugar or alcohol. *Cholesterol* is a waxy substance and basic building block of hormones like testosterone, estrogen, progesterone, vitamin D, and cortisol. On the lipid profile, cholesterol is divided into *total cholesterol*, *high-density lipoprotein* (HDL) or "good" cholesterol, and *low-density lipoprotein* (LDL), or "bad" cholesterol. Together with triglycerides, these substances comprise the lipid panel, and are measured to check primarily for heart disease and *metabolic syndrome* (MeS). Metabolic syndrome is a condition characterized by borderline-high blood pressure, insulin resistance, and elevated lipids or *dyslipidemia*—a condition in which there are unhealthy ratios of cholesterol and triglycerides, even though levels are not necessarily elevated. Additional symptoms include weight gain, particularly in the midsection, and a high *body mass index* (BMI), which is a measurement of the appropriateness of a person's body weight for his or her height. In the United States, adults over fifty years of age have a one-in-three chance of developing metabolic syndrome. Because metabolic syndrome is a significant indicator of risk for cardiovascular disease and diabetes, it is important that it be recognized as soon as possible. The lipid panel is a major diagnostic tool for identifying metabolic syndrome; early detection allows for medical intervention.

In addition to triglycerides, HDL, LDL, and total cholesterol, *homocysteine*—an amino acid byproduct—and *C-reactive protein* (CRP) are also markers of cardiovascular risk when levels become too high. While not included in a standard blood test, these two biomarkers are measured when more comprehensive blood work is required to diagnose a medical condition. You can find more information on homocysteine and CRP in Part Six, "Optional Tests" (see page 289).

In the sections that follow, reference ranges are provided for each lab value of the lipid profile. Keep in mind, though, that "normal" does not necessarily mean *ideal*. This is why a *target*, or optimal, *range* is also given. These optimal numbers can vary depending on individual factors, including weight and fitness level, genetics, presence of oxidative stress and inflammation in the body, hormone imbalances, and pre-existing medical conditions such as diabetes and liver problems. These factors should be taken into account when planning a course of treatment, which may consist of lipid-lowering or cholesterol-binding drugs, nutritional supplements, and lifestyle modifications relating to diet, exercise, and other healthy behaviors.

The information contained in this section is not intended to replace the advice of your physician. If you are concerned that you have any condition mentioned in the following pages, consult a health-care professional.

A Helpful Tip

The National Institute of Health recommends that men should have their first cholesterol test by age thirty-five, and women by age forty-five. If results are normal, follow-up tests should be conducted every five years. People who have or are genetically predisposed to diabetes, heart disease, stroke, or high blood pressure should get tested more frequently.

1. TRIGLYCERIDES

Triglycerides are the main lipid constituents in the blood and a major source of energy for the body. When you take in food, excess calories are chemically converted into triglycerides, which are stored in fat cells if they are not needed for energy. Hormones can also signal the release of triglycerides from fat cells to provide energy. Triglycerides circulate throughout the body with the help of carrier proteins known as lipoproteins, particularly *very-low-density lipoproteins,* or VLDL (see page 31). In normal amounts, triglycerides are vital for good health. However, if you consume more calories than you expend—especially from sugar and carbohydrates—your triglyceride level will become too high, causing a condition known as *hypertriglyceridemia.* Elevated triglyceride levels are a major risk factor for heart disease, diabetes, insulin resistance, metabolic syndrome, and liver disease.

Triglycerides are measured in milligrams per deciliter of blood (mg/dL). Reference ranges for triglyceride levels are provided in the table below.

REFERENCE RANGES FOR TRIGLYCERIDES

Triglycerides (mg/dL)	Category
Greater than 499	Very High
200 to 499	High
150 to199	Borderline high
Less than 150	Normal
Target Range: 50 to 100 mg/dL	

As you can see, the target range for adults is 50 to 100 mg/dL. In other words, a triglycerides level of 135 may be "normal," but it is neither ideal nor necessarily healthy. You can achieve an optimal level by adopting new lifestyle behaviors, or by taking nutritional supplements and lipid-lowering medications. And while it is possible to have a triglyceride level that is too low, high triglycerides is the far more common problem.

WHAT CAUSES HIGH TRIGLYCERIDES?

Although a high-fat diet is often blamed for elevated triglycerides (see the inset on page 23), there are a number of other factors that may cause a high level, including:

- Being overweight or obese (BMI of 25 or above)
- Certain medications, including beta blockers, diuretics, estrogen, oral contraceptives, steroids, and the breast cancer drug tamoxifen
- Chronic inflammation
- Chronic stress
- Depression (if it leads to overeating)
- Diet high in refined sugars and carbohydrates as well as unhealthy fats, such as saturated fats and trans fats
- Environmental factors, such as toxicity caused by heavy metals or pesticides
- Excessive coffee or alcohol consumption
- Inherited lipid disorders
- Insulin resistance
- Intestinal conditions
- Kidney disease
- Nutritional deficiencies
- Poorly controlled diabetes
- Pregnancy
- Regularly eating more calories than you burn
- Sex hormone imbalanace
- Underactive thyroid (hypothyroidism)

High triglycerides are a major risk factor for diabetes and insulin resistance, liver disease, metabolic syndrome, and *pancreatitis,* or inflammation of the pancreas. An elevated level also contributes to the hardening and narrowing of arteries (atherosclerosis), which is a specific type of heart disease called *coronary artery disease.* When this condition develops, the likelihood of having a heart attack or stroke is much greater. Heartbeat abnormalities (heart arrhythmias), as well as clot formation in other parts of the body (peripheral artery disease), can also occur.

WHAT ARE THE SYMPTOMS OF HIGH TRIGLYCERIDES?

High triglycerides do not by themselves produce symptoms. Conditions resulting from very high, sustained levels, however, may have physical indicators. For example, pancreatitis may develop and cause abdominal pain, loss of appetite, nausea, vomiting, and fever. And when high triglycerides are caused by a genetic disorder, *xanthomas* (fat deposits) may form under the skin. Still, most people are not aware that their levels are raised until they receive the results of their blood tests.

Fats, Food, and the Lipid Panel

In the past, it was thought that a high-fat diet posed serious health risks, from obesity and diabetes to inflammation and heart disease. However, Americans consume less total fat today than they did in the 1960s, and yet rates of heart disease and obesity are higher. Recent studies have found that a diet high in too many high-glycemic carbohydrates (see the inset on page 29) increases the risk of obesity, diabetes, and heart disease as much as, if not more than, fat intake. This is because such foods exacerbate insulin resistance, a major underlying factor of heart disease. High intake of refined sugars—which are contained in soft drinks, candy, baked goods, and other sweets—are also strongly associated with high triglycerides. Therefore, one of the best ways to improve your lipid profile is to eliminate refined sugars and flours almost completely from the diet, and instead eat whole unprocessed carbohydrates found in vegetables, beans, and raw fresh fruit. If and when grains are consumed, they should be whole and eaten in moderation.

When it comes to fats, the focus has shifted to the *type,* not the quantity, of fat that is eaten. The right fats, when consumed in moderation, are an essential component of a well-rounded, healthy diet. Four basic types of fat—saturated, monounsaturated, polyunsaturated, and trans fats—are discussed below. Knowing the "good" fats from the "bad" ones will enable you to make smarter dietary choices and, as a result, keep your lipid panel values within healthy ranges.

- **Saturated fats.** This type of fat is found primarily in animal proteins such as beef and pork, as well as full-fat dairy products like whole milk, butter, and cheese. Earlier health studies, such as the Bogalusa Health Study, found that high intake of saturated fats can somewhat increase cholesterol levels, though not necessarily in everyone. Nevertheless, you should reduce your consumption of these fats by choosing lean meats and reduced-fat dairy products, as well as by cooking with healthier oils, such as olive oil and vegetable-based oils.

- **Trans fats.** Also known as trans-fatty acids, trans fats are produced when vegetable oils are hydrogenated to become more solid and stable. The hydrogenation process also prolongs the shelf life of the oil, which is why trans fats are often used to make processed foods, fast foods, commercial baked goods, and hard margarine. In the last few years, many food manufacturers have taken steps to remove this ingredient from their products, as scientists have discovered that trans fats from partially hydrogenated oils are even more unhealthy than saturated fats. Not only do they increase the level of LDL in the body, but they also decrease high-density lipoproteins, or HDLs—the "good" cholesterol (see page 49). Avoid trans fat at all costs by staying away from hard margarine, commercially prepared baked items (cakes, cookies, donuts, muffins, etc.), and foods fried in partially hydrogenated oils. Be sure to check the nutrition label before buying any packaged food. If it contains partially hydrogenated oil, it also contains trans fats and should thus be avoided.

- **Monounsaturated fats.** This healthy fat reduces LDL levels without having any negative impact on HDL cholesterol. Monounsaturated fat is critical to the Mediterranean diet, which is reported to promote heart health, and found in olive oil, canola oil, avocados, and most nuts. Keep in mind, though, that all fats—both good and bad—are dense in calories, so even monounsaturated fats should be consumed in moderation.

- **Polyunsaturated fats.** These fats lower LDL cholesterol and are essential for good health. Two in particular, omega-3 and omega-6, must be taken in through the diet, as they are not produced by the body. Omega-6 fatty acids are plentiful in a number of foods, from nuts and seeds to vegetable oils, so most people consume sufficient amounts without even trying. Omega-3s, on the other hand, are not as abundant, found mainly in fatty fish like salmon, herring, and trout, which contain the "long-chain" fatty acids EPA and DHA. To ensure that you're getting all the omega-3s that you need, eat fish more regularly—at least two servings per week. You can also consume chia seeds, flax seeds, flax oil, or walnuts, which are concentrated sources of another omega-3 known as ALA. Fish oil and DHA/EPA supplements are also options.

Understanding the variation among fats is an important step towards achieving a wholesome diet. Triglycerides and cholesterol levels are largely influenced by excessive intake of carbohydrates and sugar, so it's a good idea to drastically lower your consumption of these foods. In addition, you should remove trans fats from your diet by choosing lean sources of protein, such as organic or grass-fed beef, and stick to reduced-fat dairy products. However, there is no need to buy dairy that is less than 2-percent fat, as your body needs medium-chain triglycerides—valuable fats that are actually good for your metabolism. Avoid processed and fast foods as often as possible, and eat more fish that are high in omega-3s and low in mercury. Olive, flax, and canola oils should be your primary selections for dressing salads and preparing low-heat dishes. When cooking, use macadamia oil, which has a high flash point and does not oxidize. Your heart will thank you for it.

HOW CAN HIGH TRIGLYCERIDES BE TREATED?

Having elevated triglycerides does not mean health problems are inevitable. There are a number of steps you can take, from medication to dietary adjustments, to reverse the trend and achieve a healthy level. Below are some ways raised levels can be safely and effectively lowered.

DRUGS

Triglyceride levels that are too high to normalize through natural means must be treated with medication. The following drugs are commonly prescribed by doctors to bring down elevated levels. If applicable, brands are provided below the drug's generic name.

DRUGS FOR HIGH TRIGLYCERIDES

Drug	Considerations
Fenofibrate *Tricor*	Side effects may include constipation, diarrhea, heartburn, nausea and/or vomiting, muscle aches, headache, retinopathy, anemia, lung problems, and pancreatitis. The drug may also deplete the body of essential nutrients, such as vitamin E, vitamin D, DHEA, and coenzyme Q_{10}. Therefore, it is recommended that you also take 100 mg of CoQ_{10} once a day, as well as a multivitamin or mineral supplement daily.
Gemfibrozil *Lopid*	Gemfibrozil may produce side effects such as constipation, diarrhea, heartburn, nausea and/or vomiting, muscle aches, headache, retinopathy, anemia, lung problems, and pancreatitis. This drug may also deplete essential nutrients from the body, including vitamin E, vitamin D, DHEA, and coenzyme Q_{10}. Therefore, it is recommended that you also take 100 mg of CoQ_{10} once a day, as well as a multivitamin or mineral supplement daily.
Niacin, extended-release	Speak to your healthcare provider before using if you are on blood thinners or diabetes medication. Extended-release usually does not cause flushing.
Omega-3 acid ethyl esters (DHA and EPA) *Lovaza*	Lovaza is a very pure form of omega-3 fatty acids, but does not differ from high-quality dietary supplements that are processed and purified to remove contaminants, such as mercury and other toxins. Do not use if you are allergic to fish or soybeans. Consult your healthcare provider before taking if you have diabetes, liver disease, a pancreatic disorder, or an underactive thyroid, or if you consume more than two alcoholic beverages per day.

The drug your doctor chooses to prescribe depends largely on individual factors, the particularities of your problem, and underlying health issues. Before beginning a regimen, you should ask about possible side effects and drug interactions to ensure safest use of the drug.

SUPPLEMENTS

There are nutritional supplements that can be helpful for lowering triglycerides while boosting your overall health. The supplements presented in the table below are those that may directly impact triglyceride levels. However, it's important to note that any substance that improves insulin sensitivity and glucose uptake can also significantly affect your level of triglycerides. Although a prescription is not required to obtain these products, you should consult a healthcare professional before using any substance in the table below. A doctor can guide you to high-quality products and recommend a dosage that fits your needs. See page 9 for a few guidelines to keep in mind when choosing supplements.

SUPPLEMENTS FOR HIGH TRIGLYCERIDES

Supplement	Dosage	Considerations
Aged garlic extract	600 mg one to three times a day.	Aged garlic extract is used to protect the heart and blood vessels, and is reported to help decrease oxidative stress markers, including those related to blood sugar regulation problems. Aged garlic has also been reported to reduce liver enzymes and fatty liver, as well as decrease the formation of advanced glycation end-products (AGEs), which are implicated in various health problems, such as heart disease, kidney problems, and cancer. Aged garlic is not reported to interfere with blood thinners.
Coenzyme Q_{10} (CoQ_{10})	30 mg three times a day or 50 mg twice a day, depending on dose per capsule.	CoQ_{10} is important for energy production, oxygen use, high blood pressure, and heart health, especially in people with kidney disorders. It can also boost endurance, improve insulin sensitivity, and lower triglycerides and blood glucose levels. This supplement is especially recommended if you are taking statin drugs, red yeast rice, and certain diabetes medications, which may result in a CoQ_{10} deficiency.
Green tea or green tea extract	3 to 6 cups (tea) or 250 mg one to two times a day (extract).	Helps improve antioxidant and lipid levels. When taken with other supplements and diet/lifestyle changes, green tea extract is reported to assist in weight loss. It can also help regulate glucose levels, lower triglycerides, and prevent kidney stones that may result from high calcium. If taking an extract, use a form standardized to 90-percent polyphenols (specifically EGCG). Tell your doctor if you are currently taking aspirin or anticoagulant drugs like warfarin (Coumadin), as green tea extract may increase the risk of bleeding.

Supplement	Dosage	Considerations
L-carnitine	1 to 3 g once a day.	Can help lower triglycerides because it helps move fat into cells for the purpose of energy production. Also supports demineralization and has been reported to reverse and prevent symptoms related to hyperthyroidism. Food sources of the substance are meat, poultry, and dairy products.
Omega-3 essential fatty acids DHA and EPA (fish oil)	1,000 mg two to three times a day.	Fish oil is one of the first supplements recommended by doctors for lowering triglycerides. In addition to its anti-inflammatory properties, fish oil is reported to lower total cholesterol levels and decrease oxidative stress, which is associated with LDL, or "bad" cholesterol. Speak to your doctor before taking if you are on blood-thinning medication, as fish oil may increase the risk of bleeding. Be sure to use only high-quality oils that have been tested for contaminants.
Probiotics	5 to 10 billion colony forming units (CFUs) two to three times a day.	Probiotics help normalize beneficial flora in the gastrointestinal tract, and are reported to decrease triglyceride and cholesterol levels. They are also reported to improve BUN levels and quality of life in people with kidney disease. It's best to use heat-stable products that do not require refrigeration. If using an antibiotic, wait three hours before taking probiotics. If diarrhea occurs, decrease your dosage. If this side effect persists for longer than 48 hours, stop taking the supplement and contact your doctor. Live cultures should be guaranteed through the date of expiration on label. For optimal results, take probiotics with meals, as food improves the survivability of the cultures.
Red yeast rice	1,200 mg one to two times a day.	This supplement acts similarly to statin drugs and lowers cholesterol levels. Some studies show it can also lower triglycerides. It is recommended that you take 100 mg of CoQ_{10} per day when supplementing with red yeast rice. Individuals who are sensitive to gastrointestinal upset may experience gas, bloating, and nausea. Take with food.

LIFESTYLE CHANGES

Adopting healthy lifestyle behaviors is the most effective way to achieve overall wellness. Even if you do not presently have high triglycerides, you should follow the dietary guidelines on pages 23 to 24 and practice the habits below to help reduce health risks. By incorporating these healthy behaviors into your daily life, you will promote your general well-being while keeping your triglycerides in check.

- Avoid inflammation-causing foods. Included in this category are foods containing trans fat, and refined and added sugars like high-fructose corn syrup, which is found in many condiments, sauces, commercially produced snack foods, and sweetened beverages. Refined carbohydrates—for example, white bread, pasta, bagels, and any food made from white flour—should be eliminated from the diet as well. If you are insulin resistant (see page 60), it is also a good idea to cut down on whole grain carbohydrates and limit your overall carbohydrate intake. Total carbohydrate consumption should amount to no more than 60 to 100 g per day.

- Cook for your heart. Use cooking oils with healthier monounsaturated fats, such as macadamia and other nut oils. Olive oil is also an acceptable alternative, but it's best to add it to food that has already been cooked. Since olive oil oxidizes (breaks down) easily when heated, it can lose some of its nutritional value. In addition, reduce your use of butter, which contains a significiant amount of saturated fat.

- Exercise. According to experts, physical activity plays an important role in lowering trigylcerides. Begin by exercising in twenty- to thirty-minute sessions at least three to four times a week, and gradually increase the duration and level of intensity. An ideal fitness routine includes both cardiovascular (aerobic) exercise and strength (resistance) training.

- Focus on fiber. A diet high in fiber has been shown to help lower triglycerides. Fiber-rich foods—which include beans, leafy green vegetables, and some whole grains like oatmeal—promote healthier eating habits in the long term. You can also boost your intake by sprinkling flax seeds and chia seeds on salads or mixing them into protein drinks.

- Incorporate omega-3s. Foods containing omega-3 fatty acids (EPA and DHA)—which are found primarily in cold-water fish oils of albacore tuna, cod, herring, mackerel, salmon, anchovies, and sardines—have an anti-inflammatory effect on the body and decrease the risk of heart disease. Omega-3s are also plentiful in chia seeds, flax seeds, and walnuts, but they should not be your only fatty-acid source; these omega-3s must first undergo chemical reactions before they can be used by the body.

- Limit your dairy intake. Until your triglycerides are within a normal range, you should eliminate full-fat butter and cream from your diet, as well as reduce your use of whole milk. Once you have reached a healthy level, you can eat dairy in moderation.

- Look for leaner cuts. Choose beef from grass-fed cows, since it contains less

Glycemic Index and Glycemic Load

Healthcare professionals often advise their patients to stay away from "high-glycemic foods," which, as recent studies have found, raise the risk of obesity, diabetes, and heart disease at least as much as unhealthy fats. Foods that contain refined sugars and/or carbohydrates—soft drinks, candy, baked goods, white bread, and pasta, for example—have a high ranking on the *glycemic index* (GI), a system that measures how quickly a carbohydrate-containing food causes a rise in blood sugar. *Glycemic load* (GL) is slightly different, reflecting not only the quality, but also the *quantity* of the carbohydrates that are consumed. GL provides a better overall picture of a particular food's impact on blood sugar levels.

Although most know that the foods listed above are filled with sugar and carbs, many people do not realize that some fruits and vegetables are also considered to be high-glycemic in relation to other foods in those categories. For instance, bananas, raisins, dates, and canned fruits have a much higher glycemic load than strawberries, cherries, and grapefruit. Similarly, carbohydrate-rich vegetables like yams and potatoes are high glycemic, whereas broccoli, kale, and spinach are not even measured because their carbohydrate content is too insignificant.

If this seems overwhelming, don't worry—both the GI and the GL of many foods have already been determined, making it easy to choose foods that will keep blood glucose at a healthy level. One of the most comprehensive books available is Shari Lieberman's *Glycemic Index Food Guide,* which lists the GI and GL of hundreds of foods and beverages. By switching to a primarily low-glycemic diet and eating whole, unprocessed carbohydrates, you will improve your lipid profile and cut your risk of chronic health problems like heart disease, metabolic syndrome, obesity, type 2 diabetes, and insulin resistance.

total fat, less saturated fat, and less cholesterol. It is also much higher in omega-3 fatty acids than conventionally raised beef. Free-range eggs, chicken, lamb, fish, and bison are also healthier. Whenever possible, buy organic meat and poultry.

- Reduce your alcohol consumption. If your triglycerides are high, it's advisable to drink only on occasion or eliminate alcohol from your lifestyle altogether. Otherwise, alcohol can be enjoyed in moderation—no more than one to two drinks per day is recommended for men, and for women, no more than five drinks per week.

- Restrict your servings of fruit and other substances containing natural sugars. Although fruits are rich in antioxidants and fiber, some are also high in sugar. This is why you should limit your fruit intake to two servings per day. Excessive consumption of fruit, fruit juice, and sources of natural sugars like honey and agave can lead to elevated trigylicerides. Be sure to choose fruits with low *glycemic load* (see the inset on page 29), which includes apricots, blueberries, and grapefruit.

- Watch your coffee habits. One researcher found that two chemicals contained in coffee, cafestol and kahweol, can raise your triglyceride levels. Fortunately, these harmful substances are removed when coffee is made in filtered drip coffeemakers. However, certain coffee habits—such as adding a lot of sugar or non-dairy creamers (coffee whiteners) containing partially hydrogenated oils—can contribute to high triglycerides. Consider swapping your morning coffee for a cup of green tea, a great source of antioxidants.

Consider This

High triglycerides indicate a major risk for heart disease, diabetes and insulin resistance, liver disease, metabolic syndrome, and inflammation of the pancreas. A 2007 study showed that the risk of heart disease and stroke for young people with the highest level of triglycerides was four times that of young people with the lowest level of triglycerides.

2. TOTAL CHOLESTEROL

Cholesterol has received a lot of negative attention in the past decade. The word alone stirs up images of a "bad" substance that is not wanted in the body. However, this is not entirely accurate; cholesterol is an essential fat that contributes to your normal biological functioning. Produced by the liver, cholesterol is required to create cell membranes as well as bile acids for fat digestion. Cholesterol is also the principal building block of many of your hormones—including estrogen, testosterone, and progesterone—and it plays a vital role in vitamin D production. Although the body naturally manufactures cholesterol, it is also acquired through dietary sources such as beef, dairy products, and eggs.

Like triglycerides, cholesterol circulates throughout the body, aided by lipoproteins in the blood. In general terms, *high-density lipoprotein,* or HDL (see page 49), is the so-called "good" cholesterol because it carries cholesterol away from the arteries to the liver, where it is eventually removed from the body. *Low-density lipoprotein,* or LDL (see page 40), on the other hand, is considered the "bad" cholesterol because it transports the substance through the bloodstream, creating the risk of clogged arteries. LDL cholesterol is the type that contributes to heart disease when levels become too high. There is also *very-low-density lipoprotein,* or VLDL, which is mostly composed of triglycerides that convert to LDL in the blood, thereby raising the level of "bad" cholesterol.

The particle size of HDL and LDL, which is measured by Vertical Auto Profile (VAP) or NMR lipid profile tests, is also important in determining cholesterol's total effect on the body (see the inset on page 50). Large HDL particles are considered more beneficial than their smaller counterparts, and are associated with a lower risk of heart disease. Recently, doctors have started to measure *oxidized LDL,* a value representing the amount of damaged cholesterol in your blood, which can lead to plaque buildup and, eventually, atherosclerosis (see the inset on page 41).

Total cholesterol is the sum of HDL, LDL, and VLDL measurements. The table on the next page lists the reference ranges used by most labs for this value.

While it is possible to have very low total cholesterol levels, this condition is rare. (See the inset on page 39 about low cholesterol.) People with abnormal cholesterol readings usually fall into in the "borderline high" or "high" categories. High cholesterol, or *hypercholesterolemia,* may be due to one or several factors.

REFERENCE RANGES FOR TOTAL CHOLESTEROL	
Total Cholesterol (mg/dL)	**Category**
Greater than 239	High
200 to 239	Borderline high
Less than 200	Desirable
Target Range: 150 to 200 mg/dL	

WHAT CAUSES HIGH TOTAL CHOLESTEROL?

There are several reasons for total cholesterol levels that are high, borderline high, or simply not ideal. If your blood test results are abnormal, your doctor will review your medical history and request additional blood work to determine the cause. Some causative factors include:

- Being overweight or obese (BMI of 25 or above)
- Bile duct obstruction
- Binge drinking or excessive alcohol consumption
- Certain medications, such as progestin and steroids
- Chronic stress
- Diet high in refined carbohydrates and sugars, as well as trans fats (partially hydrogenated oils)
- Environmental toxicity due to heavy metals, pesticides, or other contaminants
- Family medical history
- Food allergies
- Insufficient exercise or lack of exercise
- Insulin resistance
- Intestinal conditions
- Kidney disease
- Poorly controlled diabetes
- Pregnancy
- Sex hormone imbalance, particularly as regards DHEA, estrogen, and testosterone
- Smoking
- Underactive thyroid (hypothyroidism)
- Vitamin C or E deficiency

Research has also indicated that some people may experience increased cholesterol levels during the winter months. Scientists have not determined what triggers this change—alterations in blood chemistry and reduced exercise are two possibilities—but it should be taken into consideration when evaluating blood test results.

High cholesterol may lead to a number of medical complications, many of which can be life threatening if left untreated. Like high triglycerides, elevated cholesterol can cause atherosclerosis, which is usually a precursor to coronary artery disease and increases the risk of heart attack and stroke. Angina (chest pain) and *transient ischemic attacks* (TIAs), or "little strokes," are also potential complications. In addition, high cholesterol contributes to problems that affect other parts of the body besides the heart. These conditions include diabetes and insulin resistance, kidney disease, liver disease, general inflammation, and metabolic syndrome.

WHAT ARE THE SYMPTOMS OF HIGH TOTAL CHOLESTEROL?

High cholesterol alone does not produce any physical symptoms. If the risk factors for high cholesterol—such as smoking, lack of physical activity, and poor diet—apply to you, have your lipid levels tested. Do not ignore warning signs such as chest pain or shortness of breath, as they may indicate a serious problem that might be related to elevated cholesterol levels.

HOW CAN HIGH TOTAL CHOLESTEROL BE TREATED?

High cholesterol can be managed effectively with medication, but a healthy lifestyle is vital for maintaining balanced cholesterol levels. Below are some recommendations for treating the condition to discuss with your physician.

DRUGS

When cholesterol is very high, it is often necessary to prescribe a drug that will quickly bring your level within a healthy range. Your doctor may recommend one drug or a combination. Take every substance prescribed to you only as directed. If you experience any persistent side effect or symptom that concerns you, consult your medical provider. Your prescription may need to be changed.

DRUGS FOR HIGH TOTAL CHOLESTEROL

Drug	Considerations
Bile acid sequestrants (colestipol, cholestyramine) *Colestid, LoCholest, Prevalite, Questran*	Potential side effects include blurred vision, diarrhea, fatigue, headache, liver problems, loss of appetite, memory loss, nausea, and vomiting. Bile acid sequestrants can also increase your risk of bleeding and deplete the body of essential nutrients, such as beta-carotene, calcium, folic acid, iron, magnesium, phosphorus, vitamin B_{12}, vitamin D, vitamin E, and vitamin K. Therefore, it is recommended that you take a daily multivitamin or mineral supplement while using bile acid sequestrants.

Drug	Considerations
Ezetimibe *Zetia*	May cause side effects such as diarrhea, joint pain, and increase in infections. Long-term side effects, like gall stones, muscle weakness, and liver problems, are also possible. This drug can deplete essential nutrients from the body, including vitamin D. You should take 1,000 IU of vitamin D_3 daily when using ezetimibe.
Niacin (extended-release)	Speak to your healthcare provider before using if you are on blood thinners or diabetes medication. Extended-release niacin usually does not cause flushing.
Statins (atorvastatin, rosuvastatin, lovastatin, pravastatin) *Lipitor, Crestor, Mevacor, Pravachol*	Statin drugs can deplete essential nutrients from the body, including CoQ_{10}, vitamin D, and vitamin E. Take 100 mg of CoQ_{10} daily along with a multivitamin or mineral supplement to prevent nutritional deficiencies. Side effects may include headache, muscle pain, nausea, weakness, elevated liver enzymes, memory loss, and kidney problems. Inform your doctor or pharmacist if you are currently on cholesterol-lowering drugs to avoid adverse drug interactions. Do not take with grapefruit juice.

SUPPLEMENTS

Nutritional supplements are also effective for enhancing general health and well-being, and may be a better option for those who have adverse reactions to drug therapy. A prominent cardiology researcher at the University of Minnesota, for example, discovered that he could not tolerate cholesterol-lowering statins, and had to turn to diet and supplements to lower his cholesterol. The nutritional supplements listed in the table below support healthy cholesterol levels. Speak to your doctor before taking any of these substances.

SUPPLEMENTS FOR HIGH CHOLESTEROL

Supplement	Dosage	Considerations
Aged garlic extract	600 mg one to three times a day.	Aged garlic extract is used to protect the heart and blood vessels, and is reported to help decrease oxidative stress markers, including those related to blood sugar regulation problems. Aged garlic has also been reported to reduce liver enzymes and fatty liver, as well as decrease the formation of advanced glycation end-products (AGEs), which are implicated in various health problems, such as heart disease, kidney problems, and cancer. Aged garlic is not reported to interfere with blood thinners.

Supplement	Dosage	Considerations
Artichoke extract	250 mg one to three times a day.	This supplement is reported to improve cholesterol balance by reducing total cholesterol and LDL cholesterol levels. Do not use if you have an allergy to plants in the daisy family, such as aster, dandelion, goldenrod, and yarrow. If you have liver or gall bladder problems, or digestive issues, consult your medical provider before taking artichoke. Use a standardized extract.
Coenzyme Q_{10} (CoQ_{10})	30 mg three times a day or 50 mg twice a day, depending on dose per capsule.	CoQ_{10} is important for energy production, oxygen use, high blood pressure, and heart health, especially in people with kidney disorders. It can also boost endurance, improve insulin sensitivity, and lower triglycerides and blood glucose levels. This supplement is especially recommended if you are taking statin drugs, red yeast rice, and certain diabetes medications, which may result in a CoQ_{10} deficiency.
Omega-3 essential fatty acids DHA and EPA (fish oil)	1,000 mg two to three times a day.	In addition to its anti-inflammatory properties, fish oil is reported to lower total cholesterol levels and decrease oxidative stress, which is associated with LDL, or "bad" cholesterol. Speak to your doctor before taking if you are on blood-thinning medication, as fish oil may increase the risk of bleeding. Be sure to use only high-quality oils that have been tested for contaminants.
Plant sterol esters	1.7 g one to two times a day.	Plant sterol esters have been shown to improve cholesterol levels and help lower LDL cholesterol. May interact with blood thinning medications, including aspirin. Effects of plant sterols may be counteracted by ezetimibe (Zetia).
Probiotics	5 to 10 billion CFUs two to three times a day.	Probiotics help normalize beneficial flora in the gastrointestinal tract, and are reported to decrease triglyceride and cholesterol levels. They are also reported to improve BUN levels and quality of life in people with kidney disease. It's best to use heat-stable products that do not require refrigeration. If using an antibiotic, wait three hours before taking probiotics. If diarrhea occurs, decrease your dosage. If this side effect persists for longer than 48 hours, stop taking the supplement and contact your doctor. Live cultures should be guaranteed through the date of expiration on label. For optimal results, take probiotics with meals, as food improves the survivability of the cultures.

LIFESTYLE CHANGES

Although lifestyle often contributes to high cholesterol, it can also be the key to lowering it. By following the guidelines below, you will be able to reduce and control your cholesterol levels. Even if high cholesterol is not a present worry, incorporating these behaviors into your daily life will help you keep your level in check.

- Avoid inflammation-causing foods. These foods can increase oxidation of cholesterol, making it more likely to build up in the arteries and form plaque. Stay away from foods that contain refined and added sugars like high-fructose corn syrup, which is often added to condiments, sauces, commercially produced snack foods, and sweetened beverages. Refined carbohydrates (white bread, pasta, bagels, and other foods made from white flour), processed and smoked meats, and fried foods should also be eliminated from the diet.

- Break bad habits. Smoking and regular alcohol consumption are unhealthy behaviors that can contribute to health problems. Studies show that ending these habits have a positive impact on your total cholesterol level.

- Consume healthy fats. Good fats are required for nutrition, and new studies show that moderate intake has a positive impact on your health. You can incorporate these fats into your diet by cooking with high flash-point oils, such as macadamia oil and other nut oils. Add olive oil only to foods that have already been prepared, since it breaks down easily when heated. If you must use butter, switch to organic butter for a purer product; avoid margarine, which is loaded with partially hydrogenated oils. Finally, start snacking on nuts like almonds, Brazil nuts, hazelnuts, pecans, and walnuts, which are all great sources of healthy fats. However, most nuts are calorically dense, so eat them sparingly.

- Eliminate trans fats. Hard margarine, fried and processed foods, and commercially baked goods—including breads, muffins, cookies, and pastries—usually contain partially hydrogenated oils, which are the primary source of trans fat. Stay away from these foods, as trans fats have been shown to raise LDL ("bad") cholesterol levels and lower HDL ("good") cholesterol. It's important to note that foods can still contain trans fat even if its nutrition label claims otherwise. Make sure partially hydrogenated oils are not listed as ingredients before buying any packaged food item.

- Exercise. Studies have conclusively shown that physical activity plays a significant role in lowering cholesterol. Begin by exercising for twenty- to thirty-minute sessions at least three to four times a week, and gradually increase the duration and level of intensity. An ideal fitness routine includes both aerobic exercise and strength training.

- Get rid of belly fat. A large waist circumference is a tell-tale sign of high cholesterol. To lower your total cholesterol level, you must lose abdominal fat.

- Get your hormone levels checked. Low testerone levels in men are associated with hyperlipidemia and heart disease, as is the absence of the hormone estradiol in post-menopausal women. See page 251 for more about hormone testing.

- Go green. Green tea, which is rich in antioxidants and compounds known as *polyphenols*, has been found to lower total cholesterol and raise HDL levels simultaneously. Research suggests that polyphenols block the absorption of cholesterol in the digestive tract and promote its removal from the body.

- Have an egg. Forget the old ban on eggs. Contrary to popular belief, eggs do not have much impact on cholesterol levels—though some people may be more "sensitive" than others to the dietary cholesterol in eggs. Studies have shown that for the majority of people, it is excessive intake of carbohydrates, not proteins or fats, that contribute to hyperlipidemia. Therefore, it is perfectly acceptable to eat a whole egg four or five times per week with your breakfast. On the other mornings, have a protein shake or a high-protein and low-carbohydrate meal.

- Incorporate omega-3s. Omega-3 fatty acids, such as EPA and DHA, have an anti-inflammatory effect on the body and reduce the risk of heart problems. Dietary sources of omega-3 include albacore tuna, cod, herring, mackerel, salmon, anchovies, and sardines, among other cold-water fish oils. Chia seeds, flax seeds, and walnuts are also rich in omega-3 fatty acids. However, do not rely on nuts and seeds for your total intake, as their omega-3s are not immediately bioavailable, undergoing chemical reactions before they are able to be used by the body.

- Limit your intake of whole grains. Although all grains should be eaten only in moderation, you should always choose whole grains over breads, cereals, and pasta made from refined flour. Whole grains are higher in fiber and lower on the glycemic index than refined versions. Still, they contain carbohydrates that eventually must be processed by the body. Eating too many grains—even whole grains—can lead to problems with glucose and insulin regulation, in turn stimulating the formation of LDL and VLDL. Eating too many grains can also trigger intestinal inflammation, thereby causing food allergies in people who have food sensitivities. When you eat whole grains, opt for gluten-free sources like brown rice.

- Look for lean cuts. Make sure you choose meat and poultry that contain the least amount of unhealthy fats. Beef is best from cows that are grass-fed, while eggs, chicken, lamb, fish, and bison should be free-range. If you can, buy organic meat, poultry, and animal products; but if conventionally raised meats are your only option, select the leanest meats possible, as well as skinless chicken, turkey, and fish.

- Make your plate colorful. Add plenty of fresh vegetables to your daily diet, especially leafy greens like kale and spinach, which have been shown to lower cholesterol levels. Also eat more low-glycemic fruit, such as strawberries and grapefruit, but limit your intake to two servings per day.

- Reduce the amount of dairy in your diet. Most doctors recommend that people with high cholesterol switch to reduced- or low-fat milk to avoid consuming too many saturated fats, which are found in whole dairy products. In some individuals, dairy also triggers inflammation, resulting in damaged arteries. To prevent these problems, replace cow's milk with unsweetened almond milk, coconut milk, or soy milk. Rice milk, another option, may be higher in carbohydrates, so select brands with the lowest amount. When replacing cow's milk with non-dairy versions, be sure to compensate for the loss in calcium by finding other dietary sources or taking supplements recommended by your doctor. In addition, stay away from soy milk made with genetically modified soy. If your family has a history of breast or prostate cancer, or if you have food allergies or sensitivities, do not take soy without first speaking to your doctor.

- Sleep. Studies show that insufficient sleep can raise the risk of high cholesterol, and sleep disorders can increase inflammation, leading to the formation of oxidized LDL (see page 41). To prevent this, it's recommended that you get seven to eight uninterrupted hours of sleep every night.

Low Cholesterol: Is It Harmful?

Like low triglycerides, low cholesterol—or *hypocholesterolemia*—is a rare condition that usually signals an underlying medical problem. While primary hypocholesterolemia is inherited, the secondary form is typically the result of diseases such as cancer, chronic inflammation, hyperthyroidism (overactive thyroid), infection, liver disease, and malnutrition. Alcoholism can also cause low cholesterol, since it compromises the function of the liver, which produces the majority of the body's cholesterol.

Although low levels do not have a negative impact on cardiovascular health, insufficient cholesterol can adversely affect other bodily functions, including that of the brain, liver, digestive system, and sex hormone production. Cholesterol that is too low for an extended period of time increases the risk of brain hemorrhages, as blood with very low cholesterol content does not clot easily. In addition, the activity of serotonin, a mood-regulating neurotransmitter, is hindered by cholesterol deficiency. As such, low cholesterol levels have been connected to psychological disorders like anxiety and depression.

If you do not have a chronic health problem, it is unlikely that your cholesterol will drop into a potentially dangerous range. Still, it's important to realize that there is such a thing as "too low" when it comes to certain biomarkers in the blood—even cholesterol.

Did You Know?

Even though we call it the "bad cholesterol," your body needs at least some LDL cholesterol in order to function properly. According to the Mayo Clinic, low levels of LDL cholesterol can result in increased risk of cancer, depression, anxiety. In pregnant women, low LDL cholesterol can also result in preterm birth and low birth weight.

3. LDL CHOLESTEROL

Known as the "bad" cholesterol, *low-density lipoproteins*, or LDLs, carry the majority of cholesterol in the body (about 70 percent) through the bloodstream and distribute it to the cells and tissues. The main problem with LDL cholesterol is that its molecules are *oxidized*—made toxic—more frequently than other lipid particles. This oxidized form of LDL, which is even more harmful than regular LDL, becomes lodged in arteries, slowing or completely blocking the flow of blood to your heart and other parts of the body (see the inset on page 42). This sets the stage for coronary artery disease and peripheral artery disease, which can lead to heart attack, stroke, or blood clots in other parts of the body. As such, high LDL cholesterol is not something to take lightly; it may result in a major and potentially fatal health problem.

The target range for LDL values has dropped progressively lower over the last decade as scientists have learned more about the substance and the health dangers it poses. The current reference ranges are listed in the table below.

REFERENCE RANGES FOR LDL CHOLESTEROL

LDL Cholesterol (mg/dL)	Category
Greater than 189	Very high
160 to 189	High
130 to 159	Borderline high
100 to 129	Slightly above normal
Less than 100	Normal
Target Range: 80 mg/dL or lower	

People who have diabetes or a pre-existing heart condition should stay to the lower end of the target range, while those who are in generally good health can keep their LDL around 100 mg/dL. Since cholesterol is needed to make hormones and other vital compounds, very low LDL can actually be detrimental. Some studies have shown a correlative relationship between very low LDL levels and increased risk of cancer and Parkinson's disease; however, it is unclear whether very low levels precede or follow the onset of these conditions. Researchers are also unsure of the role, if any, that cholesterol-lowering statin drugs play in raising the risk of the two diseases. Men who take lipid-lowering medications, for example, have twice the risk of lowered testos-

Oxidized LDL

Scientists have long been aware of the dangers of LDL cholesterol. In recent years, however, research has found that a specific type of this bad cholesterol, oxidized LDL, may be a more serious threat. People with metabolic syndrome are known to have high levels of oxidized LDL, as well as internal inflammation. LDL that is oxidized has been "attacked" by *free radicals*—also called oxidizers or oxygen radicals—which are highly unstable and reactive oxygen molecules. In order to gain stability, free radicals react with other molecules in the body, inflicting damage on cells and tissues. When free radicals come into contact with LDL particles, the oxidized byproduct accrues in the inner lining of arteries until a thick plaque forms, slowing or completely blocking blood flow. This condition, atherosclerosis, is likely to lead to blood clots, heart attack, or stroke. In other words, a high level of oxidized LDL is a key indicator of heart disease.

Oxidized LDL has many causes, including smoking, poorly controlled blood sugar levels, and a diet high in trans fats. Not eating enough foods rich in *antioxidants*—agents that neutralize free radicals—also makes your body more susceptible to oxidative stress. Foods such as berries, beans (kidney, pinto, and small red), artichokes, apples, and russet potatoes—all of which are excellent sources of antioxidants—protect against free radicals and, therefore, oxidized LDL. Green tea also has a high antioxidant value, so consuming 250 to 500 mg daily, whether in supplement form or as a tea, will fortify your body's defenses against harmful oxidizers. (Make sure that the supplement is standardized to 90-percent polyphenols and 50-percent EGCG content.) The following nutritional supplements are also recommended for lowering oxidized LDL levels.

SUPPLEMENTS FOR HIGH OXIDIZED LDL

Supplement	Dosage	Considerations
Aged garlic extract	600 mg one to three times a day.	Aged garlic extract is used to protect the heart and blood vessels, and is reported to help decrease oxidative stress markers, including those related to blood sugar regulation problems. Aged garlic has also been reported to reduce liver enzymes and fatty liver, as well as decrease the formation of advanced glycation end-products (AGEs), which are implicated in various health problems, such as heart disease, kidney problems, and cancer. Aged garlic is not reported to interfere with blood thinners.

Supplement	Dosage	Considerations
Cocoa	900 mg two to three times a day.	Cocoa contains antioxidant flavonoids, which help to decease oxidative stress, as well as LDL and total cholesterol levels. Although high in antioxidants, some cocoa contains a small amount with caffeine. Use with caution if you have a caffeine sensitivity. If you are on medications that may interact with caffeine, consult your doctor or pharmacist before taking cocoa.
Grape seed extract	100 to 150 mg twice a day.	Grape seed has anti-inflammatory and antioxidant activity, and is reported to help decrease the oxidation of LDL cholesterol, as well as the risk of heart disease. Side effects, though uncommon, may include dizziness, headache, itchy scalp, and nausea. It may also increase the risk of blood thinning, especially if you are taking aspirin or anticoagulant drugs. If you are taking blood thinners, NSAIDS, or heart medication, take only under a doctor's supervision. Do not use if you are allergic to grapes. Use an extract that is standardized to 90-percent proanthocyanidins.
Omega-3 essential fatty acids DHA and EPA (fish oil)	1,000 mg two to three times a day.	Fish oil is one of the first supplements recommended by doctors for lowering triglycerides. In addition to its anti-inflammatory properties, fish oil is reported to lower total cholesterol levels and decrease oxidativestress, which is associated with LDL, or "bad" cholesterol. Speak to your doctor before taking if you are on blood-thinning medication, as fish oil may increase the risk of bleeding. Be sure to use only high-quality oils that have been tested for contaminants.
Plant sterol esters	1.7 g one to two times a day.	Plant sterol esters have been shown to improve cholesterol levels and help lower LDL cholesterol. May interact with blood thinning medications, including aspirin. Effects of plant sterols may be counteracted by ezetimibe (Zetia).
Pomegranate extract	100 to 500 mg two to three times a day.	Pomegranate is an antioxidant that helps to decrease oxidative stress and inflammation in the body. It is also reported to inhibit LDL oxidation and decrease the risk of heart disease. Use only under a doctor's supervision if you are taking blood thinning medication, which may interact with pomegranate. Use a standardized extract.

Supplement	Dosage	Considerations
Tocotrienols	140 to 360 mg once a day.	Tocotrienols, a subset of vitamin E, are fat-soluble antioxidants reported to help decrease oxidized LDL cholesterol and the risk of developing heart disease. May interact with blood-thinning medications, including aspirin and warfarin (Coumadin). Use only under a doctor's supervision if you are taking these drugs.

Although it's good to get your antioxidants and nutrients from dietary sources, supplements can help reinforce the healthful benefits of the foods you eat. Before using any supplement, you should speak to a health-care professional who can assist you in determining an appropriate dose based on your needs.

terone, which is associated with the progression of heart disease and diabetes. More studies are needed before scientists can say with certainty if very low LDL levels are harmful. And since few people experience this condition, this section focuses on high LDL.

WHAT CAUSES HIGH LDL CHOLESTEROL?

Since LDL cholesterol is part of your total cholesterol, the causes of high LDL cholesterol and high total cholesterol overlap. One or more of the factors below may lead to raised LDL:

- Being overweight or obese (BMI of 25 or above)
- Binge drinking or excessive alcohol consumption
- Chronic stress (elevated cortisol)
- Diets high in refined carbohydrates and sugars, trans fat, and other inflammatory foods
- Family medical history
- High blood pressure
- Hypothyroidism
- Insufficient exercise or lack of exercise
- Insulin resistance
- Kidney disease or failure
- Poorly controlled diabetes
- Pregnancy

Age is also a risk factor for elevated LDL, as men over the age of forty-five and women older than fifty-five are more likely to have raised levels. Men and women within these age groups are encouraged to have blood tests on a yearly basis to more effectively manage their LDL cholesterol.

In addition to heart problems—which include atherosclerosis, coronary artery disease, and heart attack—high LDL cholesterol is associated with increased risk of stroke, peripheral artery disease, metabolic syndrome, kidney disease, and liver disease, as well as low testosterone levels in men. And since insulin resistance and type 2 diabetes often go hand-in-hand with elevated LDL cholesterol, you may want to consider having a blood glucose test (see pages 59 to 79) if your cholesterol is high.

WHAT ARE THE SYMPTOMS OF HIGH LDL CHOLESTEROL?

While elevated LDL cholesterol does not cause symptoms on its own, heart disease is often indicated by chest pains, dizziness, and shortness of breath. Frequent leg cramps and poor circulation due to blocked arteries may also result. If you experience these symptoms, you should seek medical attention immediately.

HOW CAN HIGH LDL CHOLESTEROL BE TREATED?

Even if high LDL cholesterol shows up on your blood test results, it's not too late to lower your number and achieve a level that is ideal for you. In addition, with some changes to your lifestyle, you can prevent your level from reaching the point where medication is necessary. The following recommendations can put your LDL level on the right (downward) track.

DRUGS

The most direct way to treat an abnormal lab value is medication, particularly statin drugs—the most effective and widely used pharmaceuticals for bringing down high LDL cholesterol. These include Crestor (rosuvastatin), Lescol (fluvastatin), Lipitor (atorvastatin calcium), Mevacor (lovastatin), Pravachol (lovastatin), and Zocor (simvastatin). When using this class of drugs, 100 mg of coenzyme Q_{10} (CoQ_{10}) should also be taken, as statins are known to deplete the body of this vital nutrient, leading to severe muscle aches. Side effects such as headache, nausea, and fatigue may also occur. Speak to your health practitioner before taking a statin drug. It's important to note that unless your levels are dangerously high, it's advisable to try dietary and lifestyle modifications before taking pharmaceutical drugs.

SUPPLEMENTS

In addition to medication and lifestyle adjustments (see pages 46 to 48), you may choose to take a nutritional supplement. People who have adverse reactions to drugs may also consider natural therapies like supplementation. The substances listed in the table below have been found to support cardiovascular health and help lower LDL cholesterol. Ask your healthcare provider to recommend an appropriate dosage and suppliers of high-quality products.

SUPPLEMENTS FOR HIGH LDL CHOLESTEROL

Supplement	Dosage	Considerations
Aged garlic extract	600 mg one to three times a day.	Aged garlic extract is used to protect the heart and blood vessels, and is reported to help decrease oxidative stress markers, including those related to blood sugar regulation problems. Aged garlic has also been reported to reduce liver enzymes and fatty liver, as well as decrease the formation of advanced glycation end-products (AGEs), which are implicated in various health problems, such as heart disease, kidney problems, and cancer. Aged garlic is not reported to interfere with blood thinners.
Chromium	200 mcg once a day.	In addition to lowering triglycerides, total cholesterol, and LDL cholesterol, chromium is reported to improve insulin sensitivity and glucose tolerance.
Fiber	Check the product label for dosage guidelines. The recommendation for women is 25 g per day, and for men, 30 g per day.	Guar gum (Sunfiber) is an excellent source of soluble dietary fiber. Potential side effects include abdominal discomfort and bloating. Excess fiber may also interfere with the absorption of certain nutrients like iron and calcium.
Magnesium	250 to 500 mg twice a day.	Use magnesium aspartate, citrate, taurate, glycinate, or any amino acid chelate. Supports bone building and balances calcium intake. The ratio of calcium-to-magnesium intake should be between 1 to 1 and 2 to 1. This supplement is reported to improve blood vessel function and insulin resistance, in addition to decreasing LDL cholesterol, total cholesterol, and triglycerides. Also essential for phase-I liver detoxification. If you experience loose stools after taking magnesium, cut your dose in half and gradually increase over the course of a few months. Consult your health-care provider for dosage advice.

Supplement	Dosage	Considerations
Omega-3 essential fatty acids DHA and EPA	1,000 mg two to three times a day.	Fish oil is one of the first supplements recommended by doctors for lowering triglycerides. In addition to its anti-inflammatory properties, fish oil is reported to lower total cholesterol levels and decrease oxidative

(fish oil)		stress, which is associated with LDL, or "bad" cholesterol. Speak to your doctor before taking if you are on blood-thinning medication, as fish oil may increase the risk of bleeding. Be sure to use only high-quality oils that have been tested for contaminants.
Pantethine (pantothenic acid or vitamin B_5)	250 mg two to three times a day.	Has been reported to improve cholesterol levels by lowering total cholesterol, LDL cholesterol, and triglycerides, while increasing HDL cholesterol. You may also consider taking a good-quality multivitamin that contains pantethine.
Plant sterol esters	1.7 g one to two times a day.	Plant sterol esters have been shown to improve cholesterol levels and help lower LDL cholesterol. May interact with blood thinning medications, including aspirin. Effects of plant sterols may be counteracted by ezetimibe (Zetia).
Probiotics	5 to 10 billion CFUs two to three times a day.	Probiotics help normalize beneficial flora in the gastrointestinal tract, and are reported to decrease triglyceride and cholesterol levels. They are also reported to improve BUN levels and quality of life in people with kidney disease. It's best to use heat-stable products that do not require refrigeration. If using an antibiotic, wait three hours before taking probiotics. If diarrhea occurs, decrease your dosage. If this side effect persists for longer than 48 hours, stop taking the supplement and contact your doctor. Live cultures should be guaranteed through the date of expiration on label. For optimal results, take probiotics with meals, as food improves the survivability of the cultures.

LIFESTYLE CHANGES

Most healthcare professionals agree that diet and lifestyle changes should always be your first course of action when trying to lower your cholesterol. Even if your LDL cholesterol is not officially high, you should still take the steps needed to prevent your number from climbing upwards. There are plenty of natural approaches that will allow you to attain and maintain an optimal lab value. If you are currently taking medication for high LDL cholesterol, you should adopt these healthy behaviors to keep your medication dosages as low as possible and achieve better overall health.

The most natural way to fight high LDL cholesterol is through lifestyle modifications like quitting smoking, limiting alcohol consumption, exercising regularly, and perhaps most importantly, eating a healthy diet. In fact, a recent study published in the *Journal of the American Medical Association* suggests that diet may be more important than previously believed. According to the findings, four specific food substances—plant sterols, soy protein, soluble fiber, and nuts—can lower cholesterol by as much as 14 percent when incorporated into a healthy diet. By including these foods in your diet and following the guidelines below, you can eat your way to a healthier LDL level. Keep in mind that this type of diet also promotes the loss of body fat, which helps you lose weight. Reducing your weight by as little as five pounds can have a positive impact on LDL cholesterol levels.

- Add soy protein to your diet. Studies have shown that 25 g per day can lower your risk of heart disease. You can consume this amount easily by eating foods like edamame, tempeh, tofu, soy cheese, soy nuts, soy yogurt, and whole beans, and by replacing cow's milk with soy milk. However, be sure to stay away from genetically modified soy products, and avoid soy in general if breast or prostate cancer runs in your family. Also keep in mind that soy is a common allergen and should not be eaten in excessive quantities. If you have experienced symptoms such as unexplained achy joints, headaches, fatigue, or chronic sinus problems—common signs of food sensitivities—see your doctor. It may not be a good idea for you to consume soy protein.

- Avoid processed foods. Processed and refined foods often contain unhealthy ingredients such as high-fructose corn syrup, a harmful sugar found in condiments, sauces, snack foods, and sweetened beverages.

- Be careful with your carbohydrate choices. Most people believe that reducing fat intake is the most important factor in lowering cholesterol, but the quality and quantity of the carbohydrates that you eat has a greater impact. Choose bread, cereal, pasta, rice, and other grain products that are made from whole grains, which are rich in fiber and plant sterols. Limit your intake to one to two servings daily, as eating too many starchy carbohydrates is one of the main reasons for the current obesity epidemic in the United States. The most recent USDA dietary guidelines recommend filling no more than a quarter of your plate with whole grains. Vegetables and fruits should make up half the plate (more vegetables than fruits), and the remaining one-fourth of the plate can be filled by lean protein.

- Incorporate fish into your diet. Eating fish like herring, lake trout, mackerel, and sardines will allow you to benefit from the health-enhancing properties of omega-3 fatty acids.

- Increase your intake of fiber, especially soluble fiber. You can do this by eating foods such as apples, pears, prunes, kidney beans, barley, and oatmeal. Leafy green vegetables, including spinach and kale, are also high in fiber, not to mention plant sterols. Consuming 20 to 30 g of soluble fiber per day can decrease your LDL cholesterol.

- Purchase lean cuts of meat and poultry. Make sure they are from grass-fed and free-range animals whenever possible. Your lean protein sources should make up 34 percent of your diet if you are following a modified-carbohydrate, low-glycemic-load diet. You can also follow the USDA's dietary recommendations, which state that one-fourth of your plate should be filled by lean protein.

- Replace your fat sources. Trans and saturated fats should be swapped for healthier monounsaturated fats, which you can do easily by cooking with nut oils and eating nuts like almonds, walnuts, and hazelnuts. Nuts are also a good source of antioxidants and plant sterols, a substance that is now being added to a variety of foods.

A Helpful Tip

For lower LDL cholesterol, eat fewer foods with trans and saturated fats, and more foods with monounsaturated fats! The American Heart Association recommends that adults consume at least four servings each week of nuts, legumes, and seeds, all of which are high in monounsaturated fat, as are olive oil and sunflower oil. The AHA also advocates substituting fish, which is high in the "good fats"--Omega-3 fatty acids--for meat, which is high in "bad" saturated fat. Two or more 3.5-ounce servings of fish per week will help get you on track to your target LDL cholesterol level.

4. HDL CHOLESTEROL

The "good" cholesterol in your body is *high-density lipoprotein,* or HDL, cholesterol. It's highly desirable to have an elevated level of HDL because it carries "bad" cholesterol to the liver, where it is then removed from your system. A helpful way to think about HDL is as a maintenance or cleaning crew that searches for and expels the cholesterol that causes clogged arteries. Keeping your HDL at a favorable level significantly reduces the risk of coronary artery disease. Reference ranges for this value, which differ for men and women, are indicated in the table.

REFERENCE RANGES FOR HDL CHOLESTEROL

	At Risk	Normal	Target Range
Men	Less than 40 mg/dL	40 to 50 mg/dL	Greater than 60 mg/dL
Women	Less than 50 mg/dL	50 to 60 mg/dL	Greater than 60 mg/dL

When it comes to HDL cholesterol, most doctors agree that the higher the number, the better off you are. However, not all HDLs are created equal. Too much of the wrong type of HDL (see the inset on page 50) may mean that you are not reaping its cardioprotective benefits. An unfavorable ratio of triglycerides to HDL can also signal a problem, which is why the ratio is included on the lipid profile. A ratio of 1 to 1 is ideal, 2 to 1 is considered good, and 3 to 1 is satisfactory. If a blood test indicates that your ratio may pose heart risks, your physician will recommend an appropriate treatment. In general, a high level of HDL cholesterol is considered a key marker of good health. Low numbers, though, can raise your risk of chronic disease even if your other cholesterol levels are "normal." If your HDL level is not where it should be, getting to the root of the problem is the first step.

WHAT CAUSES LOW HDL CHOLESTEROL?

There are several causes of low HDL cholesterol, many of which are related to lifestyle. These include:

- Being overweight or obese (BMI of 25 or above)
- Chronic stress
- Diet high in refined carbohydrates and sugars, and very low in fat

- Excessive use of certain medications, such as anabolic steroids (testosterone), antipsychotics, high-dose beta blockers, high-dose thiazide diuretics, and progesterone
- High triglyceride levels

"Good" and "Bad" HDL Cholesterol

HDL cholesterol is vital for good health, but quality is just as important as quantity. First, particle size matters. Large HDL molecules (HDL-2) can transport greater quantities of bad cholesterol to the liver, which makes them more beneficial to cardiovascular health. Smaller particles (HDL-3) do not provide extra cardiovascular protection. Of equal significance is the type of protein composing the HDLs. *ApoA-I* is considered the "good" protein while *apoA-II* is "bad." Having more apoA-II HDLs than apoA-I HDLs is undesirable; this will contribute to heart disease rather than prevent it.

Luckily, there is a way to find out if a high level of HDL cholesterol is actually working in your favor. The Vertical Auto Profile (VAP) test and the nuclear magnetic resonance (NMR) lipid profile are expanded lipid panel blood tests that can identify undetected cholesterol problems. These comprehensive tests measure fifteen different blood cholesterol components, including detailed information about HDL and LDL. For instance, you can find out if your LDL cholesterol is pattern A, which is safer and can be removed more easily, or pattern B, a more dangerous type of LDL that remains in the bloodstream longer and is oxidized more easily. It also measures your level of Lp(a) cholesterol, a specific type of LDL particle. In addition, this more extensive profile will tell you the type and size of your HDL cholesterol, as well as measure VLDL, homocysteine (see page 291), and C-reactive protein (see page 299).

VAP tests and NMR lipid profiles are usually recommended for people who have diabetes, high blood pressure, atherosclerosis, or a family history of heart disease, as well as for individuals who smoke. Men over forty-five years of age and women over fifty-five should also have one of these tests, which are highly accurate and covered by most insurance providers. Numerous national and regional labs now have cutting-edge equipment developed by Atherotech, Inc., the company that created the VAP test. However, some experts believe that the NMR lipid profile may provide more accurate readings of all the important lipid fractions. Contact your local lab to find out if one or both of these tests are offered, or ask your doctor.

- Insufficient exercise or lack of exercise
- Low levels of magnesium and/or omega-3 fatty acids
- Malnutrition
- Smoking
- Testosterone deficiency (in men)

Like elevated triglycerides and cholesterol levels, heredity may also be to blame for low HDL cholesterol. Studies have shown that certain ethnic populations, such as Asian Indians, may be predisposed to low HDL. There are also rare genetic diseases that can cause low HDL levels.

Since HDL cholesterol removes the "bad" cholesterol from your body, a deficiency can increase your odds of developing serious health conditions, including atherosclerosis and coronary artery disease, heart attack, and stroke. Low HDL can also put you at high risk for blood clots, chronic inflammation, kidney disease, liver disease, metabolic syndrome, and type 2 diabetes.

WHAT ARE THE SYMPTOMS OF LOW HDL CHOLESTEROL?

Low HDL cholesterol does not produce symptoms, so a blood test is the only way to know for sure if you have this condition. However, low HDL contributes to heart disease, for which there may be warning signs such as chest pain, dizziness, leg cramps, and shortness of breath. If you experience one or more of these symptoms, medical attention is strongly advised.

HOW CAN LOW HDL CHOLESTEROL BE TREATED?

Even if your LDL cholesterol is low, it's important for your HDL to be within a desirable range. So if a blood test indicates that your HDL cholesterol is not ideal, you should take the steps necessary to raise your level. Your doctor may want to use medication for low HDL, but dietary and lifestyle measures are usually encouraged first to see if they have any impact.

DRUGS

When a blood test indicates that HDL cholesterol is too low, medication is the first course of action only if the complete lipid profile indicates very high cardiovascular risk. The drugs below are those most commonly recommended by doctors to patients who need to raise their HDL level. Take any drug that is prescribed to you only as directed by your doctor.

DRUGS FOR LOW HDL CHOLESTEROL	
Drug	**Considerations**
Fenofibrate *Tricor*	Side effects may include constipation, diarrhea, heartburn, nausea and/or vomiting, muscle aches, headache, retinopathy, anemia, lung problems, and pancreatitis. The drug may also deplete the body of essential nutrients, such as vitamin E, vitamin D, DHEA, and coenzyme Q_{10}. Therefore, it is recommended that you also take 100 mg of CoQ_{10} once a day, as well as a multivitamin or mineral supplement daily.
Gemfibrozil *Lopid*	Gemfibrozil may produce side effects such as constipation, diarrhea, heartburn, nausea and/or vomiting, muscle aches, headache, retinopathy, anemia, lung problems, and pancreatitis. This drug may also deplete essential nutrients from the body, including vitamin E, vitamin D, DHEA, and coenzyme Q_{10}. Therefore, it is recommended that you also take 100 mg of CoQ_{10} once a day, as well as a multivitamin or mineral supplement daily.
Loop diuretics (bumetanide, torsemide, furosemide) *Bumex, Demadex, Lasix*	Loop diuretics may cause depletion of calcium, magnesium, potassium, vitamin B_1, vitamin B_6, vitamin C, and zinc. Side effects may include bone loss, confusion, dry mouth, fatigue, headache, irregular heartbeat, mood changes, muscle cramps, nervousness, numbness, and poor wound healing.
Niacin (extended-release)	Speak to your healthcare provider before using if you are on blood thinners or diabetes medication. Extended-release usually does not cause flushing.
Non-steroidal anti-inflammatory drugs (NSAIDs) *Advil, Aleve, Motrin, Naprosyn*	Side effects vary among different NSAIDs, but can include constipation, diarrhea, gastrointestinal bleeding, headache, liver and/or kidney problems, and upset stomach. These drugs can also deplete the body of essential nutrients, such as DHEA, folic acid, melatonin, and zinc. You should take a quality daily multivitamin or mineral supplement while using NSAIDs. If you have trouble sleeping, taking 1 to 5 mg of melatonin one hour before bedtime may help. Start at the lowest possible dose and increase as necessary if your sleep cycle does not improve.
Phosphate salts (dicalcium phosphate, dibasic calcium phosphate)	Side effects may include upset stomach and/or vomiting.
Statins *Lipitor (atorvastatin) Crestor (rosuvastatin) Mevacor (lovastatin) Pravachol (pravastatin)*	Statin drugs can deplete essential nutrients from the body, including CoQ_{10}, vitamin D, and vitamin E. Take 100 mg of CoQ_{10} daily along with a multivitamin or mineral supplement to prevent nutritional deficiencies. Side effects may include headache, muscle pain, nausea, weakness, elevated liver enzymes, memory loss, and kidney problems. Inform your doctor or pharmacist if you are currently on cholesterol-lowering drugs to avoid adverse drug interactions. Do not take with grapefruit juice.

SUPPLEMENTS

You may want to consider taking a supplement to ensure you're getting all the nutrients your body needs to manufacture good cholesterol and ward off the bad cholesterol. Some supplements that may help boost HDL cholesterol are detailed in the table below. It's important to note that, as you may have noticed, niacin (vitamin B_3) is available as a supplement form as well as a prescription medication. However, prescription niacin—a much more concentrated form of the substance—is used only for lowering triglycerides and LDL cholesterol, and requires a doctor's supervision, as well as periodic liver enzyme testing. Most over-the-counter niacin products contain 25 to 100 mg per tablet or capsule, and are not extended release. (Extended- or sustained-release products are designed to dissolve slowly over a certain period of time.) Extended-release niacin products are available in 500-mg doses, but require regular testing of liver enzyme levels. Also, only niacin—not other forms of vitamin B_3 like niacinamide and inositol hexniacinate—is effective for hyperlipidemia. Although supplements do not require a prescription, their use should be guided by a healthcare professional. You should also consult your doctor about appropriate dosing, which may vary according to individual needs and overall health.

SUPPLEMENTS FOR LOW HDL CHOLESTEROL

Supplement	Dosage	Considerations
Aged garlic extract	600 mg one to three times a day.	Aged garlic extract is used to protect the heart and blood vessels, and is reported to help decrease oxidative stress markers, including those related to blood sugar regulation problems. Aged garlic has also been reported to reduce liver enzymes and fatty liver, as well as decrease the formation of advanced glycation end-products (AGEs), which are implicated in various health problems, such as heart disease, kidney problems, and cancer. Aged garlic is not reported to interfere with blood thinners.
Magnesium	250 to 500 mg twice a day.	Use magnesium aspartate, citrate, taurate, glycinate, or any amino acid chelate. Supports bone building and balances calcium intake. The ratio of calcium-to-magnesium intake should be between 1 to 1 and 2 to 1. This supplement is reported to improve blood vessel function and insulin resistance, in addition to decreasing LDL cholesterol, total cholesterol, and triglycerides. Also essential for

Supplement	Dosage	Considerations
Magnesium (continued)		phase-I liver detoxification. If you experience loose stools after taking magnesium, cut your dose in half and gradually increase over the course of a few months. Consult your health-care provider for dosage advice.
Niacin (vitamin B_3, extended-release)	500 to 1,000 mg once a day.	Speak to your medical provider before using if you are currently on blood thinners or diabetes medication. Extended-release niacin should not cause flushing. Have your liver enzyme levels tested regularly while taking niacin.
Omega-3 essential fatty acids DHA and EPA (fish oil)	1,000 mg two to three times a day.	Fish oil is one of the first supplements recommended by doctors for lowering triglycerides. In addition to its anti-inflammatory properties, fish oil is reported to lower total cholesterol levels and decrease oxidative stress, which is associated with LDL, or "bad" cholesterol. Speak to your doctor before taking if you are on blood-thinning medication, as fish oil may increase the risk of bleeding. Be sure to use only high-quality oils that have been tested for contaminants.
Plant sterol esters	1.7 g one to two times a day.	Plant sterol esters have been shown to improve cholesterol levels and help lower LDL cholesterol. May interact with blood thinning medications, including aspirin. Effects of plant sterols may be counteracted by ezetimibe (Zetia).
Probiotics	5 to 10 billion CFUs two to three times a day.	Probiotics help normalize beneficial flora in the gastrointestinal tract, and are reported to decrease triglyceride and cholesterol levels. They are also reported to improve BUN levels and quality of life in people with kidney disease. It's best to use heat-stable products that do not require refrigeration. If using an antibiotic, wait three hours before taking probiotics. If diarrhea occurs, decrease your dosage. If this side effect persists for longer than 48 hours, stop taking the supplement and contact your doctor. Live cultures should be guaranteed through the date of expiration on label. For optimal results, take probiotics with meals, as food improves the survivability of the cultures.

LIFESTYLE CHANGES

Like other labs on the lipid panel, maintaining a healthy HDL level—as well as preventing an *unhealthy* level—is influenced by diet and lifestyle. Although there is some debate about whether certain foods are effective for raising HDL levels, a few studies have shown that common dietary recommendations for lowering total cholesterol may also help increase HDL. The most effective dietary measures for raising HDL are the same as those used for lowering triglycerides. When triglycerides are reduced, HDL almost always increases.

First, it's most important to reduce your intake of inflammation-causing foods that elevate blood glucose, primarily sugary drinks, sweets, and foods made with white flour, like white bread and pasta. Even natural sweeteners like honey and molasses should be used sparingly. Pay attention to every source of sugar in your diet—for example, jellies, jams, ketchup, and hidden sugars in foods like yogurt and sweetened fruit—and cut back on your consumption. HDL cholesterol levels also improve when consumption of foods containing or fried in partially hydrogenated oils is decreased. As you already know, these oils are loaded with trans fat, a substance that contributes to internal inflammation, heart disease, and other health problems. Instead, take in more monounsaturated fats, which enhance the anti-inflammatory properties of HDL, by using nut oils when cooking or by snacking on raw unsalted nuts. Nuts, along with cranberries and fish high in omega-3s, also help support a better LDL-to-HDL ratio. Boosting fiber intake by eating more leafy green vegetables, beans, low-glycemic fruit, and some whole grains is strongly encouraged as well; you should aim for at least two servings of fiber-rich foods per day. In addition to providing your body with fiber, these foods are excellent sources of antioxidants, which reduce inflammation. Finally, one or two glasses of red wine per day have been reported to have a positive impact on HDL levels. However, drinking more than this amount is not recommended.

In addition to adjusting dietary intake, adopting a few healthy habits will also favorably affect your HDL cholesterol. Aerobic workouts—exercise that increases your heart rate—are especially beneficial for raising HDL numbers, so do some form of cardio in thirty-minute sessions four or five times a week. Running, walking, bicycling, swimming, and sports such as tennis are all great options. Physical activity will also help you lose weight, which is crucial for healthy cholesterol levels as well. If you smoke, quitting can raise your HDL level by 10 percent.

CONCLUSION

You are now familiar with the full lipid panel. These four biomarkers—triglycerides, total cholesterol, LDL, and HDL—along with homocysteine and C-reactive protein (see pages 291 and 299), are closely connected, so treating one abnormal lab value may positively affect one or more of the others. When reading your lipid panel blood test results, keep in mind that "normal" and "target" numbers are not always the same for everyone. Your unique biochemistry, genetics, and other individual factors play a role in determining lab values, as well as your risk of heart disease, metabolic syndrome, and other medical conditions. You should strive for your *personal best* number, which should be as close to the target range as possible. When a blood test indicates that treatment is necessary, you should work with a health practitioner—preferably one who is familiar with your medical history—to correct the problem with medication, lifestyle changes, or both.

A Helpful Tip

Before taking a blood test including a lipid panel, you typically will be asked to abstain from all food or drink for ten to twelve hours before the test is scheduled. You are permitted to drink water and take any other prescribed medicines during the fast, unless your doctor tells you otherwise.

PART 2

The Basic Metabolic Panel

The basic metabolic panel (BMP) tests for various indicators of metabolic functioning, including blood sugar (glucose) level, electrolyte and fluid balance, and kidney operation. Glucose, calcium, sodium, potassium, carbon dioxide, chloride, urea nitrogen, creatinine, and the glomerular filtration rate (GFR) are also included in the BMP, which is primarily used to detect and diagnose conditions such as diabetes and kidney disease. Doctors may also order this panel of tests to determine if a medication is working properly or throwing certain lab values out of balance. For example, diuretics used to treat high blood pressure may affect electrolyte balance and the kidneys, so a BMP test is frequently recommended for patients taking these drugs. Some BMP tests require fasting for at least eight hours prior to having your blood drawn, so be sure to ask your health practitioner for pretesting instructions.

One of the biggest problems with BMP tests is that "trending" lab values—numbers that technically fall within the normal range but are headed in the wrong direction—are rarely discussed with patients. In other words, "low normal" and "high normal" lab values are not typically treated as health concerns. Instead, the usual approach is to watch and wait for a trending lab to finally become abnormal. By this time, a disease or other medical condition has very often already developed.

A Kaiser Permanente Study that tracked over 46,000 people for a decade demonstrated the limitations of this approach. According to the study, for every one-point rise in fasting blood sugar over 84 mg/dL, an individual's risk of diabetes increases by about 6 percent. This may seem like only a slight increase, but by the time blood glucose levels reach 90 to 94 mg/dL, the risk of developing diabetes increases by 49 percent. And if blood glucose levels reach the highest normal range of 95 to 99 mg/dL, the risk of diabetes is more than doubled.

Why is this so shocking? Because the "normal" range for fasting blood glucose levels is 65 to 99 mg/dL, which means that lab values which may actually warrant further consideration are treated as normal. More alarming is the fact that when fasting blood sugar reaches a level of 90 mg/dL—a value technically within the "normal" range—vascular and kidney damage can begin to develop in the body. For the most part, doctors do not inform patients about concerns regarding their blood glucose until their level reaches 100 mg/dL, when—according to the Kaiser Study—their diabetes risk has already climbed to a staggering 84 percent. These statistics are a testament to the critical importance of blood tests and why you should become knowledgeable about your labs and always inquire about your results, even when you are told they are normal. Monitoring and managing trends is just as important as treating abnormal blood values. In the case of BMP tests, reversing a trend with diet, lifestyle changes, and even supplements can help prevent the development of diabetes and kidney disease, among other medical conditions.

Did You Know?

As discovered by Dr. Karl Landsteiner in 1901, there are four major blood groups, each based on the presence or absence of two specific antigens (molecules that stimulates immune responses): A, B, AB, and O. Blood group O is considered the "universal donor" because it lacks both A and B antigens and can thus be donated to any other group; blood group AB is considered the "universal recipient" because it possesses both antigens and can thus accept donations from any group.

5. GLUCOSE

Glucose is a type of sugar that acts as the body's chief source of energy. During digestion, foods rich in carbohydrates (starches and sugars) are broken down into three simple sugars—*fructose, galactose,* and *glucose.* Upon entering the bloodstream, glucose is transported to each of your cells. In response to the rise in glucose in the body, the pancreas releases *insulin,* a hormone that attaches to cell membranes to allow glucose to be taken out of the blood and carried to the cells, where it is used for energy production.

However, excessive carbohydrate and sugar consumption can disrupt normal glucose metabolism, triggering blood sugar imbalances. Excessive insulin release and *insulin resistance* can cause poor blood sugar control, leading to chronic high blood sugar, or *hyperglycemia.* Blood glucose levels may also "crash," or drop suddenly, resulting in low concentrations of blood glucose in a condition known as *hypoglycemia.* Hypoglycemia occurs because too much insulin is released, which may be due to defective insulin receptors or a deficiency of one or more of the trace minerals needed for blood glucose regulation—B vitamins, chromium, magnesium, vanadium, and zinc. Low vitamin D can also be a cause, since the vitamin plays an important role in insulin production and sensitivity. A disproportionate amount of insulin in the blood causes glucose to be carried out of the bloodstream and into the cells, resulting in a drop in blood sugar. This can trigger symptoms such as anxiousness, agitation, dizziness, sweating, and weakness.

Besides nutritional deficiencies and defective insulin receptors, blood sugar imbalance may also be related to environmental toxins, low thyroid hormones, low sex hormones, and chronic stress. Both high blood glucose and low blood glucose are associated with diabetes (see the inset on page 63), heart disease, and kidney failure, among other medical issues. Poorly controlled blood sugar is also directly linked to Alzheimer's disease, Parkinson's disease, and autoimmune disorders.

If a routine lab test indicates that your blood glucose level is abnormal, your doctor will most likely order a *fasting blood sugar* (FBS) test, which requires you to abstain from food and beverages besides water for about eight hours beforehand. This blood test, which is typically used to check for diabetes, can provide a better picture of your glucose level, since it is unaffected by food and drink. Your doctor may also recommend a *hemoglobin A1C (HbA1c) test,* which reflects average blood sugar over the past two or three months. Specifically, the test measures the amount of damage done to red blood cells (RBCs), which occurs when glucose molecules become attached to hemoglobin (a protein found in RBCs), or *glycated*. Other options are the two-hour *postprandial* (after eating) *blood sugar test* and the *oral glucose tolerance test*, which is typically ordered for pregnant women suspected to have *gestational* (pregnancy-induced) *diabetes*.

The reference ranges for fasting blood glucose are provided in the table.

REFERENCE RANGES FOR BLOOD GLUCOSE	
Fasting Blood Glucose (mg/dL)	**Category**
Higher than 125	Diabetes
100 to 125	Prediabetes (impaired fasting glucose)
65 to 99	Normal
Lower than 65	Low (hypoglycemic)
Target Range: 70 to 84 mg/dL	

In addition to blood sugar, it's also important to monitor your levels of insulin, especially if you have one or more risk factors for type 2 diabetes. *Insulin resistance* (IR), is a condition in which the hormone insulin does not bind to cells and activate the insulin receptors, so blood sugar is not lowered. Typically, IR precedes type 2 diabetes and lasts for at least a decade before diabetes develops. This destructive process is associated with a host of medical issues, including Alzheimer's disease, breast cancer, hypertension, kidney disease, and obesity. Insulin resistance is a defining characteristic of metabolic syndrome, which increases the risk of heart disease, stroke, and non-alcoholic fatty liver disease.

One way to test for this condition is a two-hour postprandial blood test, in which glucose and insulin levels are measured two hours after eating a meal containing 75 g of carbohydrates, such as a bagel with jelly. Results of this test indicate the efficiency with which the body processes glucose and secretes insulin. Reference ranges for insulin levels are provided in the table below.

REFERENCE RANGES FOR INSULIN	
Insulin (mg/dL)	**Category**
50 or above	High alert
25 to 49	High, trending towards insulin resistance
17 to 25	Acceptable
Target Range: 5 to 17 mg/dL, with blood glucose less than 90 mg/dL	

As indicated by the target range above, the relationship between insulin and blood glucose levels is significant. If both blood glucose and insulin are high, you are at the peak of insulin resistance. If blood glucose is high and insulin is very low (2 mg/dL, for example), your body is likely in the process of developing diabetes, even if your fasting blood glucose level is considered normal. And if your blood glucose level is somewhere between low and normal, and your insulin level is high, you are in the process of becoming insulin resistant.

High insulin can be caused by a number of factors, including a diet high in refined sugars and carbohydrates, insufficient exercise or lack of exercise, obesity, and genetics. Fructose and galactose intolerance, which are hereditary conditions, can also be at the root of high insulin, as can antibiotics, corticosteroids, and oral contraceptives, among other medications. If left untreated, type 2 diabetes is the usual result. Low insulin levels are also problematic and can be a sign of type 1 diabetes, *hypopituitarism* (underactive pituitary glands), or diseases of the pancreas. An insulin level of 2 mg/dL or lower in combination with a very high blood glucose reading requires extensive testing.

While insulin is not included on the basic metabolic panel, testing for insulin resistance is crucial. This section, however, concentrates on the causes, associated medical concerns, and recommended treatments for abnormal blood glucose levels, which will allow you to take the appropriate action based on the outcome of your lab test.

WHAT CAUSES HIGH BLOOD GLUCOSE?

When the body does not produce enough insulin or cannot use insulin properly, the result is high blood sugar, or hyperglycemia. This condition is a symptom of *prediabetes,* which raises the risk of heart disease and related health problems, even though diabetes has not fully developed. Some causes of high blood glucose include:

- Acromegaly, a disorder characterized by the overproduction of growth hormone
- Cancer (liver and pancreatic)
- Chronic stress
- Diet high in simple carbohydrates and/or refined sugars
- Environmental toxicity
- Hormonal changes or imbalances (estrogen in women, testosterone in men)

- Hypothyroidism
- Insulin resistance
- Kidney disease or kidney failure
- Medications including birth control pills, corticosteroids, diuretics, epinephrine, estrogen, lithium, tricyclic antidepressants, and salicylates
- Nutritional deficiencies, especially of B vitamins, chromium, magnesium, vanadium, and/or zinc, which help regulate blood glucose
- Physical trauma, such as injury or heart attack
- Weight gain (leading to insulin resistance)

Borderline-high blood sugar should not be ignored, since insulin resistance and type 2 diabetes are likely consequences. Diabetes and insulin resistance are linked to a host of medical conditions, including cancer, dementia and Alzheimer's disease, eye disorders, heart disease, high blood pressure, kidney disease, neuropathy (nerve damage) and stroke.

WHAT ARE THE SYMPTOMS OF HIGH BLOOD GLUCOSE?

A blood test is the only way to confirm the presence of high blood sugar, but there are a few symptoms that may be present and prompt you to seek medical attention. Fatigue, increased hunger, excessive thirst, frequent urination, and slow healing of wounds are symptoms of elevated blood sugar and, potentially, diabetes. It is also common for people with type 2 diabetes to gain weight, especially around the waist. Belly fat can lead to insulin resistance, which contributes to further weight gain. In general, if you have excessive belly fat, it is likely that you will at least be insulin resistant.

People who have diabetes must regularly monitor their blood glucose levels and be aware of the signs of hypoglycemia, such as anxiety, blurred vision, confusion, and trembling or shaking. Hypoglycemia can occur due to changes in eating patterns, exercise, or medication. Diabetics can also develop hypoglycemia in response to some type of stress. In severe circumstances, very high blood sugar can lead to *ketoacidosis*, or diabetic coma. Some warning signs of this potentially fatal state include shortness of breath, stomach pain, fruity-smelling breath, and vomiting. Hypoglycemic episodes require immediate intervention to prevent serious conditions like ketoacidosis, as well as other dangerous problems.

Diabetes—A National Health Crisis

Diabetes, a chronic disease characterized by high levels of glucose in the blood, is escalating at an alarming rate in the United States, where more than 11 million people have been diagnosed with the disease and another 7 million live with it unknowingly. The disease can be diagnosed at any age and create serious medical complications affecting the nerves, eyes, gums, and teeth. According to the National Diabetes Information Clearinghouse (NDIC), people with diabetes are twice as likely to have a stroke and develop heart disease, and four times as likely to get certain cancers. Moreover, one of the most common causes of kidney damage and failure is diabetes; dialysis clinics are popping up everywhere in response to a growing number of diabetes patients with chronic kidney failure. (See the inset on page 74.) For these reasons and more, it is crucial to manage diabetes before it spirals out of control.

There are several indicators of diabetes, but a blood glucose test (see pages 59 to 60) is required before a diagnosis can be made. Some symptoms include:

- Blurred vision
- Dry, itchy skin
- Excessive hunger and thirst
- Fatigue
- Frequent urination
- High blood pressure
- Memory decline
- Recurring bladder, nail, and/or skin infections
- Slowly healing bruises, cuts, and sores
- Tingling or loss of feeling in the feet (neuropathy)

There are two main types of diabetes, type 1 and type 2. *Type 1 diabetes,* formerly known as juvenile diabetes, is caused by a dysfunction of the immune system in which the body attacks *beta cells*—the insulin-producing cells of the pancreas. When these cells are destroyed, the body can no longer produce insulin. The disease, which occurs most often in children, can be triggered by a wide range of factors, including viruses, infections, vaccinations, and allergies to cow's milk. Until the development of injectable insulin, type 1 diabetes was fatal.

Type 2 diabetes is the more common type. In fact, about 95 percent of people with diabetes in the United States have type 2, which was once known as *adult-onset diabetes.* However, this term is no longer applicable, since the obesity epidemic has caused many children under the age of eighteen to develop this chronic condition as well. The precursor to type 2 diabetes is insulin resistance (see the inset on page 74). Over time, the excessive release of insulin—the body's attempt to manage blood sugar—burns out the beta cells, destroying their ability to make insulin and control glucose levels. Type 2 diabetes has fully developed when blood sugar levels cannot be lowered due to poor insulin release or utilization. People who have type 2 diabetes tend to be overweight; in fact, the disease was at first believed to be caused by a poor diet and lifestyle. Yet new research has shown that hormonal changes, chronic stress, environmental pollutants, and nutritional deficiencies (especially magnesium) can contribute to the development of type 2 diabetes.

It's worth mentioning that there is also a third type of diabetes, *gestational diabetes,* which occurs only during pregnancy. Most women who develop gestational diabetes no longer need to take insulin after they give birth, but they are at a higher risk of becoming diabetic later in life. Babies born to women with gestational diabetes tend to have a higher birth weight, and are also at an increased risk of developing weight problems or diabetes during their lifetime.

Treating both type 1 and type 2 diabetes can involve taking medication (including insulin injections), following a healthy diet low in simple carbohydrates and sugars, and engaging in regular physical activity. Luckily, when type 2 diabetes is caught early, it can be controlled through diet and exercise in many cases. Regular blood testing is essential for diabetes detection and management. If one or more of the symptoms listed above apply to you, notify your doctor. Poor insulin and glucose control is the number one factor associated with shortened lifespan, so it's important to stop the problem before it starts, or to treat the problem before it leads to other dangerous health issues.

HOW CAN HIGH BLOOD GLUCOSE BE TREATED?

High blood sugar requires treatment, whether it's due to mild hyperglycemia or full-blown diabetes. This section highlights medical treatments for diabetes as well as general lifestyle strategies that can help lower elevated blood sugar levels.

DRUGS

Although it cannot be cured, diabetes can be effectively controlled through lifestyle change, which may include modifying your diet, getting sufficient amounts of the right nutrients, and exercising regularly. If lifestyle modification alone cannot lower levels, though, there are medications you can take to normalize your blood sugar and manage the condition. The table below lists pharmaceutical drugs that are commonly prescribed to improve glucose metabolism and lower blood glucose levels. These drugs are generally used to treat people with diabetes, but more doctors are beginning to prescribe them for insulin resistance and borderline-high glucose levels as well. It's important to note that the medication prescribed usually differs depending on what type of diabetes you have.

DRUGS FOR DIABETES (HIGH BLOOD GLUCOSE)

Drug	Considerations
Alpha-glucosidase inhibitors (acarbose, miglitol) *Glyset, Precose*	Since these drugs slow the breakdown and absorption of glucose, they may cause low blood sugar levels (hypoglycemia). You should not skip meals or go for long periods without eating while taking these drugs.
Amylin (pramlintide) *Symlin*	This drug slows the movement of food through the stomach, so tell your doctor if you have ever had *gastroparesis,* a condition in which food passes very slowly from the stomach to the intestine. Consult a healthcare professional before taking if you are using pain medication, or are pregnant or breastfeeding.
Biguanides (metformin, rosiglitazone, glipizide) *Avandamet, Glucophage, Metaglip*	Metformin may cause deficiencies of nutrients such as vitamin B_{12}, folic acid, and CoQ_{10}. Side effects can include anemia, fatigue, increased hunger and/or fluid buildup, muscle weakness, nausea and vomiting, tremors, and heart palpitations.
Dipeptidyl peptidase-4 (DPP-4) inhibitors (sitagliptin) *Januvia*	Consult your health practitioner before using if you have ever had pancreatitis, gallstones, kidney disease, or high triglycerides.
Glucagon-like peptide (GLP-1) agonists (exenatide) *Byetta*	Byetta is usually taken within the hour before the morning and evening meals. It should not be taken after meals. If you use oral contraceptives, do not take at the same time as Byetta. Contact your medical provider if you experience symptoms associated with high or low blood sugar.
Insulin (injection) *Humulin, Novolin, Humalog, Novolog, Lente, Ultralente*	Dosage varies depending on the type of insulin prescribed.* Insulin is typically taken before a meal, but timing differs by product. Take only as directed by your physician.

*Please note that insulin can be rapid-acting, short-acting, intermediate-acting, or long-acting. It is also available in a pre-mixed form, which is a combination of short- and intermediate-acting insulin. The type prescribed depends on age, blood sugar management goals, lifestyle (diet, exercise habits, etc.), and other factors.

Drug	Considerations
Rapid insulin releasers (repaglinide, nateglinide) *Prandin, Starlix*	Before using, tell your doctor if you have or have ever had kidney disease, liver disease, hormonal disorders, or type 1 diabetes. Inform your medical provider immediately if you experience symptoms of either high or low blood sugar.
Sulfonylureas (glyburide, glipizide, tolazamide) *Diabeta, Glycron, Glucotrol, Tolinase*	Sulfonylureas can lead to the depletion of nutrients like CoQ_{10}. Additional side effects may include drowsiness, fatigue, anxiety, weight gain, gas and/or bloating, muscle weakness, tremors, sleep problems, depression, and heart palpitations.
Thiazolidinediones, or TZDs (pioglitazone, rosiglitazone) *Actos, Avandia*	Check with your doctor before using these drugs if you have or have ever had heart problems or abnormalities, high blood pressure, or liver disease. Women who are breastfeeding should not take thiazolidinediones.

You should be aware that the Action to Control Cardiovascular Risk in Diabetes (ACCORD) Study, along with similar research, reported that increasing the dosage and/or number of diabetes medications in an attempt to implement more aggressive glucose control can increase the risk of mortality. This is why doctors prefer that diabetes patients also make the necessary lifestyle changes to control their blood sugar naturally. If fewer medications are used, but you do not put any effort into adjusting your diet and overall lifestyle, the result will still be poor glucose control in combination with higher hemoglobin A1C. This can cause organ and tissue damage, leading to medical complications over time. Ultimately, the future of your health depends on the decisions you make to control your insulin resistance and diabetes, and this requires lifestyle modification (see pages 70 to 73).

Another issue related to diabetes medication is that several commonly prescribed drugs cause nutrient depletion, which can produce other symptoms and conditions. For example, metformin, a very popular drug used to manage type 2 diabetes, has been shown to deplete vitamin B_{12}, which increases the risk of diabetic neuropathy. Other drugs may diminish the body's supply of CoQ_{10}, which is essential for maintaining cardiac tissues. Shortages can lead to an enlarged heart and, eventually, congestive heart failure. The drugs presented in the following table have been linked to nutrient depletion. If you have been prescribed one of these medications, you should speak to your doctor about taking a dietary supplement.

Drug therapy can be used and prescribed responsibly, but it should not be solely relied upon to control the disease. Lifestyle modification should always be part of a management program for high blood glucose. Without it, higher

NUTRITIONAL DEFICIENCIES CAUSED BY BLOOD-SUGAR LOWERING MEDICATIONS

Drug	Nutrients Depleted	Associated Symptoms and Health Problems
ACE inhibitors (captopril, enalapril, fosinapril, lisnopril, quinapril, ramipril, trandolapril)	Sodium and zinc	Symptoms include decreased immunity, slow wound healing, smell and taste disturbances, anorexia, depression, night blindness, joint pain, involuntary eye movements (nystagmus), and changes to the skin, nails, or hair. Women may experience menstrual irregularities.
Metformin *Glucophage*	CoQ_{10}, folic acid (vitamin B_9), and vitamin B_{12}	CoQ_{10} depletion can lead to blood sugar imbalances, heart problems, low energy, muscle weakness, and decreased immunity. Folic acid depletion can result in blood sugar dysregulation, cervical dysplasia, increased risk of cancer, muscle weakness, and decreased immunity. It can also cause birth defects. Depletion of vitamin B_{12} may lead to anemia, depression, fatigue, increased cardiovascular risks, skin tingling and numbness (paresthesia), and general weakness.
Sulfonylureas, second generation (glipizide, glyburide)	CoQ_{10}	Symptoms include blood sugar imbalance, heart problems, low energy, muscle weakness, and decreased immunity.

drug dosages are necessary, which only increases the risk of side effects and complications. Medication has beneficial effects, but it needs to be supported by a healthy lifestyle.

SUPPLEMENTS

Finally, you may want to consider taking a nutritional supplement to enhance your diet. There are several substances that can effectively lower your blood glucose levels. Some of these are highlighted in the table below. Although these substances can be obtained without a prescription, they should be taken only under the supervision of a healthcare professional so that you are aware of any risks, side effects, and negative interactions. If you are currently on medication for blood sugar control, you need to notify your doctor if you choose to take a supplement, as your prescription may need to be adjusted. Otherwise, your blood sugar may drop to very low levels.

SUPPLEMENTS FOR HIGH BLOOD GLUCOSE

Supplement	Dosage	Considerations
Aged garlic extract	600 mg one to three times a day.	Aged garlic extract is used to protect the heart and blood vessels, and is reported to help decrease oxidative stress markers, including those related to blood sugar regulation problems. Aged garlic has also been reported to decrease the formation of advanced glycation end-products (AGEs), which are implicated in various health problems, such as heart disease, kidney problems, and cancer. Aged garlic is not reported to interfere with blood thinners. Reported to reduce liver enzymes and fatty liver.
Alpha-lipoic acid	600 mg one to two times a day.	Reported to help with blood sugar uptake and use in the body. Also helps detoxify the body, protect the kidneys, and improve cholesterol levels. Make sure that the raw material provider for the product is from Europe to guarantee effectiveness.
Bilberry	80 mg two to three times a day.	Has been shown to protect against eye problems that may result from blood sugar imbalance. Although not reported in studies, bilberry may increase your risk of bleeding. If you are taking aspirin or other anticoagulant medications, always talk to your doctor before supplementing with bilberry or any dietary supplement.
Bitter melon	250 to 500 mg three times a day.	Use a standardized extract that contains 10-percent charantins. When combined with chromium and glutathione (called Glucokine), bitter melon is reported to lower blood sugar and hemoglobin A1c, as well as facilitate weight loss.
Cinnamon	250 mg twice a day.	Studies have shown that cinnamon improves insulin sensitivity and acts as an antioxidant. If you are taking a medication for blood sugar control, make sure to alert your doctor before taking cinnamon. Use a standardized extract such as Cinnulin PF.
Fiber	Check the product label for dosage guidelines. The recommendation for women is 25 g per day, and for men, 30 g per day.	Guar gum (Sunfiber) is an excellent source of soluble dietary fiber. Potential side effects include abdominal discomfort and bloating. Excess fiber may also interfere with the absorption of certain nutrients like iron and calcium.

Supplement	Dosage	Considerations
GTF (Glucose Tolerance Factor) chromium	200 to 400 mcg once a day.	Chromium is important for blood sugar and insulin regulation. Additionally, people who have a diet high in refined carbohydrates like sugar may also be low in chromium. Use under a doctor's supervision if you are diabetic, as it may affect medication dosage. Do not use if you have kidney or liver problems, chromate or leather contact allergy, or a behavioral psychiatric condition such as schizophrenia or depression.
Magnesium	250 to 500 mg twice a day.	Use magnesium aspartate, citrate, taurate, glycinate, or any amino acid chelate. Supports bone building and balances calcium intake. The ratio of calcium-to-magnesium intake should be between 1 to 1 and 2 to 1. This supplement is reported to improve blood vessel function and insulin resistance, in addition to decreasing LDL cholesterol, total cholesterol, and triglycerides. Also essential for phase-I liver detoxification. If you experience loose stools after taking magnesium, cut your dose in half and gradually increase over the course of a few months. Consult your health-care provider for dosage advice.
Multivitamin	Take as directed on the label.	A multivitamin/mineral supplement contains essential nutrients that help metabolism and blood sugar regulation. It also can be used to replace the nutrients that may be depleted due to blood sugar medications or a poor diet. Use only high-quality products. See page 11 for a list of essential nutrients to look for in a daily multivitamin.
N-acetyl cysteine (NAC)	500 mg two to three times a day.	NAC is an antioxidant that is reported to help protect against blood vessel damage and clots due to insulin resistance, diabetes, and other blood sugar regulation problems. It also helps improve the body's capacity to decrease the harmful effects of toxins. NAC has been reported to improve kidney function in laboratory and human studies, and support glutathione production in the kidneys. It is generally well tolerated when taken in recommended dosages.
Omega-3 essential fatty acids DHA and EPA (fish oil)	1,000 mg two to three times a day.	Excessive inflammation is common in people who are insulin resistant and diabetic, and can lead to other health problems like immune imbalances, sleep problems, and heart disease. Fish oil acts as an antioxidant and decreases inflammation in the body, in addition to supporting heart and blood vessel health. Speak to your doctor before taking if you are on blood-thinning medication, as fish oil may increase

Supplement	Dosage	Considerations
Omega-3 *(continued)*		the risk of bleeding. Be sure to use only high-quality oils that have been tested for contaminants.
Vanadium	250 mcg once a day.	Studies have shown that vanadium has insulin-like properties in humans and can help regulate blood sugar levels.
Zinc	25 to 50 mg once a day.	Zinc is important in immunity and acts as an antioxidant. It is also reported to help regulate blood sugar. May also be used by men to treat low testosterone and support prostate health. Take zinc in the form of an amino acid chelate or citrate. Check with your doctor before using.

LIFESTYLE CHANGES

The importance of making healthy food choices, exercising regularly, losing excess weight, getting adequate sleep, and managing stress cannot be emphasized enough when it comes to treating and correcting blood sugar disturbances. Time and time again, it has been proven that lifestyle change is the most effective method for controlling high blood sugar and type 2 diabetes. One of the most important elements in a holistic approach to diabetes management is diet. In addition to controlling the amount of refined sugars and carbohydrates you eat, following these basic guidelines should help improve blood glucose control and lower your fasting glucose level.

- Add cinnamon to your daily intake. One-quarter teaspoon (1 g) of cinnamon per day can go a long way in lowering your blood sugar. According to reports, this one small dose can bring down your blood glucose level by 18 to 29 percent. Get your 1-g serving by sprinkling ground cinnamon on whole grain toast, mixing it in a protein shake, or by using a standardized cinnamon extract. (See the table on page 68.)

- Choose low-glycemic foods. Familiarize yourself with the glycemic index (see the inset on page 29) and build your diet around low-glycemic foods. Avoid carbohydrate-rich foods like potatoes, rice, pasta, and sweets, as well as products containing artificial sugars like high-fructose corn syrup. Make sure that the most of the carbohydrates you eat are low on the glycemic index, like beans, peas, zucchini, grapefruit, and berries. And although many fruits are low-glycemic, some—including bananas, dried fruits, pineapple, and watermelon—contain more carbohydrates and, therefore, should be eaten less frequently and in smaller amounts. Limit how much fruit juice you drink as well. Meats, fish, poultry, and other animal-based proteins do not contain carbohydrates and, therefore, have very little impact on insulin levels. The same goes for fats. In fact, protein and fats can help lower the glycemic effect of a meal.

- Don't fall into the low-fat food trap. Many foods that are marketed to dieters, such as low-fat or fat-free cookies and ice cream, are often loaded with carbohydrates. Sugar-free versions of snack foods and dessert items are often high in carbs as well, due to the flours and other starches that are used as ingredients. You should also be careful about eating foods sweetened with sugar alcohols, which contain flours and other carbohydrates. These products can be eaten in moderation as long as doing so does not cause you to exceed your total daily carbohydrate limit, which should be low enough to keep your blood sugar levels within a healthy range. Keep in mind, though, that these sweeteners can cause gas, cramping, and diarrhea.

- Increase your vegetable servings. Try to eat between five and nine servings of vegetables per day. However, be sure to choose vegetables that are low in starch so that your carbohydrate consumption is kept under control. Asparagus, avocados, cabbage, green beans, lettuces, leafy greens, and sprouts are all great options. Starchy vegetables, like potatoes and corn, should be eaten sparingly and must be worked into your total daily carbohydrate intake (see below), as they count towards your carbohydrate servings.

- Keep your carbohydrate consumption under control. Limit your intake of bread, cereal, pasta, and rice, especially in the morning. A registered dietitian can help you determine an appropriate total daily allowance of carbohydrates. The goal is to eat a sufficient amount to meet your nutritional needs while keeping blood sugar and weight under control. More and more medical research is showing that low-carbohydrate diets are effective for managing diabetes, as well as weight. If your blood sugar is trending high, try to eat low-carb breakfasts; eating many carbohydrates in the morning can cause an insulin increase, which leads to a subsequent drop in blood sugar. Low blood sugar, of course, creates the need to consume more carbohydrates, and the vicious cycle that results keeps insulin levels high and contributes to weight gain. If you do not want to give up carbohydrates in the morning, make sure you combine them with protein and healthy fats so that you slow down the rate at which the glucose is released into the bloodstream.

- Limit fast foods. Studies have shown that people who frequently eat fast food establishments are at a higher risk for weight gain and insulin resistance.

That being said, many fast food restaurants have taken significant steps to improve their menus, offering more fruit and salad options, as well as buns made from whole grains. The soft drink consumption involved in dining at fast food restaurant may pose just as great a risk—if not greater—as the food. A 32-ounce (or "large") soft drink contains about thirty teaspoons of sugar. Coffee drinks sold by fast food restaurants are also loaded with sugar. Although fast food is not recommended, you can eat it on occasion, provided that you stick with healthy options, and avoid their soft drinks and other sweetened beverages.

• Stay hydrated. Studies have shown that drinking adequate water may reduce appetite and facilitate weight loss, both of which can help you better manage high blood sugar. Additionally, meeting your daily water requirement assists the kidneys in filtering the blood and flushing toxins out of the body. One study found that drinking more water over time led to lower rates of chronic kidney disease compared to people who drank the least amount of water. Protecting the kidneys is extremely important in people with diabetes, since the disease can lead to chronic kidney disease (see the inset on page 000). Experts generally advise drinking two to three liters of water per day depending on your size, physical activity, climate, and health goals.

• Stock your kitchen with organic foods. When possible, buy foods that are certified organic. Pesticides and other toxins that are often found in nonorganic foods have been linked to insulin resistance, the precursor to type 2 diabetes.

• Take in adequate minerals. Chromium, magnesium, and zinc are essential minerals that support blood sugar balance and insulin regulation. However, studies show that many Americans do not take in sufficient amounts through their diet, which tends to be high in sugar. High sugar levels in the blood will deplete these nutrients more quickly, as they are used up to help the body respond to the surge of glucose. Therefore, to avoid a deficiency, restrict your sugar intake, and be sure to eat foods rich in each of these nutrients. Chromium can be found in small quantities in most foods, with the highest concentrations in beef, liver, chicken, dairy products, eggs, and seafood. Magnesium is plentiful in artichokes, beans, nuts, oat bran, seeds and spinach. (See page 312 in Part Six, "Optional Tests," for more information on magnesium.) While zinc is not always easy to obtain from the diet, it is contained in shellfish, beef, and fortified cereals that contain 25-percent of the Daily Value (DV) for zinc. One of the best ways to ensure adequate intake of these minerals is by taking a dietary supplement, especially if you already have problems with blood sugar management (see the table on pages 77 to 78).

• Up your fiber consumption. Because it is not absorbed by the body, fiber does not raise blood sugar levels. In fact, fiber helps to slow down the release of sugar into the bloodstream following a meal. Fiber-rich foods also make you feel full more quickly, which is further incentive to meet your daily requirement of at least 25 to 30 grams per day. Legumes, leafy green vegetables, and flax seeds are all excellent sources of fiber. Another good source is guar gum, a fiber supplement that helps to stabilize blood sugar by slowing the transit time, or absorption, of sugar in the intestine.

One of the most important ways to reduce your blood sugar is regular exercise, which has been shown to improve insulin sensitivity by as much as 23 percent. Plan to do some kind of physical activity for thirty to sixty minutes at least three or four times a week. A combination of aerobic exercise and strength training is ideal, but even a low-impact activity like walking is sufficient. Try going for a walk or taking a bike ride three days a week, and then do some form of strength training two days a week. Regular exercise can also help you shed pounds, which almost always aids in reducing insulin resistance and lowering blood glucose levels. Medical experts agree that weight loss is one of the best ways to prevent prediabetic conditions from developing into diabetes. Losing even 10 percent of your weight in body fat significantly reduces health risks associated with being obese or overweight, diabetes included.

Along with diet and exercise, strive to spend some more time in the sun. Research indicates that thirty minutes of full sunlight exposure three times a week can help lower blood glucose by boosting your body's production of vitamin D, which is essential for proper insulin utilization. Do not shower immediately after being in the sun, however, since showering removes the body oils in which vitamin D is formed and, therefore, limits how much vitamin D is absorbed by the body. You should have a blood test to check your level of vitamin D. If it is low, you will most likely need to take a vitamin D_3 supplement to maintain an optimal blood level.

WHAT CAUSES LOW BLOOD GLUCOSE?

Low blood glucose, or hypoglycemia, is typically defined as a blood glucose level lower than 50 mg/dL in men, 45 mg/dL in women, and 40 mg/dL in infants and children. However, many people can experience symptoms of hypoglycemia when their level is still in the low 60s. "True" hypoglycemia, as it is medically defined, affects only 5 to 10 percent of individuals who have experienced symptoms of the condition. In other words, some people may have temporarily felt the effects of low blood sugar (after skipping a meal, for example), but are not clinically hypoglycemic.

Diabetes and Chronic Kidney Disease

The kidneys are essential for your health because they filter toxins, excess salts, and other harmful substances out of the blood. However, insulin resistance and diabetes can compromise kidney function, as high blood sugar levels damage the blood vessels in the kidneys, impairing their ability to filter the blood. In addition, diabetes can damage the nerves responsible for emptying the bladder, causing urine to build up and put more pressure on the kidneys. Furthermore, when kidney function is not optimal, proteins like albumin (see page 155) can leak into the urine and are lost from the body, and harmful waste products may accumulate in the blood. The internal oxidation and inflammation that occurs in people with diabetes also takes a toll on the kidneys. Lastly, diabetes may affect the body's levels of certain minerals and amino acids, which can alter blood flow rate and electrolyte balance that is normally regulated by the kidneys.

The gradual loss of kidney function over time is known as *chronic kidney disease* (CKD), which affects nearly one-third of diabetes patients and may—but does not always—lead to kidney failure. This is one of the biggest health crises in the United States right now, and dialysis centers are springing up everywhere because of the increased demand. Undoubtedly, the record rates of obesity, insulin resistance, and diabetes are contributing to this growing problem. And because chronic kidney disease develops in stages, people rarely experience symptoms until the kidneys have ceased to work. When this happens, some of the following signs may be observed:

- Albumin in the urine
- Dry, itchy skin
- Frequent urination
- High blood pressure
- Leg cramps
- Less need for insulin and diabetes medication, as the kidneys are unable to metabolize it
- Loss of appetite
- Morning sickness and/or general nausea
- Pale skin
- Swelling of the ankles and/or legs (edema)
- Weakness
- Weight loss, particularly from loss of lean muscle

A blood test can be used to detect kidney dysfunction before it becomes complete kidney failure. High levels of blood urea nitrogen (BUN) and creatinine (see pages 123 and 130), two waste products, are key indicators of a kidney problem. As noted above, the presence of albumin in the urine also signals kidney damage. Finally, a close watch should be kept on blood pressure, especially in people with diabetes—high blood pressure and diabetes are the two main medical conditions that increase the risk of kidney disease. Regular checkups and lab tests can help you maintain kidney health, which is critical to your general well-being.

Hypoglycemia frequently occurs in people with diabetes as a result of too much insulin or blood-sugar-lowering medications. However, people who do *not* have diabetes can also have hypoglycemia. The condition may stem from:

- Critical illnesses or infections
- Eating disorders like anorexia
- Excessive alcohol intake
- Fasting
- Hereditary fructose intolerance
- Hormonal imbalances
- Insulinoma (a tumor in the pancreas that causes too much insulin to be produced)
- Kidney disease or kidney failure
- Liver disease or liver failure
- Medications, including blood sugar-lowering drugs, aspirin (in large doses), pentamidine, quinine, salicylates, and sulfa medications

Low blood glucose can also occur in people with diabetes when they skip a meal, or take too much insulin or medication and then do not eat enough to compensate. The result is an excess of insulin in the blood, which then processes and removes too much glucose from the bloodstream. Diabetic hypoglycemia requires medical attention, but it should not be overtreated, as this can cause blood sugar to rise to an excessively high level. People who have diabetes must take the necessary measures to prevent spikes in blood sugar, as this can increase the risk of medical complications.

Both diabetic and non-diabetic hypoglycemia should not be ignored. As already mentioned, severe episodes of hypoglycemia can cause medical emergencies such as falls, seizures, and loss of consciousness. Low blood sugar and levels that trend slightly low are concerns because the body cannot properly function without sufficient glucose. Furthermore, the brain, which cannot produce glucose on its own, requires an adequate amount for normal cognitive function. Low blood sugar levels are linked to insomnia, since a drop in blood sugar at night triggers the release of adrenaline to break down glycogen (stored sugar) into glucose. The release of adrenaline also stimulates the brain, causing you to wake up.

If a blood test shows that your blood sugar is low, you should speak to your doctor about how to reverse the trend and treat the underlying cause. You should also consider consulting a dietitian to help you develop an eating plan that can stabilize your blood sugar levels. A typical nutritional plan for problems with low blood sugar involves eating foods very low in refined sugars and high in fiber, as well as including a little bit of protein in each meal. Checking your blood sugar with an in-home meter—which you should already be doing if you have diabetes—can help you track the highs and lows that occur after you eat, allowing you to adjust your dietary habits accordingly. Testing your blood regularly will also help you avoid spikes and drops in your glucose levels.

WHAT ARE THE SYMPTOMS OF LOW BLOOD GLUCOSE?

The physical indicators of low blood sugar appear when blood sugar drops to around 60 mg/dL or lower. Depending on the severity, hypoglycemia can be a minor annoyance or extremely dangerous. Symptoms may include anxiety, confusion, dizziness, fatigue, headache, heart palpitations, intense hunger, memory loss, nervousness, sweating or clammy skin, and trembling. In severe cases, this condition may cause seizures and loss of consciousness.

HOW CAN LOW BLOOD GLUCOSE BE TREATED?

Immediate treatment is needed when a person experiences a hypoglycemic attack. For diabetics who experience hypoglycemia, the general recommendation is to take 15 to 20 g of quick-acting carbohydrates (simple sugars) from sources like glucose gels or tablets, non-diet soda, or hard candies. This usually relieves symptoms and raises blood sugar. However, in more extreme circumstances, a person may not respond to these attempts and, therefore, medical intervention is required. If glucose tablets or another source of quick-acting sugar does not stimulate a response after one or two tries, call an ambulance.

If you have severe or frequent hypoglycemic attacks, you must be evaluated by a physician. For most people, rapid drops in blood sugar are brought on by poor eating habits, too much exercise, or stress. Fortunately, there are a number of ways to control the condition so that hypoglycemic episodes are kept to a minimum, if not eliminated.

DRUGS

The drugs below are to be used only under the supervision of a doctor, and are not intended for transient (temporary) or exercise-induced hypoglycemia.

DRUGS FOR LOW BLOOD GLUCOSE	
Drug	**Considerations**
Dextrose (IV)	Dextrose must be administered by a doctor or trained medical personnel.
Diazoxide *Proglycem*	May cause changes in taste, appetite loss, upset stomach, headache, and tiredness. Inform your medical provider if you have low potassium, diabetes, high blood pressure, or heart, kidney, or liver disease.
Glucagon *GlucaGen*	Acts as first aid in severe cases of hypoglycemia resulting in unconsciousness. A doctor may also prescribe glucagon so that it is on hand in case of an emergency. Make sure that you know exactly how to self-administer the drug.
Streptozotocin *Zanosar*	Tell your physician if you have kidney or liver disease, or problems with blood clotting. Women who are pregnant or breastfeeding should not use this drug.

SUPPLEMENTS

Your healthcare provider may also recommend taking a nutritional supplement for better blood sugar control. The supplements listed in the table below support healthy blood glucose balance.

SUPPLEMENTS FOR LOW BLOOD GLUCOSE		
Supplement	**Dosage**	**Considerations**
GTF (Glucose Tolerance Factor) chromium	200 to 400 mcg once a day.	Chromium is important for blood sugar and insulin regulation. Additionally, people who have a diet high in refined carbohydrates like sugar may also be low in chromium. Use under a doctor's supervision if you are diabetic, as it may affect medication dosage. Do not use if you have kidney or liver problems, chromate or leather contact allergy, or a behavioral psychiatric condition such as schizophrenia or depression.

Supplement	Dosage	Considerations
Magnesium	250 to 500 mg twice a day.	Use magnesium aspartate, citrate, taurate, glycinate, or any amino acid chelate. Supports bone building and balances calcium intake. The ratio of calcium-to-magnesium intake should be between 1 to 1 and 2 to 1. This supplement is reported to improve blood vessel function and insulin resistance, in addition to decreasing LDL cholesterol, total cholesterol, and triglycerides. Also essential for phase-I liver detoxification. If you experience loose stools after taking magnesium, cut your dose in half and gradually increase over the course of a few months. Consult your health-care provider for dosage advice.
Zinc	25 to 50 mg once a day.	Zinc is important in immunity and acts as an antioxidant. It is also reported to help regulate blood sugar. May also be used by men to treat low testosterone and support prostate health. Take zinc in the form of an amino acid chelate or citrate. Check with your doctor before using.

LIFESTYLE CHANGES

Treatment for hypoglycemic episodes can differ slightly depending on whether hypoglycemia is *diabetic* or *reactive* (non-diabetic). As mentioned above, diabetics should immediately ingest a source of quick-acting carbohydrates when they experience an attack. People who have reactive hypoglycemia can also keep glucose tablets or hard candies on hand, but these should be consumed only to prevent an imminent hypoglycemic episode—they should not be eaten regularly. It is better to use a long-term strategy to treat reactive hypoglycemia, such as eating small, well-balanced meals and/or snacks every three hours. And if you experience any symptom that indicates a drop in blood sugar, eat a well-balanced snack that includes protein, healthy fat, and carbs. If the drop is more acute, though, you may need to resort to fast-acting sugars.

Long-term treatment of hypoglycemia, particularly reactive hypoglycemia, requires dietary modification. It's essential to avoid refined sugars and eat foods that help slow the release of sugar into the bloodstream after meals. Here are additional dietary tips for stabilizing blood sugar levels:

- Drink less alcohol, coffee, and other caffeinated beverages. Depending on how sensitive you are to caffeine, you may need to switch to decaffeinated coffee or tea. Also, remember that coffee, espresso, and chai tea drinks served at many chains and coffee houses are loaded with sugars, and should be avoided. When it comes to alcohol, stay away from cocktails that contain fruit juice, and stick to one drink only.

- Eat plenty of vegetables and fruits in a proportionate amount. Ideally, you should eat vegetables and fruits in a ratio of 3 to 1. (For every three servings of vegetables, have one fruit serving.) Again, choose fruits that are low in glycemic load, like apples, berries, and grapefruit, and limit your intake to two servings per day.

- Eliminate or limit refined sugars, and avoid excessive intake of carbohydrates. Foods containing refined sugars and carbs can make hypoglycemia worse. In addition, avoid soft drinks, and be aware that even artificially sweetened beverages can cause blood sugar levels to drop in some people.

- Pair sources of protein and/or fat with carbohydrates. This food combination helps to slow the release and absorption of glucose, in turn preventing blood sugar from dropping too low.

- Try to incorporate fiber into every meal and snack, since it helps balance blood sugar. Fiber-rich foods include beans, nuts, berries, leafy green vegetables, and modest amounts of whole grains. Aim for 25 g or more per day, and remember to stay hydrated in order to prevent uncomfortable bloating or digestion issues.

Physical activity also needs to be considered. Although exercise lowers blood sugar levels, most people with reactive hypoglycemia can still tolerate normal exercise, which is important to overall health. An ideal exercise routine is one that includes both cardio and strength training, but the workout does not need to be rigorous in order to be beneficial. Begin with a low-impact form of exercise, such as walking, for thirty minutes four or five times a week, gradually increasing the level of intensity. If exercise makes your blood sugar drop too low, make sure you have a small snack beforehand, and replenish your sugars and proteins during and after exercise. One way to do this is to add a packet of Propel powder, which is enriched with vitamins and antioxidants, to your water, plus a small scoop of protein powder. One of these drinks provides 10 to 15 g of protein, and it's recommended that you drink one for every twenty to thirty minutes of training. Although most brands use dextrose or sucrose as a sweetener, more and more companies like Gleukos are making their sports drinks with glucose , which is more effective for replacing sugar in the bloodstream.

6. CALCIUM

Calcium is the most abundant mineral in the body. An average healthy male contains 2.5 to 3 pounds of calcium, while an average healthy female contains about 2 pounds. Approximately 99 percent of the body's calcium supply is found in the bones and teeth, leaving only about 1 percent in the cells and body fluids. Calcium is essential for not only strong teeth and bones, but also for proper nerve impulse transmission, enzyme function, blood clotting, and energy production. The level of calcium in the body is regulated by a complex *feedback loop*—a pathway that controls a certain physiological function—involving parathyroid hormone (PTH), vitamin D, and calcitonin. The amount of magnesium and phosphorus in the body also affects calcium levels.

It's important that you consume an adequate amount of calcium, which is found mainly in dairy products (milk, cheese, and yogurt, for example), fish that have bones (such as salmon and sardines), sesame seeds, and leafy green vegetables. As you age, be sure to maintain adequate intake of the mineral, since both high and low levels can increase your chances of developing conditions relating to the bones, heart, kidneys, nerves, and teeth. *Hypercalcemia* (high calcium) can put you at risk for kidney problems, for example, while long-term *hypocalcemia* (low calcium) typically leads to *osteoporosis*—the gradual thinning of bone tissue and loss of bone density.

A blood calcium test (also called an *ionized calcium test*) indicates the amount of calcium in the blood, not the bones. This amount is reflected in the results of a *total calcium test*, which measures both free (circulating) and bound forms of calcium in the blood. The reference ranges for blood calcium levels, which are measured in milligrams per deciliter (mg/dL), are provided below. Results that fall within the normal range generally mean that calcium is being properly metabolized, so there is no specific target range.

REFERENCE RANGES FOR CALCIUM

Calcium (mg/dL)	Category
Greater than 12	Very high (Moderate to severe hypercalcemia)
10.2 to 12	High (Mild hypercalcemia)
8.6 to 10.2	Normal
Less than 8.6	Low (Hypocalcemia)

A urine calcium test may also be ordered if, for instance, a person is exhibiting classic symptoms of kidney stones. Men should produce less than 300 mg of urine calcium per day, and women, less than 250 mg per day. Amounts greater than 300 mg per day can indicate that too much calcium is being consumed or, alternatively, being pulled from the bones. High urine calcium levels may also mean that too much calcium is being absorbed from the intestines, which occurs in certain diseases like sarcoidosis. Leaking, or the loss of calcium due to compromised kidney function, may also be to blame. In general, 100 to 300 mg per day can be considered normal, depending on the individual. If a calcium test indicates that your level is abnormal, work with your physician to determine the source of the problem and begin treatment.

WHAT CAUSES HIGH CALCIUM?

The medical term used to describe too much calcium in the blood is *hypercalcemia,* a condition that affects less than 1 percent of the population. In most cases (about 98 percent), hypercalcemia is caused by parathyroid disease, or *hyperparathyroidism,* which occurs when an excess of parathyroid hormone is continually released by the parathyroid glands. The number one cause of this disease is the growth of benign tumors in the parathyroid glands, which are responsible for controlling the levels of calcium and phosphorus in the blood. Kidney disease can also cause the parathyroid glands to become overactive, as it disturbs blood calcium and phosphorus levels and, therefore, disrupts feedback to the parathyroid glands. Additional causes of hypercalcemia include:

- Adrenal gland failure
- Advanced liver disease
- Certain cancers, including breast cancer, lung cancer, leukemia, and prostate cancer (with bone metastasis)
- Dehydration
- Diet very high in calcium (more than 2,000 mg per day)
- *Familial hypocalciuric hypercalcemia,* a hereditary condition that hinders the body's ability to regulate calcium properly
- High levels of vitamin A and/or vitamin D
- Hyperthyroidism
- Kidney disease or kidney failure

- Medications, such as calcium-containing antacids, lithium, and thiazide diuretics
- Prolonged immobilization
- Sarcoidosis (disease leading to inflammation in various organs)
- Tuberculosis

Since hypercalcemia can be detected and, in most cases, effectively treated, long-term complications are unlikely. But there are several health problems that may be connected to hypercalcemia, including heart arrhythmias (irregular heartbeat), high blood pressure, intestinal disorders (such as peptic ulcer disease), kidney stones, kidney failure, thyroid disease, vitamin D toxicity, and occasionally vitamin A toxicity. You may also show low levels of iron, magnesium, vitamin K, and/or zinc, which share absorption sites with calcium in the intestines and, therefore, do not absorb as easily when calcium intake is high. In addition, high calcium levels are associated with changes in the nervous system, resulting in confusion and dementia. And although osteoporosis (bone thinning) is more commonly linked to low calcium levels, it is also possible to develop this condition, as well as other bone diseases, as a result of long-term hypercalcemia. If high blood calcium is caused by the bones' release of calcium into the blood, bone density loss occurs over time. This is why it is important to detect and reverse hypercalcemia before it has a chance to damage the body.

WHAT ARE THE SYMPTOMS OF HIGH CALCIUM?

Mild hypercalcemia usually does not have symptoms, but moderate or severe cases may cause abdominal pain, constipation, depression, fatigue, headaches, nausea, and vomiting. Loss of appetite may occur as well, while thirst and the urge to urinate increases considerably. Remember, though, that these physical indicators can stem from a number of health conditions, not just hypercalcemia. If you experience a symptom that persists or worsens, a visit to your doctor is in order.

HOW CAN HIGH CALCIUM BE TREATED?

The method used to treat high calcium levels is dependent upon the underlying source of the condition, which must be determined by a full medical examination. Hypercalcemia should be treated medically and only under the supervision of a physician. For hypercalcemia that is caused by hyperparathyroidism, doctors may recommend parathyroid surgery, while treatment for cancer-induced cases varies according to the overall goals of cancer therapy. But the most common approach to treatment is medication and/or lifestyle modification.

DRUGS

Usually, medication is prescribed only for severe cases of hypercalcemia. The choice of drug depends on the cause of the condition, as well as the overall health of the patient. The drugs listed in the table below help stabilize calcium metabolism and absorption, normalize parathyroid gland function, and increase calcium excretion. Always ask your physician about potential risks, side effects, and interactions before taking any drug. If you experience a side effect that persists or intensifies, you should notify your medical provider.

DRUGS FOR HIGH CALCIUM

Drug	Considerations
Bisphosphonates (alendronate, ibandronate, pamidronate, zolendronic acid) *Aredia, Boniva, Fosamax, Zometa (administered intraveneously)*	Bisphosphonates can deplete calcium and phosphorus from the body. Potential side effects may include abdominal pain, nausea and/or vomiting, gas or bloating, bone loss, ulcers, and irregular heartbeat.
Calcimimetics (cinacalcet) *Sensipar*	Tell your treating doctor if you have a history of liver disease or seizures, or if you are pregnant or breastfeeding. Seek medical attention if side effects such as upset stomach, dizziness, weakness, and chest pain persist or worsen.
Calcitonin (injection or nasal spray) *Calcimar, Cibacalcin, Miacalcin*	Side effects can include bone pain, nausea and/or vomiting, and runny nose.
Gallium nitrate *Ganite*	This drug is used to treat only cancer-related hypercalcemia and is given intravenously under medical supervision.
Loop diuretics (bumetanide, furosemide, torsemide) *Bumex, Demadex, Lasix*	Loop diuretics may cause depletion of calcium, magnesium, potassium, vitamin B_1, vitamin B_6, vitamin C, and zinc. Side effects may include bone loss, confusion, dry mouth, fatigue, headache, irregular heartbeat, mood changes, muscle cramps, nervousness, numbness, and poor wound healing.
Phosphate salts (dicalcium phosphate, dibasic calcium phosphate)	Side effects may include upset stomach and/or vomiting.

SUPPLEMENTS

The supplements listed in the following table may also be effective for improving conditions that can cause high calcium levels. Remember, nutritional supplements can be obtained without a prescription, but you should not take any supplement without consulting a healthcare professional. Health risks are possible when using a substance of any kind.

SUPPLEMENTS FOR CONDITIONS RELATED TO HIGH CALCIUM

Supplement	Dosage	Considerations
Green tea or green tea extract	3 to 6 cups (tea) or 250 mg one to two times a day (extract).	Green tea is reported to decrease kidney stone formation, which may be due to high calcium levels, as well as improve bone density in elderly women. If taking an extract, use a form standardized to 90-percent polyphenols (specifically EGCG). The supplement may increase blood thinning, especially if you are taking aspirin or anticoagulant drugs.
Magnesium	250 to 500 mg twice a day.	Use magnesium aspartate, citrate, taurate, glycinate, or any amino acid chelate. Supports bone building and balances calcium intake. The ratio of calcium-to-magnesium intake should be between 1 to 1 and 2 to 1. This supplement is reported to improve blood vessel function and insulin resistance, in addition to decreasing LDL cholesterol, total cholesterol, and triglycerides. Also essential for phase-I liver detoxification. If you experience loose stools after taking magnesium, cut your dose in half and gradually increase over the course of a few months. Consult your health-care provider for dosage advice.
Shatavari	250 to 500 mg twice a day.	Similar to the asparagus growing in your garden, Shatavari has been used for centuries in Ayurvedic medicine. Studies have found that it is a good source of phytoestrogens, which improve calcium-regulating processes in the body. It is also reported to balance cholesterol, improve immunity, and have antioxidant and gastrointestinal-protective properties. Should not be consumed by people with kidney or heart problems, or by women who are pregnant or breastfeeding, unless under the supervision of a doctor.

LIFESTYLE CHANGES

Lifestyle approaches to treating hypercalcemia depend on the underlying cause of the condition. When hyperparathyroidism or cancer is the cause, you should follow the advice of your doctor for adjusting your diet and lifestyle. If you have elevated calcium due to failing kidneys, decreasing calcium intake is necessary. The following recommendations may also help hypercalcemia related to impaired kidney function:

- Consider supplementing with magnesium. Magnesium helps prevent kidney stones, which are sometimes a cause of chronic kidney failure. It also improves insulin action in the body, aids in controlling high blood pressure, and is needed to utilize calcium in the bones more efficiently. See the table on page 84 for dosage recommendations and considerations. More information on magnesium can also be in found in Part Six, "Optional Tests" (see page 312).

- Control your homocysteine levels. Homocysteine, an amino acid byproduct, can damage the kidneys when high amounts are present in the blood. See the homocysteine chapter in Part Six, "Optional Tests" (page 000) to learn lifestyle strategies for keeping your levels in check.

- Decrease your consumption of milk and dairy products. Better yet, cut them out of your diet entirely. Substitute cow's milk with almond or soy milk, and choose products that do not use dairy ingredients.

- Detoxify your kidneys. Eating foods like artichokes, asparagus, celery, melons, and parsley—all of which have detoxifying properties—will cleanse your kidneys effectively.

- Drink more water. Sufficient water intake improves the kidneys' ability to filter toxins and other substances that can cause kidney stones.

- Incorporate low-calcium foods into your daily diet. This food group includes apples, asparagus, beets, cantaloupe, chicken, cottage cheese, eggplant, grapes, pineapple, pinto beans, strawberries, and tomatoes.

- Limit your use of analgesics (painkillers). Drugs like ibuprofen and naproxen sodium can cause kidney failure with overuse.

- Manage any health conditions that are related to your failing kidneys. Poorly managed diabetes and high blood pressure are two of the biggest causes of kidney failure. If you have high blood pressure, ask your doctor about taking an ACE inhibitor. These drugs have been found to prevent the loss of protein in the kidneys, and thus may help you avoid kidney failure.

- Reduce or eliminate your intake of soft drinks. These beverages contain phosphoric acids (phosphates), which can cause calcium depletion in your bones. In addition, studies have found that drinking colas can raise the risk of kidney stones, and that drinking two or more soft drinks per day more than doubles your risk of chronic kidney disease.

Of course, it's wise to follow the guidelines above even if your hypercalcemia is not due to kidney problems. Additionally, it's important to stay out of the sun when you have hypercalcemia, since excess vitamin D can contribute to the condition. When venturing outside, wear sunscreen with an SPF of at least 30, and wear long pants and sleeves to cover exposed skin until your calcium levels return to normal. Exercise is also recommended, since regular physical activity promotes healthy bone density. Weakened bones are a common result of hypercalcemia, as high blood calcium levels mean that it is being lost in the bones. Seek out the advice of a fitness professional or doctor to ensure you choose safe exercises that stimulate bone calcium production.

WHAT CAUSES LOW CALCIUM?

There are numerous causes of hypocalcemia, or low blood calcium, but the most common is a condition known as *hypoalbuminemia* (see page 158). Albumin is a protein in the blood that acts as a carrier for calcium, so when levels are low, blood calcium also sharply decreases. This condition is usually seen in patients who have been hospitalized with acute injuries, illness, or malnutrition. Other causes of hypocalcemia include:

- Age
- Diet low in fat and high in fiber
- Excessive alcohol or caffeine consumption
- High intake of phosphorus, which is found primarily in carbonated beverages, meats, seafood, cheese, milk, whole grain bread, and many snack foods
- Hypoparathyroidism (underactive parathyroid glands)
- Intestinal malabsorption conditions, such as Celiac's disease
- Kidney disease or kidney failure
- Low intake of magnesium, protein, and/or vitamin D
- Malnutrition

- Medications (See the inset below)
- Pancreatitis (inflammation of the pancreas)
- Pregnancy

Medications and Hypocalcemia

Sometimes, low blood calcium is not caused by diet or an underlying health issue, but by prescription medication. The following drugs may affect the level of calcium in your body and lead to hypocalcemia.

- Aluminum and magnesium antacids
- Antacids or anti-ulcer drugs, such as proton-pump inhibitors (PPIs) like Prilosec and histamine receptor blockers like Tagamet (cimetidine)
- Antibiotics, including aminoglycosides, fluoroquinolones, tetracycline, and isoniazid
- Anticonvulsants such as carbamazepine (Tegretol), phenytoin (Dilantin), and phenobarbital (Solfoton)
- Antiretroviral drugs, which are used in the treatment of HIV
- Bile acid sequestrants, like cholestyramine (Questran), to lower cholesterol
- Bisphosphonates, such as alendronate (Fosamax)
- Colchicine, a gout medication
- Corticosteroids
- Digoxin, which is used to treat congestive heart failure and associated symptoms
- Diuretics, loop (furosemide, or Lasix) and potassium-sparing (triamterene, or Dyazide and Maxide)
- EDTA, a chelating agent
- Levothyroxine, a hormone replacement to treat an underactive thyroid
- Mineral oil
- Phosphate enemas
- Salicylates

Low blood calcium is linked to a number of health issues, so treatment is usually necessary. Reduced levels can lead to irregular heartbeat, or heart arrhythmia, which may increase the risk of a cardiovascular event, including congestive heart failure. It can also lead to seizures and lung spasms. The condition that is most strongly correlated with chronic low-grade hypocalcemia is osteoporosis, or the gradual thinning of bone and bone tissue. This problem mainly affects women, especially as they age, so it's essential that older women get enough calcium in their diet. Complications of osteoporosis include curvature of the spine, loss of height, and brittle bones, which may result in frequent fractures.

WHAT ARE THE SYMPTOMS OF LOW CALCIUM?

Symptoms may not occur with hypocalcemia, especially in the early stages. As the condition worsens, people may experience abdominal discomfort, anxiety, tingling sensations in their fingers, and muscle cramps or spasms. Irritability, lethargy, and frequent bone fractures—a symptom of osteoporosis—are also possible. Such symptoms should be brought to a doctor's attention so that the appropriate tests can be ordered.

HOW CAN LOW CALCIUM BE TREATED?

A doctor must evaluate any case of hypocalcemia, as even slightly low levels can signal that something is amiss in the body. Various treatments for the condition are highlighted in this section.

DRUGS

In moderate and severe cases of hypocalcemia, calcium injections or intravenous drips are the usual forms of treatment. Your doctor will prescribe the appropriate treatment depending on your needs.

SUPPLEMENTS

Nutritional supplementation has proven to be an effective approach for treating mild hypocalcemia when guided by a physician. While calcium supplements are beneficial, there are a few other substances that may be needed to help boost your calcium level. The importance of consulting a health-care professional about nutritional supplements cannot be stressed enough. Before using any substance listed in the table below, ask your medical provider about potential side effects and interactions. In addition, you should have your blood tested before taking any substance so that your doctor can determine a dose appropriate to your health needs and goals.

SUPPLEMENTS FOR LOW CALCIUM		
Supplement	**Dosage**	**Considerations**
Calcium	500 mg one to three times a day.	Take a highly absorbable form of calcium, such as calcium aspartate, citrate, or hydroxyapatite. If using calcium to help sleep problems, take one 500-mg dose at bedtime.
Magnesium	250 to 500 mg twice a day.	Use magnesium aspartate, citrate, taurate, glycinate, or any amino acid chelate. Supports bone building and balances calcium intake. The ratio of calcium-to-magnesium intake should be between 1 to 1 and 2 to 1. This supplement is reported to improve blood vessel function and insulin resistance, in addition to decreasing LDL cholesterol, total cholesterol, and triglycerides. Also essential for phase-I liver detoxification. If you experience loose stools after taking magnesium, cut your dose in half and gradually increase over the course of a few months. Consult your health-care provider for dosage advice.
Vitamin D (Vitamin D_3, or cholecalciferol)	1,000 to 4,000 IU once a day.	Vitamin D is necessary for proper calcium absorption. Inform your doctor if you are taking any drug that can deplete vitamin D, such as anticonvulsants, cholesterol-lowering medications, anti-ulcer drugs, or mineral oil. People with kidney disease or atherosclerosis should not take vitamin D. Excessive intake can increase the risk of hardened arteries and high blood calcium levels. People with sarcoidosis, tuberculosis, hyperparathyroidism, and lymphoma should use vitamin D only as directed by a physician. The tolerable upper limit for vitamin D intake is 4,000 IU per day. Higher dosages may be used to treat vitamin D deficiencies, but must be short-term and medically supervised.

LIFESTYLE CHANGES

Whether hypocalcemia is mild or acute, there are certain dietary guidelines that should be closely followed for better blood calcium management.

- Avoid foods that are high in fiber, including beans, collards, chocolate, rhubarb, soybeans, spinach, and sweet potatoes. Such high-fiber foods contain *oxalates* (oxalic acid) and *phytates* (phytic acid), which bind to calcium and inhibit its absorption in the body.

- Consume more calcium-rich dairy products, such as milk, buttermilk, cheese, cottage cheese, and yogurt. Choose organic products that do not contain hormones and antibiotics typically found in regular brands.

- Eliminate caffeinated drinks, including coffee and tea, from your diet. As noted on page 86, excessive caffeine intake is associated with hypocalcemia.

- Lower your consumption of dietary phosphates (phosphoric acids). These are commonly found in carbonated beverages, cheese, milk, meats, seafood, whole grain bread, and many snack foods. Your total daily intake should be no more than 400 to 800 mg per day, so pay attention to nutrition labels on foods that you buy.

- Snack on nuts and seeds, which are good sources of calcium and magnesium.

Additionally, if bone health is a concern, you should cut out refined sugars and carbohydrates, as they increase blood acidity and can cause bone calcium depletion. Also, increase your intake of fruits and vegetables, especially green leafy vegetables. These foods are excellent sources of calcium and potassium (see page 91), a vital mineral that reduces blood acidity and protects calcium in the bones.

You should also make sure that your overall lifestyle is just as healthy as your diet. This means exercising, getting out in the sun, managing stress effectively, and throwing away your cigarettes if you're a smoker. Remember, sunlight exposure boosts vitamin D levels, which are essential for optimal calcium absorption. Additionally, a combination of weight-bearing and aerobic exercises strengthens your bones, slowing down any bone loss that may result from low blood calcium. Finally, adopt strategies—for example, yoga, meditation, or other relaxation exercises—to reduce your stress level. Chronic stress often interferes with hormone regulation, which can lead to bone problems, particularly if estrogen or cortisol levels become imbalanced. Low estrogen is connected to bone loss, while high cortisol in the blood can hinder the function of *osteoblasts*—cells responsible for making and maintaining the bones.

Consider This

Although many people associate calcium with dairy products—milk, cheese, and yogurt—other food substances are also rich in calcium. Kale (100 mg per raw serving), bok choy (74 mg per raw serving), and broccoli (21 mg per raw serving) are all great sources of calcium, as are sardines (324 mg per 3-ounce serving), baked beans (124 mg per 1-cup serving), and fortified oatmeal (350 mg per packet).

7. POTASSIUM

Potassium is an essential mineral and *electrolyte*—a mineral that dissolves in water and carries an electrical charge—that helps control fluid balance in the body. It is required for nerve impulse transmission and muscle contraction, among other vital functions. Potassium helps maintain nerve and muscle growth, heart function, and balanced pH, and assists in the cellular metabolism of carbohydrates and proteins. Intake of potassium can significantly affect your risk of high blood pressure and stroke. In addition, a recent study showed that if your potassium level is chronically in the low-normal range, you are more likely to develop diabetes within the next decade of life.

Since potassium is found in so many foods, especially fruits and vegetables, most people take in a sufficient amount. But there are many factors, including illness and diet, that may cause your level to become too high (hyperkalemia) or low (hypokalemia). The numeric ranges for high, low, and normal blood potassium levels, which are measured in milliequivalents per liter (mEq/L), are provided in the table below.

REFERENCE RANGES FOR POTASSIUM

Potassium (mEq/L)	Category
Greater than 7.0	Extremely high (Severe hyperkalemia)
6.1 to 7.0	Very high (Moderate hyperkalemia)
5.5 to 6.0	High (Mild hyperkalemia)
3.5 to 5.4	Normal
3.1 to 3.4	Low (Mild hypokalemia)
2.5 to 3.0	Very low (Moderate hypokalemia)
Less than 2.5	Extremely low (Severe hypokalemia)
Target Range: 3.5 to 4.5 mEq/L	

A blood potassium test can help detect adrenal, digestive, heart, kidney, and muscle disorders, as both high and low levels are potentially detrimental.

WHAT CAUSES HIGH POTASSIUM?

Very often, high potassium levels, or *hyperkalemia,* stem from disorders that affect the ability of the kidneys to remove excess potassium from the body. An undesirable cellular release of potassium also causes blood levels to become elevated; this process may be triggered by physical trauma, tumors, or gastrointestinal bleeding. Following a low-sodium diet can raise blood potassium, as a proper ratio of these two minerals is needed for electrolyte balance. The most common causes of hyperkalemia are listed below.

- Adrenal disorders, such as Addison's disease (chronic adrenal insufficiency)
- Cancer
- Cellular release of potassium into the blood, which can be triggered by burns, heart attack, rhabdomyolysis, physical trauma, or chemotherapy, among other factors
- Chronic diseases, including lupus and sickle cell disease
- Diabetes or insulin resistance
- Diet low in sodium, including vegetarian diets
- Excessive intake of potassium through either diet or supplements, including the herbs alfalfa, dandelion, horsetail, and nettle
- Genetic diseases such as Gordon's syndrome, a built-in resistance to the hormone aldosterone
- Hormone deficiency (particularly in aldosterone, an adrenal hormone that regulates potassium and sodium levels)
- Kidney disease or kidney failure
- Medications (See the inset on page 93.)
- Metabolic acidosis, a condition in which the pH of the body's fluids is too acidic
- Toxicity caused by the drug digoxin, which is used to treat irregular heartbeat
- Urinary tract obstructions (obstructive uropathy)

Since potassium plays such a vital role in heart and skeletal muscle function, a high level can disturb the electrical rhythm of the heart as well as muscle activity. When it progresses past the mild stages, hyperkalemia increases the risk of heart arrhythmia and heart attack.

WHAT ARE THE SYMPTOMS OF HIGH POTASSIUM?

Hyperkalemia rarely produces physical symptoms but, on occasion, people may experience nausea, fatigue, muscle aches and weakness, and an increased respiratory rate. Moderate cases of hyperkalemia can cause changes in heart rhythm, which may be detected by an electrocardiogram (ECG or EKG). Still, the condition frequently goes unnoticed until a routine blood test shows an abnormality. Additional testing is usually needed to determine the source of the problem; cortisol levels may be measured to gauge adrenal function, while blood urea nitrogen (BUN) and creatinine levels (see pages 123 and 130) should be checked to assess kidney function. The results of these tests are needed in order to plan a course of treatment and prevent medical complications.

Medications and Hyperkalemia

Hyperkalemia, or elevated blood potassium, occurs in approximately 8 percent of hospitalized patients. A chief cause is prescribed drugs, which may produce adverse side effects and interactions that lead to high potassium levels. Below is a list of medications that have been shown to have this effect. If you are taking any of these drugs, speak to your physician about your risk of developing high potassium levels. A blood test may be in order.

- ACE (angiotensin-converting enzyme) inhibitors like captopril (Capoten), enalapril (Renitec, Vasotec), and fosinopril (Monopril)
- Antibiotics such as pentamidine (Nebupent) and trimethoprim-sulfamethoxazole (Septra)
- Anticoagulants, such as heparin
- ARBs (angiotensin-receptor blockers), such as losartan (Cozaar) and valsartan (Diovan)
- Beta blockers, including metoprolol (Lopressor, Toprol) and propranolol (Inderal)
- COX-2 inhibitors, such as celecoxib (Celebrex)
- Cyclosporine (Sandimmune)
- Ketoconazole (Nizoral), an antifungal medication
- Nonsteroidal anti-inflammatory drugs (NSAIDs) like ibuprofen (Advil, Motrin)
- Potassium-sparing diuretics, such as triamterene (Dyazide) and triamterene-HCTZ (Maxzide)

HOW CAN HIGH POTASSIUM BE TREATED?

Treating high potassium levels depends on the underlying cause, which is usually kidney failure or medication. Mild hyperkalemia that is related to diet or the use of certain medications or supplements can be reversed simply by reducing potassium intake and discontinuing the use of the problematic substance. However, prescription and regimen adjustments should be made only under the supervision of a doctor. Moderate and severe cases of hyperkalemia require immediate treatment. This may involve intravenous medication or, when the problem is kidney related, a restricted diet or even dialysis. Whatever the case may be, long-term solutions are needed to keep potassium levels within a normal range. This section covers the various drugs, supplements, and lifestyle changes that can be implemented to promote a healthy potassium level.

DRUGS

The drugs in the table below are used to treat moderate to severe cases of hyperkalemia. They usually must be administered by a doctor and used only under medical supervision. If your doctor prescribes one of the drugs listed above, be sure to discuss proper dosing, as well as potential risks and side effects.

DRUGS FOR HIGH POTASSIUM LEVELS

Drug	Considerations
Beta-agonists (isoproterenol, albuterol) *Isuprel, Proventil*	Beta-agonists are given only to patients who have very high potassium levels. This drug must be administered by a doctor or trained medical personnel.
Calcium chloride/ gluconate (calcium salts)	Injectable calcium must be administered by a doctor or trained medical personnel.
Dextrose (IV)	Dextrose must be administered by a doctor or trained medical personnel.
Fludrocortisone acetate *Florinef*	Must be prescribed by a health-care professional. Follow the recommendations of your doctor, especially if you have or have ever had diabetes, underactive thyroid, osteoporosis, ulcers, or kidney, liver, or heart disease.
Furosemide *Lasix*	May cause depletion of certain nutrients, including calcium, magnesium, potassium, sodium, thiamine, vitamin B_6, vitamin C, and zinc.

Drug	Considerations
Insulin (injection) *Humulin, Novolin, Humalog, Novolog, Lente, Ultralente*	Injectable insulin is used along with glucose in emergency situations of hyperkalemia, and must be administered by a doctor or trained medical personnel.
Magnesium sulfate (injection)	Intravenous magnesium must be administered by a doctor or trained medical personnel.
Sodium bicarbonate (injection)	Intravenous sodium bicarbonate must be administered by a doctor or trained medical personnel.
Sodium polystyrene sulfonate *Kayexalate*	This drug is used only to treat very high potassium levels, and must be administered by a doctor or trained medical personnel.

SUPPLEMENTS

Supplementation may be an option in non-emergency situations, but this decision is one best made by your physician.

LIFESTYLE CHANGES

In nonemergency situations, a low-potassium diet is usually recommended for reducing potassium levels. Since most foods contain potassium in some amount, the key is to eat more foods with lower concentrations while limiting the serving size of foods with higher potassium content. Foods that are rich in potassium and, therefore, should be kept to a minimum include acorn squash, artichokes, bananas, dried beans, citrus and dried fruits, dark leafy greens, dairy products, fruit juice (especially grapefruit, orange, prune, and tomato juice), legumes, nuts, prunes, potatoes, sweet potatoes, soy products, and tomatoes. Fish, particularly cod and salmon, are also a significant source of potassium, and beef and dark turkey meat contain moderate amounts as well. As you decrease your intake of these foods, increase your consumption of foods that contain potassium in lower amounts, such as:

- Cabbage
- Carrots
- Cauliflower
- Cucumbers
- Eggs
- Lemons
- Onions
- Peanuts
- Plums
- Ricotta cheese

Additionally, consider taking rice protein, a powder that can be mixed into liquid and consumed as a beverage. Although rice protein does not directly lower potassium, it can be beneficial for people with high levels—especially when they are due to kidney failure—because of its low potassium content in comparison to other high-protein foods.

Another way to avoid high potassium levels is to eliminate salt substitutes from your diet, since adequate sodium is needed to keep your potassium level balanced and within a normal range. Adequate rest is also important, since lack of sleep can lead to blood sugar disturbances, in turn altering potassium excretion. Therefore, you should aim to get seven to eight hours of restful sleep per night. In addition, ask your physician about what type and amount of exercise you should do. If you are given medical approval, start a workout regimen that combines aerobic activity, like walking or biking, with strength training that uses some weights. This combination is considered optimal.

WHAT CAUSES LOW POTASSIUM?

As already mentioned, low blood potassium, or *hypokalemia,* is typically defined as any lab value lower than 3.5 mEq/L. There are numerous reasons for a drop in potassium levels, some of which are:

- Adrenal disorders, such as hyperaldosteronism (too much aldosterone is produced) or chronic adrenal stress
- Diabetes insipidus, a condition resulting in water loss due to lack of antidiuretic hormone (ADH) or the inability of the kidneys to respond to it
- Diarrhea
- Diet high in sodium and very low in potassium
- Digestive problems
- Diseases affecting the ability of the kidneys to hold on to potassium, including Bartter syndrome, Cushing syndrome, Fanconi syndrome, and Liddle syndrome
- Excessive vomiting due to illness or eating disorders such as bulimia
- Hormonal imbalances, including insulin, sex hormones, and thyroid hormones
- Kidney disease or kidney failure
- Magnesium deficiency

- Medications (See the inset on page 98.)
- Overuse of laxatives
- Pituitary disorders
- Water loss through sweating or excessive urination

While a slight drop in blood potassium usually does not pose major health risks, chronic hypokalemia is associated with muscle aches, cramps, and weakness. In severe cases, heart arrhythmias, cardiac weakness, or heart attack can occur. Changes in the central nervous system, such as delirium or psychosis, are also possible when potassium levels drop too low for an extended period of time.

Additionally, people taking the drug digoxin, which is used to treat abnormal heartbeat and congestive heart failure, should keep a close eye on their blood potassium, as low levels may increase the likelihood of digoxin toxicity. In general, people taking this drug need to keep their potassium at a normal level to prevent undesirable side effects. Diabetes patients should also monitor their potassium, as a deficiency can trigger hyperglycemia.

WHAT ARE THE SYMPTOMS OF LOW POTASSIUM?

Like hyperkalemia, hypokalemia is typically asymptomatic, especially when blood potassium is only slightly low. When hypokalemia is moderate or severe, constipation, fatigue, muscle cramps and weakness, and heart palpitations may occur. Determining the cause of your low potassium level is necessary in order to alleviate these symptoms and avoid future medical problems.

HOW CAN LOW POTASSIUM BE TREATED?

Treatment of hypokalemia must target the source of the condition, such as medications, excessive vomiting (caused by disorders like bulimia, for example), overuse of laxatives, or kidney disorders. This section covers the different types of treatment that might be employed in cases of low potassium.

DRUGS

In acute or emergency situations, intravenous potassium may be administered by a doctor or trained medical professional. Additionally, the medications K-Dur or Klor-Con (timed-release potassium chloride) may be prescribed to people who have chronically low potassium levels due to another health issue.

Medications and Hypokalemia

Pharmaceutical drugs are a common cause of low blood potassium levels. In fact, as much as 20 percent of hospitalized patients are affected by hypokalemia. Below is a list of medications that can lower potassium to an unhealthy level.

- Anti-asthmatic drugs, including most beta-agonists (such as albuterol) and theophylline
- Antibiotics, including penicillin, nafcillin, foscarnet, gentamicin, and tobramycin
- Antiretroviral drugs
- Colchicine, a gout medication
- Diuretics, both loop (furosemide, or Lasix) and thiazide (hydrochlorothiazide, or HCTZ, and methylclothiazide)
- Indapamide (Lozol) and metolazone (Zaroxolyn), drugs used to treat fluid retention caused by heart disease and other conditions
- Laxatives available over the counter, such as cascara sagrada, mineral oil, and senna
- Levodopa (L-DOPA, Sinemet), a medication for Parkinson's disease
- Salicylates such as aspirin
- Steroids, including cortisone (Cortef), prednisolone (Pediapred), prednisone (Deltasone), and dexamethasone (Decadron).

If you are taking any of the medications listed above and experience symptoms of hypokalemia, notify your medical provider.

SUPPLEMENTS

While potassium supplements can help restore more optimal levels, they should be used with caution and taken only under the supervision of a healthcare professional. Potassium supplements, which may be taken as potassium citrate or potassium gluconate, can have gastrointestinal side effects such as nausea, abdominal discomfort, and diarrhea. Moreover, excessive use occasionally leads to weakness, mental confusion, low blood pressure, and irregular heartbeat. Unless otherwise instructed by your doctor, potassium supplements should not be taken if you have a digestive disorder or kidney problems, or if you are currently taking blood pressure medication or diuretics. An appropriate dose for most people is 99 mg twice a day, but check with your doctor to make sure that this amount is appropriate for your needs.

LIFESTYLE CHANGES

For mild cases of low potassium, your doctor will probably tell you to maintain adequate fluid intake, increase your consumption of potassium-rich foods, and reduce the amount of sodium in your diet. Here are some other adjustments you can make to your life to ensure balanced blood potassium in the long term:

- Decrease sodium intake. Recommendations for sodium intake are continually being lowered, since Americans take in far too much sodium, a leading contributor to high blood pressure. It is currently recommended that you consume less than 2,300 mg per day. To ensure that you do not exceed this limit, avoid processed foods and meats like ham, bacon, hot dogs, and jerky, which are very high in sodium. Also cut out fast food and prepackaged meals, or look for versions that contain less than 500 mg for the whole meal. Do not add salt to your food; a single teaspoon contains 2,500 mg of sodium. Instead, flavor your food with herbal seasonings—good brands include Mrs. Dash and Mr. Pepper—or other garlic pepper blends.

- Fill your diet with high-potassium foods. Potassium is found in most foods, but the best sources include acorn squash, artichokes, dried beans, beets, citrus and dried fruits, dairy products, fish (cod and salmon), fruit juices, mushrooms, nuts (almonds, peanuts, and pistachios), pumpkin, soy products, spinach, and tomatoes. Although many fruits and fruit juices are high in potassium, they can also contain a significant amount of natural sugars and, therefore, should be consumed in controlled amounts. This is especially important if you are insulin resistant or have blood sugar problems.

- Lower your stress level. Excessive release of cortisol, the hormone produced during stress, can put too much burden on the adrenal glands. Adrenal exhaustion may alter sodium levels and create other imbalances in the body that lead to low potassium.

- Read nutrition labels. When buying packaged foods, choose products that say "Low Sodium" or contain less than 140 mg per serving. Be aware that labels that read "No Salt Added" do not necessarily mean sodium free, as many foods naturally contain sodium. If your doctor recommends a sodium-restricted diet, ask about products that use acceptable salt substitutes.

- Use electrolyte replacement fluids. Many of these fluids now contain little or no sugar. Depending on your specific situation, your doctor may recommend that you consume them on a regular basis, particularly if your low potassium level is due to acute diarrhea or colitis. Electrolyte replacement is essential for people who exercise regularly.

It's necessary to mention that while exercise is vital for good health, it should be done cautiously (and with your doctor's permission) if you have low potassium. This is because intense exercise can result in potassium loss through sweating. Additionally, low potassium weakens the muscles, thereby making rigorous exercise difficult. If you suffer from hypokalemia, do not exercise unless your doctor gives approval. Once your potassium reaches a normal level, reintroduce exercise to your lifestyle in gradual, moderate amounts.

Did You Know?

If you suffer from low potassium, there are many potassium-rich foods you can eat that will help boost your levels. Many athletes are accustomed to eating a banana before or after their workouts, but there are even better sources available. According to the USDA, one cup of cooked white beans, or navy beans, contains 708 mg of potassium. That's almost double the amount found in a banana!

8. SODIUM

Although it is not generally thought of as beneficial, sodium is an essential nutrient and electrolyte. Along with potassium, sodium works to balance fluids in the body. It also influences blood pressure regulation, heart rhythm, muscle contraction, and nerve impulse transmission. Since sodium is so important, the body has built-in mechanisms for keeping blood levels within a fairly tight range. Blood sodium is regulated by the kidneys and hormones produced by the adrenal glands and the pituitary gland.

Abnormal blood sodium levels may indicate an underlying medical condition like Cushing's syndrome (overactive adrenal glands) or Addison's disease (underactive adrenal glands). Sodium imbalances are also very often related to the body's hydration status, meaning dehydration or overhydration. When there is an excess of water in the body, sodium becomes diluted, resulting in low blood sodium levels, or *hyponatremia*. It is rare, but possible, for hyponatremia to be caused by drinking too much water. Cases of this have been seen as a result of water-drinking contests, a hazing ritual used by some fraternities. On the other hand, when the body is water-deficient or dehydrated, there is a relative surplus of sodium in the blood, which is known as *hypernatremia*. This condition may occur as a result of not drinking enough water or excessive sweating. It is seen most frequently among the elderly, since the thirst mechanism—which is normally triggered by low fluid intake—declines with age. Therefore, elderly people are urged to drink water even if they do not feel thirsty to avoid becoming dehydrated and developing hypernatremia, which can be fatal in very severe cases.

Although "salt" and "sodium" are often used interchangeably, they are not the same. Table salt is actually sodium chloride, a specific type of sodium obtained through the diet rather than produced naturally by the body. In addition to sodium chloride, there are other types of dietary sodium—sodium nitrate, sodium phosphate, and sodium acetate, for example—that are added to most prepackaged foods, with the highest concentrations in fast food, condiments, and canned and processed meats. Diets high or low in salt can promote hypernatremia or hyponatremia, but they are rarely the cause, since the body can usually naturally compensate for variances in intake.

Sodium levels are measured on a routine basic metabolic panel test, but a separate blood sodium test may also be ordered if a person displays symptoms of hypernatremia or hyponatremia (see pages 103 and 107). Reference ranges for blood sodium, which are measured by testing laboratories using either milliequivalents or millimoles per liter, are listed below. While milliequivalents per liter (mEq/L) is the unit of measurement used in the United States, millimoles per liter (mmol/L) is the unit more commonly used by the rest of the world.

REFERENCE RANGES FOR SODIUM	
Sodium (mEq/L or mmol/L)	**Category**
Greater than 155	Very high (Critical level of hypernatremia)
144 to 155	High (Hypernatremia)
134 to 143	Ideal
120 to 133	Low (Hyponatremia)
Less than 120	Very low (Critcal level of hyponatremia)

If a blood test shows an abnormal sodium level, a urine test may be used to determine the cause of the imbalance.

WHAT CAUSES HIGH SODIUM?

Elevated blood sodium, or hypernatremia, is usually due to inadequate water intake or excessive water loss through diarrhea, sweating, urination, vomiting, or some other problem. This condition occurs in approximately 1 percent of hospitalized patients, as well as in 2 percent of debilitated elderly people and breastfed infants. Hypernatremia is more common in older adults because the thirst mechanism becomes weaker with age, making them more susceptible to dehydration. The condition is also seen in infants because they can become dehydrated more easily due to their small body size. Moreover, breastfeeding makes it difficult to measure how much or how little liquid an infant has consumed. Mothers who are breastfeeding are advised to monitor their babies' urine output to ensure they are adequately hydrated. High sodium levels may also be related to factors such as:

- Cushing's syndrome (overactive adrenal glands)
- Cystic fibrosis
- Diabetes insipidus
- Diet low in potassium
- Drinking high-sodium water, usually from a water softener

- Elevated levels of cortisol due to chronic stress
- Excessive salt intake
- Head trauma
- Loss of body fluids due to vomiting, diarrhea, or sweating induced by a high fever
- Medical administration of IV fluids
- Medications that may cause adrenal gland imbalance, such as oral contraceptives and steroids
- Pituitary tumors, which alter antidiuretic hormone levels

Acute hypernatremia, or sodium levels that rise very quickly, may cause convulsions and even comas. Early treatment is therefore essential in preventing dangerous medical complications.

WHAT ARE THE SYMPTOMS OF HIGH SODIUM?

The symptoms that usually appear first in hypernatremia are similar to the signs of dehydration, and include dry mouth and mucous membranes, dizziness, nausea, and vomiting. A mild elevation in blood sodium can also result in fluid retention and raised blood pressure. When the condition worsens, irritability, mental confusion, lethargy, and muscle twitching can occur.

HOW CAN HIGH SODIUM BE TREATED?

The goal of treatment for high sodium is usually to restore normal fluid levels. This can be achieved through increasing fluid intake, oral rehydration therapy, or correcting the underlying problem. Various short-term and long-term solutions for hypernatremia are detailed in this section.

DRUGS

The drugs listed in the table below may be used to treat high sodium levels in the blood. They are given only under medical supervision. If your high sodium level cannot be treated using any of these medications, your doctor will determine a course of treatment that better fits your needs. Speak to a medical professional about potential side effects, risks, and interactions of any drug that you are prescribed.

DRUGS FOR HIGH SODIUM	
Drug	**Considerations**
Desmopressin acetate *DDAVP, Minirin, Stimate*	This drug is used to treat hypernatremia related to ADH imbalance. It is given only under the supervision of a medical professional.
Saline solution, 0.9% sodium chloride (IV)	This drug is given only under the supervision of a medical professional.
Vasopressin *Pitressin*	This drug is given only under the supervision of a medical professional.

SUPPLEMENTS

Supplements are not recommended for people with high sodium levels. Hypernatremia must be treated medically.

LIFESTYLE CHANGES

Although hypernatremia is usually caused by dehydration, excessive dietary intake of sodium can also be a problem, even when blood levels are kept stable by the body. Consuming a large amount of sodium forces the kidneys to retain more water in order to keep blood sodium at a proper level. More water in the blood increases blood volume, in turn raising blood pressure and putting a strain on the heart. This is why the Food and Nutrition Board advises no more than 2,300 mg of sodium per day for adults. Keeping your daily intake under this amount helps to keep sodium levels within a healthy range and reduce your risk of high blood pressure. Moreover, it is recommended that people who are over fifty years of age or have diabetes, high blood pressure, or kidney disease consume no more than 1,500 mg per day in order to lower the risk of kidney damage. It's interesting to note that, over the past five years, attention has also been given to the role of chloride (see page 109) in salt-induced hypertension.

Below is some general advice for controlling sodium intake and retention. If you have kidney disease or kidney failure, follow your doctor's directions for reducing your consumption of sodium.

- Avoid meats that are canned, cured, pickled, or smoked. These meats, which include ham, hot dogs, and jerky, have high sodium content. On average, a single serving of cured meat contains 350 mg of sodium. By comparison, there is approximately 75 mg of sodium per serving of fresh meats and poultry.

• Cut out fast food and prepackaged meals. Pre-prepared foods, such as frozen dinners and canned soups, are very high in sodium—one frozen dinner can contain up to 1,000 mg and 1 cup of most canned soup brands has approximately 800 mg. In contrast, a serving of fresh vegetables has only about 35 mg of sodium, and fruits, 10 mg. At the very least, read nutrition labels and choose products that have the lowest sodium content or are unsalted.

• Decrease your stress level. In response to stress, the adrenal glands produce hormones like cortisol, as well as epinephrine and norepinephrine, which cause blood vessel constriction. The combined effects of these hormones and aldosterone, an adrenal hormone that promotes sodium and water retention, can cause blood pressure to increase.

• Do not drink water treated with a water softener. This appliance replaces calcium and magnesium ions in water with sodium ions, thereby increasing the water's sodium content. People on sodium-restricted diets are usually advised not to drink water from a water softener, as it is difficult to determine how much sodium you are actually getting from the water.

• Eat more high-potassium foods. As already mentioned, one way to maintain healthy sodium levels in the blood is to increase your potassium intake, as potassium helps push sodium out of the body. Fruits and vegetables, which are naturally low in sodium, are also the best sources of potassium, particularly acorn squash, apples, artichokes, beets, blueberries, citrus fruits, dark leafy greens, grapes, peaches, and tomatoes. Fruit juices (especially grapefruit, orange, prune, and tomato), dried beans, and nuts also contain significant amounts of potassium.

• Eat the recommended amount of fiber. A meta-analysis of studies on fiber found that increased intake of dietary fiber is correlated with reduced blood pressure. However, it's unclear whether this can be attributed to fiber alone, since many high-fiber foods are also very high in potassium. Still, adults should consume between 25 and 35 g of fiber per day, so fill your diet with foods like leafy greens, cooked or dried beans, whole grains, and raw fresh fruit.

• Minimize the amount of cheese you eat. Processed cheese is high in sodium, so stick to cheeses such as Monterey Jack, mozzarella, and ricotta, which tend have a lower concentration of sodium. You can also choose low-salt products, but continue to eat them only in moderation.

• When using salt substitutes, check the ingredients. If you're following a sodium-restricted diet, you may want to eat foods that use salt substitutes.

However, you should be aware that some salt-alternative products still use a small amount of salt to improve the taste. In addition, they often contain potassium chloride, which should not be used by people who are taking certain medications or have particular medical conditions. Therefore, you should ask a healthcare professional to recommend salt-alternative products, and make sure you receive your doctor's approval before adding such products to your diet.

As stated in previous sections, regular exercise is an essential part of a healthy lifestyle. But since hypernatremia can be caused by dehydration, it's important that you maintain proper fluid intake while exercising. The general recommendation is two to three 8-ounce glasses of water two hours before exercising, and 4 to 8 ounces of water per every fifteen to thirty minutes of physical activity. If you exercise for longer than ninety minutes, you should also consume an 8-ounce sports drink to replace your electrolytes. Continue to replenish your fluids after exercising as well, as you lose water through perspiration. Weigh yourself after exercising to monitor your fluid loss, and drink 20 ounces of water for every pound lost.

WHAT CAUSES LOW SODIUM?

Like high blood sodium, low sodium levels are connected to the relative amount of water in the body. Hyponatremia occurs when the sodium in the blood becomes diluted due to excess water, or when there is a sharp decrease in electrolytes because of fluid loss. The vast majority of hyponatremia cases occur because of conditions such as:

- Addison's disease (chronic adrenal insufficiency)
- Cirrhosis of the liver
- Congestive heart failure
- Excessive alcohol consumption, especially of beer
- Hypothyroidism
- Kidney disorders, kidney disease, or kidney failure
- Loss of body fluids due to vomiting, diarrhea, or sweating induced by a high fever
- Medications, including ACE inhibitors, colchicine (a gout medication), loop and thiazide diuretics, salicylates, and tricyclic antidepressants
- Overhydration

- Physical traumas, such as burns
- Syndrome of inappropriate antidiuretics hormone hypersecretion (SIADH), which is seen conditions such as in pneumonia, brain tumors, tuberculosis, and some cancers

Drug interactions—between ACE inhibitors and angiotensin receptor blockers (ARBs), for example—can also cause sodium levels to drop. It's crucial to treat the condition before it worsens, since irregular heartbeat, low blood pressure, and neurological impairment may develop. Sudden drops in sodium levels (acute hyponatremia) are especially worrisome, as cerebral edema is a possible consequence. This condition can cause *brainstem herniation*—the movement of brain tissues, blood vessels, and cerebrospinal fluid—and is potentially life-threatening. If your doctor prescribes you these medications, your blood sodium level will be closely monitored.

WHAT ARE THE SYMPTOMS OF LOW SODIUM?

The symptoms of chronic (long-term) low sodium are not as severe as the signs of acute hyponatremia and can vary depending on underlying medical condition. Elderly people with mild chronic hyponatremia may experience generalized weakness and, therefore, be more prone to falling, while individuals with congestive heart failure may have edema. If your low sodium level is due to adrenal insufficiency, you might experience salt cravings, dizziness upon standing (postural hypotension), and general lethargy. Symptoms are usually nonspecific and can include headache, muscle spasms or cramps, fainting, fatigue, appetite loss, nausea, and stomach cramps. These symptoms are also seen in over-hydrated athletes. However, when sodium levels drop quickly (acute hyponatremia), a state of confusion and decreased consciousness can set in, sometimes resulting in convulsions, seizures, or coma.

HOW CAN LOW SODIUM BE TREATED?

Hyponatremia is most commonly seen in hospitalized patients, either as a result of an underlying medical condition or the administration of IV fluids. Treatment is based on the severity of the condition and its cause. Patients who are ambulatory (able to walk), are typically advised to decrease fluid consumption and, when necessary, to stop taking medications, such as diuretics, that might be depleting the body of sodium. In emergency situations in which levels are very low and must be raised quickly, drugs, such as 3-percent hypertonic saline solution, may be administered.

DRUGS

There are also drugs that can be prescribed for low sodium levels that are caused by specific disorders. The medications in the table below may be used under a doctor's supervision. To ensure the drugs are working properly, frequent blood testing is necessary.

DRUGS FOR LOW SODIUM	
Drug	**Considerations**
Conivaptan (IV) *Vaprisol*	Treats hyponatremia by reducing the body's level of antidiuretic hormone (ADH). This drug is given only under medical supervision.
Tolvaptan *Samsca*	Take this medication with a full glass of water (8 ounces), as dehydration can occur. Notify your doctor if you have severe liver disease or cirrhosis before taking. Do not use if you are dehydrated or unable to urinate.

Since a medical condition is usually the cause, all cases of hyponatremia should be treated medically. In rare cases, hyponatremia may occur as a result of low sodium intake in combination with regularly drinking large amounts of water. When this happens, it's generally recommended that you increase sodium consumption while reducing your water intake. Accidental hyponatremia, which most commonly affects athletes who exercise intensely without drinking enough water, can usually be remedied with proper rehydration. Athletes are now advised to eat salty foods prior to long bouts of exercise in order to prevent hyponatremia. However, chronic hyponatremia cannot be treated with lifestyle changes, dietary modification, or nutritional supplementation. A doctor's care is always necessary.

A Helpful Tip

While it's important to drink fluids while exercising, excessive drinking of water alone can lead to low sodium levels in extreme cases. Because your body loses not only water but also sodium when you sweat, it is better to hydrate with a glucose- or maltodextrin-based sports drink. Doctors now also recommend that athletes eat a salty food before an extended workout in order to prevent low sodium afterwards.

9. CHLORIDE

Along with potassium and sodium, chloride is an electrolyte that helps to balance fluids inside and outside of your body's cells. Chloride is also instrumental in maintaining proper blood volume, blood pressure, and *pH*—the ratio of acids to bases in the body—in addition to playing an important role in metabolism. Chloride is usually taken into the body via the consumption of table salt (sodium chloride) and foods such as celery, rye, olives, and lettuce. Most of the chloride that enters your system is absorbed by the gastrointestinal tract, and the kidneys regulate the amount of chloride in the blood. Excess chloride is excreted in the urine.

A proper level of chloride is essential in order for the body to carry out basic functions. A disturbance in your blood chloride level often signals a problem with your kidneys, hormones, acid-alkaline balance, or electrolyte levels. Elevated blood chloride is called *hyperchloremia,* while a very low blood chloride level is known as *hypochloremia.* Reference ranges for high, low, and normal blood chloride values, which are measured in millimoles per liter (mmol/L), are provided below. You should note that there is no target range for chloride, as the normal range is already somewhat narrowly defined.

REFERENCE RANGES FOR CHLORIDE

Chloride (mmol/L)	Category
Greater than 108	High (Hypercholremia)
97 to 108	Normal
Less than 97	Low (Hypocholremia)

A blood chloride test is rarely ordered by itself. Instead, chloride may be measured along with other electrolytes if a person exhibits symptoms that may indicate an imbalance.

WHAT CAUSES HIGH CHLORIDE?

As you will notice on the list below, the causes of high blood chloride levels (hyperchloremia) overlap with the causes of high sodium (hypernatremia). As explained on page 101, sodium and chloride come together in the form of table salt. High intake of table salt can increase both sodium and chloride levels in someone who does not have healthy kidneys, which are needed to properly excrete substances the body does not need. When the kidneys are properly functioning, though, excessive consumption of table salt will not alone raise blood chloride or sodium levels. Contributing factors to elevated chloride include:

- Cushing's syndrome
- Cystic fibrosis
- Diabetes insipidus
- Excessive salt intake
- Hyperparathyroidism (overproduction of parathyroid hormone)
- Hyperthyroidism
- Kidney disorder known as renal tubular acidosis (types 1 and 2)
- Loss of body fluids due to vomiting, diarrhea, or sweating induced by a high fever
- Medical administration of IV fluids
- Medications that may cause adrenal hormone imbalance, including oral contraceptives and steroids
- Metabolic acidosis (acid buildup in the body leading to pH imbalance)
- Physical traumas, including burns and head injuries
- Pituitary tumors
- Respiratory alkalosis (rapid breathing that raises blood pH) and related conditions that may cause it, such as hyperventilation and cystic fibrosis

When left untreated, high chloride can negatively affect oxygen transport. In people with diabetes, elevated chloride often leads to poor blood sugar control.

WHAT ARE THE SYMPTOMS OF HIGH CHLORIDE?

A high level of chloride in the blood does not necessarily produce symptoms. But if dehydration is the cause, intense thirst, decreased urinary output, and dry mucous membranes (of the eyes, lips, and mouth, for example) may result. Elevated blood chloride can also cause a person to feel agitated and confused, as well as experience breathing difficulty and muscle tension, twitching, or spasms.

HOW CAN HIGH CHLORIDE BE TREATED?

Hyperchloremia is almost always related to a medical condition and, therefore, should never be self-treated. Effective treatment of high blood chloride depends on correcting the underlying cause. If dehydration is the root of the problem, for example, fluid intake must be increased and maintained. In general, a physician or or specialist must always evaluate and treat elevated chloride levels.

DRUGS

Severe cases of hyperchloremia may call for oral rehydration therapy or intravenous administration of fluids. High levels caused by medical conditions like kidney disease may require the use of specific therapies or medications. In this case, a specialist will decide upon an appropriate treatment.

SUPPLEMENTS

Proper electrolyte balance depends on adequate intake of *all* electrolyte minerals. While sufficient amounts of potassium can be obtained through plant foods, it's difficult to acquire enough magnesium and calcium through dietary sources alone. Taking one or more of the supplements in the table below can help support a healthy balance of electrolyte minerals. Nutritional supplements do not require a prescription, but you should check with your doctor before taking any supplement to ensure that you use it appropriately and safely.

SUPPLEMENTS FOR HIGH CHLORIDE

Supplement	Dosage	Considerations
Calcium	500 mg one to three times a day.	Take a highly absorbable form of calcium, such as calcium aspartate, citrate, or hydroxyapatite. If using calcium to help sleep problems, take one 500-mg dose at bedtime.
Magnesium	250 to 500 mg twice a day.	Use magnesium aspartate, citrate, taurate, glycinate, or any amino acid chelate. Supports bone building and balances calcium intake. The ratio of calcium-to-magnesium intake should be between 1 to 1 and 2 to 1. This supplement is reported to improve blood vessel function and insulin resistance, in addition to decreasing LDL cholesterol, total cholesterol, and triglycerides. Also essential for phase-I liver detoxification. If you experience loose stools after taking magnesium, cut your dose in half

Supplement	Dosage	Considerations
Magnesium *(continued)*		and gradually increase over the course of a few months. Consult your health-care provider for dosage advice.
Potassium	99 mg twice a day.	Use potassium citrate or gluconate. May cause gastrointestinal side effects such as nausea, abdominal discomfort, and diarrhea. Excessive use of this supplement could potentially lead to weakness, mental confusion, low blood pressure, and irregular heartbeat. Do not use if you have a digestive disorder or kidney problems, or are currently taking blood pressure medication or diuretic drugs, unless directed by your doctor.

LIFESTYLE CHANGES

If your level falls into the "high-normal" range, there are a number of lifestyle adjustments you can make to ensure that your level returns to or remains within a healthy range. Diet is an important factor when it comes to chloride, and since chloride and sodium levels are closely related, a low-sodium diet is usually highly beneficial. Here are some ways you can promote electrolyte balance and boost your overall health:

- Avoid foods with high sodium content. This group includes prepackaged meals, condiments, and salty snacks, as well as meats that are canned, cured, pickled, or smoked. Reducing your intake of processed foods will cut your consumption of sodium chloride (added salt). When buying packaged foods, look for products that labeled "low sodium." This should not be confused with foods labeled as having "reduced sodium," "light sodium," or "no salt added," which are not necessarily better for you.

- Do not use a water softener. Softened water is high in sodium ions, so drinking or bathing in it can add to your body's total sodium level and, in turn, cause blood chloride to become elevated.

- Eat the recommended amount of fiber. It's recommended that adults consume between 25 and 35 g of fiber per day. This goal can be met by filling your diet with leafy green vegetables, cooked or dried beans, whole grains, and raw fresh fruit. Taking in a sufficient amount of fiber helps prevent some chronic conditions that can lead to abnormal blood chloride levels. In addition to helping to control blood glucose, fiber also promotes bowel regularity.

- Experiment with salt-free seasonings and salt substitutes. Instead of flavoring your food with table salt (sodium chloride), try spice-based seasonings or garlic pepper blends. These flavorings are pleasing to the palate but much healthier. As a bonus, you'll be learning how to cook with spices and herbs like rosemary, turmeric, basil, chives, chili powder, and curry powder, which are high in antioxidants and other beneficial phytonutrients. If you want to use salt substitutes, however, check with your doctor before adding any salt-alternative product to your diet. Some salt substitutes contain potassium chloride, which should not be combined with certain medications or used by people with medical conditions like kidney disease.

- Include more nutrient-rich low-sodium foods in your diet. In general, fruits and vegetables are naturally low in sodium and high in potassium, so making them staples will help you maintain pH balance and fluid balance in the body. Additionally, increasing your consumption of foods that are rich in potassium and calcium, like broccoli, kale, unsalted nuts, sweet potatoes, and apricots, will help keep your sodium and chloride levels in balance. Green vegetables, such as spinach and kale, are also good sources of calcium and magnesium.

WHAT CAUSES LOW CHLORIDE?

Blood chloride values less than 97 mmol/L are considered to be low, indicating hypochloremia. This condition occurs with any disorder that also causes low sodium (see pages 106 to 107). Most cases of hypochloremia occur in acute care (hospital) settings as a side effect of gastric suctioning, diuretic therapy, or the administration of IV fluids. Other reasons for low blood chloride include:

- Addison's disease (chronic adrenal insufficiency)
- Congestive heart failure
- Hypothyroidism
- Kidney disease or kidney failure
- Loss of body fluids due to vomiting, diarrhea, or sweating caused by high fevers
- Medications, including ACE inhibitors, colchicine, loop diuretics, salicylates, thiazide diuretics
- Metabolic alkalosis (loss of acid from the body, resulting in pH imbalance)
- Physical traumas
- Respiratory acidosis (shortness of breath resulting in lowered blood pH), which can be caused by chronic lung diseases like emphysema
- SIADH (syndrome of inappropriate antidiuretics hormone hypersecretion)

If blood test indicates your chloride level is low (and you are not hospitalized), your doctor will order further testing to check for disorders of the kidneys, liver, adrenal glands, and thyroid. Adrenal dysfunction can be detected by measuring your level of cortisol along with other adrenal hormones. Thyroid hormone levels (TSH, free T3, T4, and thyroid antibodies) can be measured in order to rule out thyroid dysfunction. Determining the cause is essential, as prolonged chloride deficiency affects blood pressure and heartbeat, and in severe cases, can induce convulsions or seizures.

WHAT ARE THE SYMPTOMS OF LOW CHLORIDE?

The signs of low chloride are nonspecific and, in many cases, nonexistent. Some people may experience confusion, dizziness, fainting, fatigue, headache, and muscle weakness, as well as loss of appetite, nausea, and stomach cramps. These symptoms, especially lethargy and confusion, may require immediate medical attention. You should also seek medical care if you have an acute illness that causes excessive vomiting and diarrhea, as your physician can tell you how to prevent a potentially dangerous drop in electrolyte levels.

HOW CAN LOW CHLORIDE BE TREATED?

Since nearly every case of hypochloremia is related to an underlying health condition, it must be treated medically. If the condition is related to a kidney disorder or hormone imbalance, a specialist will determine the best course of treatment for you.

DRUGS

If your underlying medical condition can be treated with pharmaceuticals, your doctor will determine which drug is right for you. Sometimes, low chloride may also stem from medications you are already taking. If this is the case, changing your prescription should help bring your level within a normal range. It's important to monitor your blood levels while undergoing therapy.

10. CARBON DIOXIDE

Carbon dioxide, or CO_2, is a gaseous waste product of cellular metabolism. At the same time that oxygen is inhaled, the blood carries carbon dioxide to the lungs, where it is exhaled. Approximately 90 percent of carbon dioxide in the blood is in the form of bicarbonate (HCO_3), while the other 10 percent exists either as dissolved carbon dioxide gas or carbonic acid (H_2CO_3). In other words, a blood CO_2 test, which is often ordered along with either other electrolyte blood tests or blood gas tests, essentially measures the amount of bicarbonate in your blood. Although carbon dioxide is typically thought of as having a negative influence on health, bicarbonate is actually very important, especially for maintaining balanced blood pH—blood that is neither too acidic nor too basic (alkaline). Levels of carbon dioxide that are higher or lower than normal may be indicative of pH imbalance or electrolyte imbalance, conditions that stem from a wide range of dysfunctions. Elevated carbon dioxide in the blood is known as *hypercapnia,* and a low carbon dioxide level is *hypocapnia.* Reference ranges for carbon dioxide lab values, which are measured in millimoles per liter (mmol/L), are provided below.

REFERENCE RANGES FOR CARBON DIOXIDE

Carbon Dioxide (mmol/L)	Category
Greater than 33	High (Hypercapnia)
21 to 33	Normal
Less than 21	Low (Hypocapnia)
Target Range: 23 to 29 mmol/L	

WHAT CAUSES HIGH CARBON DIOXIDE?

High levels of carbon dioxide in the blood, or hypercapnia, can develop for a number of reasons. Some common causes of elevated carbon dioxide include:

- Alcoholism
- Ankylosing spondylitis, a chronic disease causing inflammation of the joints in the spine, in turn hindering the ability of the lungs to fully inhale and exhale
- Dehydration, and conditions that may cause it, such as severe vomiting
- Elevated blood calcium (hypercalcemia)

- Guillain-Barré syndrome, a rare disorder in which the immune system attacks the peripheral nervous system
- High rate of carbohydrate infusion during *total parenteral nutrition* (TPN) *therapy,* which is administered to patients unable to swallow food
- Hormonal disorders, including Cushing's syndrome and hyperaldosteronism
- Hypoventilation, which is very often due to respiratory illnesses like chronic obstructive pulmonary disease (COPD), emphysema, pneumonia, asthma, and any condition preventing full exhalation
- Medications, especially antacids, barbiturates and other Central Nervous System depressants, narcotics, steroids, and thiazide diuretics, as well as supplements like licorice root
- Motor neuron diseases, such as Lou Gehrig's disease
- pH imbalance, which may be caused by conditions such as metabolic alkalosis
- Sleep apnea
- Tobacco chewing

Of the causes listed above, the most common is respiratory illnesses that affect the ability to fully exhale. Metabolic alkalosis is also a fairly common cause. In fact, this condition accounts for nearly 50 percent of patients who are hospitalized with pH-related disorders. Severe metabolic alkalosis—when blood pH is greater than 7.55 on a scale from 0 to 14—is a serious medical issue that can be fatal without treatment. This is also true for hypercapnia, which can result in other serious health issues like high blood pressure, rapid heart rate, irregular heartbeat, and death if left untreated. The most common cause of high carbon dioxide in non-hospitalized individuals, though, is sleep apnea, which hinders the proper utilization of oxygen in the body.

WHAT ARE THE SYMPTOMS OF HIGH CARBON DIOXIDE?

In mild cases of hypercapnia, people may not experience symptoms, especially if the condition develops gradually over time. When symptoms occur, they are usually nonspecific and may include headache, drowsiness, or difficulty thinking clearly. More severe cases of the condition, however, may induce muscle twitching, quickened pulse, flushed skin, dizziness and disorientation, and rapid breathing. Very high carbon dioxide levels can also trigger neuromuscular weakness, convulsions, and diminished consciousness.

HOW CAN HIGH CARBON DIOXIDE BE TREATED?

Like other conditions discussed in this section, treating high carbon dioxide levels depends on the underlying problem. Some general treatment strategies are discussed below.

DRUGS

There are no pharmaceutical drugs that are designed specifically for lowering carbon dioxide levels. Rather, treatment for high CO_2 levels usually involves the use of oxygen therapy or some form of mechanical ventilation, such as continuous positive airway pressure (CPAP) devices—which are used for sleep apnea—bilevel positive airway pressure (BIPAP), and intubation.

SUPPLEMENTS

Although there are no nutritional supplements that specifically target elevated carbon dioxide, there are a few substances that promote healthy metabolism, cellular respiration, and antioxidant status, which are important for managing and avoiding high carbon dioxide levels. The supplements in the table below are useful for preventing conditions that may lead to hypercapnia. Be sure to consult your physician about proper dosing, as well as potential risks and side effects, before using any substance.

SUPPLEMENTS FOR HIGH CARBON DIOXIDE

Supplement	Dosage	Considerations
Astragalus	250 to 500 mg three to four times a day.	This herb may help improve oxygenation of the body. While it generally aids immune function, astragalus should be used with caution if you have an autoimmune disease, such as lupus or multiple sclerosis. Avoid use if you are pregnant or breastfeeding.
B-complex vitamins (containing at least 50 mg B_6)	1 tablet or capsule once a day, or as directed on the product label.	Typically listed as a B-25, B-50, or 5-100 supplement. Quality B-complex vitamins generally contain vitamins B_1 (thiamin), B_2 (riboflavin), B_3 (niacin), B_5 (pantothenic acid), B_6 (pyridoxine), folic acid, and B_{12} (cyanocobalamin). Betaine (TMG) should also be added for increased protection. B vitamins can be found in quality multi-vitamins and mineral supplements as well. Speak to your health-care provider before taking if you have a medical condition, including anemia, diabetes, and liver problems.

Supplement	Dosage	Considerations
Calcium	500 mg one to three times a day.	Take a highly absorbable form of calcium, such as calcium aspartate, citrate, or hydroxyapatite. If using calcium to help sleep problems, take one 500-mg dose at bedtime.
Coenzyme Q_{10} (CoQ_{10})	30 mg three times a day or 50 mg twice a day, depending on dose per capsule.	CoQ_{10} is important for energy production, oxygen use, high blood pressure, and heart health, especially in people with kidney disorders. It can also boost endurance, improve insulin sensitivity, and lower triglycerides and blood glucose levels. This supplement is especially recommended if you are taking statin drugs, red yeast rice, and certain diabetes medications, which may result in a CoQ_{10} deficiency.
Cordyceps	525 mg two to three times a day.	Helps with lung function by increasing oxygen to the cells, and has shown to improve BUN and creatinine levels in in laboratory studies. It is especially recommended for people who have conditions like diabetes and high blood pressure, which increase the risk of kidney failure. Also reported to support liver function. While some medical literature suggests that cordyceps rebalances immune activity, it should be used with caution if you have an autoimmune disease, such as lupus or multiple sclerosis, as it may cause the immune system to become more active.
L-theanine	100 to 200 mg one to three times a day.	This supplement alleviates mental and physical stress, and decreases the level of phenethylamine (PEA) in the brain, a stimulatory neurotransmitter. Some medical sources say no side effects have been observed, but others warn that dizziness, headaches, and upset stomach are possible. Women who are pregnant or breastfeeding should avoid use.
Magnesium	250 to 500 mg twice a day.	Use magnesium aspartate, citrate, taurate, glycinate, or any amino acid chelate. Supports bone building and balances calcium intake. The ratio of calcium-to-magnesium intake should be between 1 to 1 and 2 to 1. This supplement is reported to improve blood vessel function and insulin resistance, in addition to decreasing LDL cholesterol, total cholesterol, and triglycerides. Also essential for phase-I liver detoxification. If you experience loose stools after taking magnesium, cut your dose in half and gradually increase over the course of a few months. Consult your health-care provider for dosage advice.
Melatonin	1 to 3 mg once a day, an hour before bedtime.	This is a natural hormone that improves sleep patterns and acts as an antioxidant in the body. It also resets the cortisol release pattern. Possible but rare side effects include dizziness and headache. People who are taking anticoagulants, immunosuppressants, oral contraceptives, or diabetes medication must use with caution and only under the supervision of a health professional. Doses higher than the recommended amount can be taken only under the advice and guidance of a doctor.

LIFESTYLE CHANGES

There is no single lifestyle factor that directly prevents or helps to reverse high carbon dioxide in the blood. However, if the cause of the problem is sleep apnea, pH imbalance, or electrolyte imbalance, there are some adjustments you can make to your diet and lifestyle to improve your condition and promote healthier CO_2 levels. Following the guidelines below will enable you to breathe properly, achieve restful sleep, and maintain your body's internal stability. If you are overweight, it's also a good idea to start a weight-loss program to shed excess pounds, as there is a direct link between obesity—particularly belly fat—and sleep apnea.

- Eat for acid-alkaline balance. If your high carbon dioxide level is due to pH imbalance, it may be helpful to increase your intake of acid-forming foods. Eating more pork, turkey, veal, fish, beans, and dairy products will support proper pH. However, keep in mind that the best treatment for conditions like metabolic alkalosis is oxygen therapy, which, of course, requires medical supervision.

- Exercise, but not too late in the day. Even small amounts of exercise promote restful sleep and controlled respiration while sleeping. Plan to exercise four or five times a week in thirty-minute sessions. Ideally, your routine should combine aerobic activity and strength training. Try not to work out too late in the evening or right before you plan to go to sleep, since your sleep patterns may be disturbed. For the same reason, you should eat your last meal of the day before 7:00 PM.

- Stick to complex carbohydrates. Sleep apnea is often caused by being overweight or obese. If this is the case for you, restrict the amount of carbohydrates you eat during the day, especially simple carbohydrates—breads, pastas, and high-starch vegetables like potatoes and corn. These types of foods keep insulin levels elevated, in turn blocking the body's ability to burn fat. However, an evening meal that includes complex carbohydrates, such as brown rice, can be a powerful sleep aid. This is because complex carbs stimulate the production of serotonin, a brain chemical that influences the sleep-wake cycle, allowing you to sleep more deeply and restfully.

- Try to follow a low-allergen diet. Food allergies and sensitivities, which often go undetected, can cause sinus congestion, leading to inflamed airways. People who have been diagnosed with sleep apnea should consider trying an elimination diet—starting with grains (not gluten-free) and dairy products—to see if congestion decreases. It may take up to four weeks to notice a difference.

WHAT CAUSES LOW CARBON DIOXIDE?

A CO_2 deficiency in the blood, or *hypocapnia,* is defined as any value less than 21 millimoles per liter (mmol/L). Potential causes of low carbon dioxide levels include:

- Addison's disease
- Asthma
- Cirrhosis
- Diabetic ketoacidosis
- Excessive use of aspirin
- Heart failure
- Heat exhaustion
- High altitude
- Hyperthyroidism
- Hyperventilation
- Liver failure
- Lung cancer
- Medical treatments such as acetazolamide (Diamox) and ventilators (assisted-breathing devices)
- Pain
- pH imbalance, which may be caused by conditions such as metabolic acidosis
- Respiratory illnesses, such as emphysema, chronic bronchitis, and pneumonia
- Smoking

Severe hypocapnia can cause *cerebral hypoxia,* a state of reduced oxygen in the brain. This condition, in turn, can lead to dizziness, visual disturbances, anxiety, and black-outs. Low carbon dioxide levels can also affect your body's balance of electrolytes and nutrients, particularly calcium, potassium, and phosphorus.

WHAT ARE THE SYMPTOMS OF LOW CARBON DIOXIDE?

Low carbon dioxide levels may produce symptoms that range in severity. Dizziness, headaches, diarrhea, muscle cramps, and tingling sensations in the hands and feet are the more mild physical indicators. Severe cases may cause abdominal pain, chest pain, heart palpitations or a fast heartbeat (tachycardia), mental confusion, muscle contractions (tetany), nausea and vomiting, and ultimately, cardiac or respiratory arrest, resulting in death.

HOW CAN LOW CARBON DIOXIDE BE TREATED?

A CO_2-deficient state can be remedied by treating the underlying medical condition, which may entail the use of medications, supplements, lifestyle modifications, or a combination of approaches.

DRUGS

Drug therapy varies according to the underlying medical issue. For example, if metabolic acidosis is the problem, sodium bicarbonate solution may be intravenously administered. If a person has anxiety that induces hyperventilation—a common cause of low carbon dioxide—doctors may prescribe anti-anxiety medications such as lorazepam (Ativan), alprazolam (Xanax), and diazepam (Valium). However, these drugs can cause mental and physical dependency issues and melatonin depletion, which can interfere with sleep patterns.

SUPPLEMENTS

There are supplements you can take to support metabolism, cellular respiration, and antioxidant status, all of which are important when it comes to normalizing carbon dioxide levels. The nutritional supplements in the table below do not directly treat hypocapnia, but may aid in preventing conditions that can cause low CO_2. Be sure to ask your doctor about risks, side effects, and proper dosage amounts before supplementing with any substance.

SUPPLEMENTS FOR LOW CARBON DIOXIDE

Supplement	Dosage	Considerations
B-complex vitamins (containing at least 50 mg B_6)	1 tablet or capsule once a day, or as directed on the product label.	Typically listed as a B-25, B-50, or 5-100 supplement. Quality B-complex vitamins generally contain vitamins B_1 (thamin), B_2 (riboflavin), B_3 (niacin), B_5 (pantothenic acid), B_6 (pyridoxine), folic acid, and B_{12} (cyanocobalamin). Betaine (TMG) should also be added for increased protection. B vitamins can be found in quality multivitamins and mineral supplements as well. Speak to your health-care provider before taking if you have a medical condition, including anemia, diabetes, and liver problems.
Calcium	500 mg one to three times a day.	Take a highly absorbable form of calcium, such as calcium aspartate, citrate, or hydroxyapatite. If using calcium to help sleep problems, take one 500-mg dose at bedtime.
L-theanine	100 to 200 mg one to three times a day.	This supplement alleviates mental and physical stress, and decreases the level of phenethylamine (PEA) in the brain, a stimulatory neurotransmitter. Some medical sources say no side effects have been observed, but others warn that dizziness, headaches, and upset stomach are possible. Women who are pregnant or breastfeeding should avoid use.

Supplement	Dosage	Considerations
Magnesium	250 to 500 mg twice a day.	Use magnesium aspartate, citrate, taurate, glycinate, or any amino acid chelate. Supports bone building and balances calcium intake. The ratio of calcium-to-magnesium intake should be between 1 to 1 and 2 to 1. This supplement is reported to improve blood vessel function and insulin resistance, in addition to decreasing LDL cholesterol, total cholesterol, and triglycerides. Also essential for phase-I liver detoxification. If you experience loose stools after taking magnesium, cut your dose in half and gradually increase over the course of a few months. Consult your health-care provider for dosage advice.
Melatonin	1 to 3 mg once a day, an hour before bedtime.	This is a natural hormone that improves sleep patterns and acts as an antioxidant in the body. It also resets the cortisol release pattern. Possible but rare side effects include dizziness and headache. People who are taking anticoagulants, immunosuppressants, oral contraceptives, or diabetes medication must use with caution and only under the supervision of a health professional. Doses higher than the recommended amount can be taken only under the advice and guidance of a doctor.
Relora	250 mg two to three times a day.	This supplement helps alleviate stress. Since it may cause drowsiness, do not take before driving an automobile or working with or around heavy machinery.

LIFESTYLE CHANGES

Modifying your diet can help you avoid some of the leading causes of low CO_2 in the blood, including metabolic acidosis. First and foremost, you should avoid acid-forming foods in order to counteract acidity in the body and maintain a balanced pH. At the same time, increase your intake of fruits and vegetables such as apples, apricots, berries, cantaloupe, asparagus, broccoli, kale, peppers, and sprouts. Eating a vegetable-rich diet will provide the right nutrients to support the buffering capacity of the blood. In addition, eat nuts like almonds, Brazil nuts, and cashews—as they are low in acidity—along with sea vegetables and lean proteins like chicken. In addition to a balanced diet, restful sleep, stress management, and regular exercise are also important.

11. BLOOD UREA NITROGEN

Typically referred to as BUN, blood urea nitrogen is a form of nitrogen in urea, a waste product produced during protein metabolism. The nitrogen by-products are first made into ammonia, and the liver converts it into urea. Urea is then transported through the bloodstream to the kidneys, which filter the substance from your blood and remove it from the body. Therefore, if BUN levels are higher or lower than normal, the problem usually has to do with the kidneys (see the inset on page 125). Suspected kidney dysfunction is the most common reason for a BUN test, which is usually administered in combination with a creatinine blood test (see page 130). BUN levels might also be measured to help diagnose medical conditions such as heart or liver failure, urinary tract obstruction, and gastrointestinal bleeding.

Although optimal BUN levels can vary according to a person's age and gender, the generally accepted "normal" range is 6 to 20 milligrams per deciliter (mg/dL). Values less than 6 mg/dL are considered low, and values over 20 mg/dL are considered high. There is no optimal value for this lab.

WHAT CAUSES HIGH BUN LEVELS?

Elevated BUN, which is known as *azotemia,* is usually a sign of impaired kidney function, which can occur for any number of reasons, from diabetes complications to chronic use of medications such as acetaminophen, aspirin, and arthritis drugs. High BUN levels may also result from conditions that adversely affect the kidneys. Congestive heart failure, for instance, inhibits blood flow to the kidneys, and dehydration greatly reduces urination. Listed below are some additional factors that can cause BUN levels to increase:

- Bile duct dysfunction
- Congestive heart failure
- Dehydration
- Diet high in protein
- Gastrointestinal bleeding
- Kidney disease or kidney failure
- Prostate enlargement
- Rheumatoid arthritis or gout
- Total parenteral nutrition (TPN) therapy and other forms of hyperalimentation—the intravenous administration of large quantities of nutrients
- Urinary tract obstruction

Age and gender also influence BUN levels, which tend to be higher in men and elderly people. In addition, a number of medications can raise BUN, such as:

- Aminoglycoside antibiotics such as gentamicin (Garamycin), kanamycin (Kantrex), and tobramycin (Nebcin)
- Anti-fungal and -bacterial medications, such as amphotericin B (Fungizone) and nafcillin
- Chemotherapy agents that are nephrotoxic (toxic to the kidneys), like carboplatin (Paraplatin) and cisplatin (Platinol)
- Corticosteroids
- Diuretics, including furosemide (Lasix), chlorothiazide (Diuril) hydrochlorothiazide (HydroDIURIL), triamterene with hydrochlorothiazide (Dyazide)
- Immunosuppressants such as azathioprine (Imuran) and cyclosporin (Sandimmune)
- Tetracycline antibiotics

Since elevated BUN is strongly correlated with health issues like kidney disease, it's important to have your levels measured as part of your routine physical. A creatinine test (see page 130), as well as a BUN/creatinine ratio test (see page 137), should also be done to get a more complete picture of kidney health.

WHAT ARE THE SYMPTOMS OF HIGH BUN LEVELS?

There are usually no outward signs or symptoms of elevated BUN until kidney failure is fairly advanced, which is why it's so important to monitor your levels. In general, symptoms of kidney dysfunction are generalized and difficult to detect, and include fatigue, lack of appetite, poor concentration, and trouble sleeping. People may experience mid-back pain (the approximate location of the kidneys) and develop edema (fluid retention), especially in the eyes and face, abdomen, thighs, and ankles. Urinary production can also begin to diminish. When elevated BUN is caused by another underlying condition, such as dehydration, symptoms may differ. People with high levels often experience itchy skin, body odor, and breath that has a urine-like odor.

HOW CAN HIGH BUN LEVELS BE TREATED?

If your BUN level is currently elevated or trends high, your doctor will likely recommend that you modify your lifestyle by incorporating a few key habits. Supplements can also be taken to balance BUN levels and reinforce the benefits of a healthy lifestyle.

BUN, Creatinine, and Your Kidneys

Chronic kidney disease, or CKD, is a growing public health concern in the United States, affecting an estimated 26 million adults nationwide. Of primary concern is the rising rate of kidney failure, a debilitating condition that is difficult to manage and eventually leads to a dialysis—a procedure that dramatically affects a person's ability to live a normal life.

The rapid increase in kidney failure is largely due to the high rates of related conditions like high blood pressure, obesity, and especially diabetes. Dialysis centers have sprung up all over the country to meet the needs of kidney patients, whose number is continually escalating—and yet the disease remains mostly overlooked. Furthermore, most people are unaware of the significance of blood tests—especially ones measuring BUN, creatinine (see page 130), and glomerular filtration rate, or GFR (see page 140)—in identifying and diagnosing kidney problems. Many more do not take the steps necessary to correct detected abnormalities because the importance of these labs is not properly explained. All of this adds up to a serious problem for the American population.

As mentioned above, dialysis is the most common treatment for kidney failure. Dialysis involves getting hooked up to a machine for hours as it filters wastes and excess water out of your blood. Although this process is life saving, the machines do not have the same filtering capacity as your kidneys. Even with this treatment, it's hard to achieve and maintain normal levels of certain substances like potassium and phosphorus, which tend to run high after kidney failure has occurred. Therefore, in addition to undergoing dialysis and managing the conditions that caused kidney failure in the first place, patients must also adjust their diet by carefully controlling their intake of potassium, sodium, and even fluids. Dialysis can also be done at home without a machine, but this method has its own set of potential side effects and challenges. In other words, dialysis—regardless of the method used—is not easy, and it is not a cure.

The bottom line is this: If you have a medical condition like diabetes or high blood pressure, do everything in your power to manage the disease. If you are at risk for these conditions, do everything you can to make sure they do not develop by following the dietary and lifestyle recommendations provided in this book. Be sure to have your BUN, creatinine, and GFR levels tested, and more importantly, pay attention to your blood test results. If you have diabetes, high blood pressure, or a related condition, you should make sure that your creatinine level does not begin to trend high, as this can be a sign of impaired kidney function. Very often, improving disease management, especially of diabetes, will allow levels to return to normal. Still, always ask your doctor about any abnormal value—even if they are just trending high or low. Kidney disease and kidney failure are not always possible to reverse, but they *can* be helped.

SUPPLEMENTS

The supplements below have shown to be effective for keeping BUN levels in balance and supporting kidney function. Speak to your medical provider about proper dosing before taking supplements.

SUPPLEMENTS FOR HIGH BUN LEVELS		
Supplement	**Dosage**	**Considerations**
Cordyceps	525 mg two to three times a day.	Helps with lung function by increasing oxygen to the cells, and has shown to improve BUN and creatinine levels in laboratory studies. It is especially recommended for people who have conditions like diabetes and high blood pressure, which increase the risk of kidney failure. Also reported to support liver function. While some medical literature suggests that cordyceps rebalances immune activity, it should be used with caution if you have an autoimmune disease, such as lupus or multiple sclerosis, as it may cause the immune system to become more active.
Goldenrod	15 to 20 drops two to three times a day.	Helps the kidneys remove wastes and excess fluid. People who have high blood pressure or fluid retention (edema) related to heart or kidney disease should not use goldenrod. The supplement should not be taken with diuretics, as this may cause the loss of too much fluid. Women who are pregnant or breastfeeding should avoid using.
Probiotics	5 to 10 billion CFUs two to three times a day.	Probiotics help normalize beneficial flora in the gastrointestinal tract, and are reported to decrease triglyceride and cholesterol levels. They are also reported to improve BUN levels and quality of life in people with kidney disease. It's best to use heat-stable products that do not require refrigeration. If using an antibiotic, wait three hours before taking probiotics. If diarrhea occurs, decrease your dosage. If this side effect persists for longer than 48 hours, stop taking the supplement and contact your doctor. A good-quality product is Renadyl, formerly marketed under the name Kibow Biotics. This specialized supplement processes and removes nitrogen wastes from the body.

LIFESTYLE CHANGES

First, you may be advised to temporarily decrease your protein intake, since the excessive breakdown of proteins (catabolism) can raise levels. When your level reaches a normal range, you can begin to incorporate more proteins into your diet. You can also promote normal BUN levels by maintaining adequate fluid intake, drinking approximately 2 to 3 liters of filtered water per day if your BUN level is high. In addition, always rehydrate during and after exercise.

WHAT CAUSES LOW BUN LEVELS?

Although women and children naturally have lower BUN levels than men, very low BUN may be indicative of a medical condition. Potential causes of abnormally low levels include:

- Advanced metabolic acidosis
- Celiac disease
- Insufficient protein in the diet
- Liver disease (severe)
- Malnutrition
- Overhydration

It's important to note that, unlike kidney disease, BUN is not the primary lab used to diagnose liver disease or malnutrition. However, BUN is an important factor when assessing these conditions.

WHAT ARE THE SYMPTOMS OF LOW BUN LEVELS?

The symptoms typically associated with low BUN levels arise from the conditions causing the low level in the first place. Liver disease, for example, commonly causes confusion, while edema may result from a lack of protein in the diet. In general, people who have low BUN levels are very weak and, therefore, may experience labored breathing.

HOW CAN LOW BUN LEVELS BE TREATED?

As with elevated levels, low levels can be effectively treated with supplements and lifestyle adjustments.

SUPPLEMENTS

The supplements in the table below may be beneficial for improving protein intake and, therefore, normalizing low BUN levels caused by poor nutrition. Keep in mind that all the supplements listed may not be equally effective or suited to your needs. Consult your doctor or health practitioner before using any product.

SUPPLEMENTS FOR LOW BUN LEVELS

Supplement	Dosage	Considerations
Creatine	5 g twice a day for one week, continuing with 5 g a day.	Creatine is typically used to enhance athletic performance and increase muscle mass, which can raise BUN and creatinine levels. It may also be useful for treating congestive heart failure, hyperlipidemia, and neuromuscular disease. Supplements are safe when taken in recommended dosages, but may cause stomach cramps, muscle cramps, or muscle breakdown, which can lead to muscle tears and discomfort. Weight gain, increased body mass, heat intolerance, fever, dehydration, and electrolyte imbalances may also occur. Consult your medical provider before using.
Probiotics	5 to 10 billion CFUs two to three times a day.	Probiotics help normalize beneficial flora in the gastrointestinal tract, and are reported to decrease triglyceride and cholesterol levels. They are also reported to improve BUN levels and quality of life in people with kidney disease. It's best to use heat-stable products that do not require refrigeration. If using an antibiotic, wait three hours before taking probiotics. If diarrhea occurs, decrease your dosage. If this side effect persists for longer than 48 hours, stop taking the supplement and contact your doctor. A good-quality product is Renadyl, formerly marketed under the name Kibow Biotics. This specialized supplement processes and removes nitrogen wastes from the body.
Whey protein	20 to 30 g (1 to 2 scoops added to a beverage) one to two times a day.	Studies have shown that whey protein is a form of protein that is both easily digested and superior to other proteins for muscle building. It has also been reported to improve immunity and work as an antioxidant in the body. However, high doses can cause increased bowel movements, nausea, thirst, bloating, cramps, reduced appetite, fatigue, and headaches. Avoid use if you are pregnant or breastfeeding.

LIFESTYLE CHANGES

Protein is the single most important dietary factor when it comes to raising and lowering BUN levels. If your BUN level is low or trends low, you may be advised to increase your consumption of healthy proteins such as beans, fish, nuts, seeds, as well as bison, chicken, and turkey. However, patients with liver failure must instead be treated with specialized protein products, as they cannot process and utilize branched-chain amino acid chains found in regular dietary protein. Excessive intake of protein in any form is not a long-term solution and should not be done for longer than is recommended by a doctor.

Consider This

BUN levels typically indicate how well or poorly your kidneys are working. Your kidneys are essential to proper bodily functioning; they filter your blood for excess water and wastes, producing urine in the process. Unfortunately, kidney disease is a growing problem worldwide; 20 million Americans suffer from one form or another, and many more are at risk due to diabetes, high blood pressure, heart disease, or a family history of kidney disease. Get your BUN levels tested today!

12. CREATININE

Creatinine is a chemical waste product of muscle metabolism. It is generated by *creatine,* a compound manufactured by the liver that serves as a source of energy for the muscles. Approximately 95 percent of the body's total creatine is located in skeletal muscle. As a natural part of metabolism, some creatine is spontaneously converted into creatinine, which is transported through the bloodstream to the kidneys and removed from the body in urine. Therefore, a blood creatinine test serves as a reliable measure of kidney function, especially when evaluated alongside the results of a BUN test.

The amounts of creatine and creatinine in the blood are determined by muscle mass, so men usually have higher levels than women. Creatine is now available as a dietary supplement that is often used to enhance athletic performance. Tell your doctor if you take these supplements, since they usually raise your creatinine levels. The normal ranges for creatinine in adult men and women, as well as children under twelve years of age, are provided in the table.

REFERENCE RANGES FOR CREATININE

Category	Normal Range (mg/dL)
Men	0.6 to 1.2
Women	0.5 to 1.1
Children (twelve years of age or younger)	0.3 to 0.7

Sometimes, creatinine levels in urine are measured alongside blood creatinine levels in order to calculate a value called *creatinine clearance.* This number reflects how well your kidneys are filtering the substance out of your system. For men forty years old or younger, a normal creatinine clearance reading is 90 to 140 milliliters per minute (mL/min), or 1.78 to 2.32 milliliters per second (mL/sec). Normal creatinine clearance values for women forty years old or younger are 87 to 107 mL/min, or 1.45 to 1.78 mL/sec. Normal readings in older adults are lower, as creatinine clearance values decline with age.

WHAT CAUSES HIGH CREATININE?

Most cases of high creatinine levels are caused by kidney problems, especially chronic kidney disease and kidney failure, which are often caused by long-term diabetes, high blood pressure, or obesity. The risk of kidney failure increases when diabetes and high blood pressure are poorly managed. Kidney dysfunction may occur as a result of damaged or swollen blood vessels (glomerulonephritis); bacterial infections, including malaria and streptococcus; or reduced blood flow caused by congestive heart failure, dehydration, or complications of diabetes. Some other causes of elevated blood creatinine include:

- Autoimmune diseases like IgA nephropathy, which affects the kidneys
- Congestive heart failure
- Dehydration
- Diabetes
- Excessive protein intake
- Heavy metal toxicity
- High blood pressure
- Hyperthyroidism
- Hypothyroidism
- Kidney disease or kidney failure
- Muscle disorders, including dermatomyositis, muscular dystrophy, myasthenia gravis, and polymyositis

The following medications may also increase creatinine levels:

- ACE inhibitors and angiotensin receptor blockers (ARBs), especially when used at the same time
- Aminoglycoside antibiotics, including gentamicin and tobramycin
- Certain cephalosporin antibiotics, such as cefoxitin (Mefoxin)
- Cimetidine (Tagamet), an antacid
- Fibrates like femfibrozil (Lopid), which are used to lower cholesterol
- Heavy metal chemotherapy drugs like cisplatinum (Cisplatin)
- Methyldopa (Aldomet), which is prescribed for high blood pressure
- NSAIDs, a group that includes acetaminophen, aspirin, ibuprofen, and naproxyn
- Sulfamethoxezole/trimethoprin (Bactrim), an antibacterial medication
- Vancomycin (Vancocin), a glycopeptide antibiotic
- Vitamin C supplements

Blood creatinine levels may also be temporarily elevated due to burns, muscle injuries, and strenuous exercise.

WHAT ARE THE SYMPTOMS OF HIGH CREATININE?

Elevated creatinine does not cause symptoms on its own. However, if you suffer from one of the conditions listed on page 131, you may experience symptoms associated with that specific disorder. As it becomes more advanced, kidney dysfunction can cause confusion, fatigue, and shortness of breath, along with other nonspecific symptoms. Always consult your physician if you experience any symptom that does not go away after a two or three days.

HOW CAN HIGH CREATININE BE TREATED?

Most doctors express concern when they see high creatinine levels, which may be a sign that kidney failure is imminent or already present. Moreover, high levels that are sustained for an extended period of time can eventually lead to kidney damage. Still, you shouldn't panic right away if your level is high—it may be due to a less severe condition such as excessive protein intake, dehydration, or side effects of medication. Your doctor will assess each of these areas and, depending on the problem, advise you to step up your fluid intake, eliminate any unnecessary medications that may raise creatinine, or adjust your diet. The drugs, supplements, and lifestyle modifications discussed below may help balance your level.

DRUGS

High creatinine levels that are caused by medical issues can be normalized by treating the underlying cause. Therefore, treatments for lowering creatinine vary widely. When a high creatinine level is the result of high blood pressure, for example, antihypertensive medications— including ACE inhibitors and angiotensin receptor blockers (ARBs)—may be prescribed. There is strong evidence that these drugs help protect the kidneys, which is why they are also prescribed to diabetes patients, even if their blood pressure is not very high. Additionally, new evidence suggests that atorvastatin (Lipitor), a statin drug normally taken to lower cholesterol, improves kidney blood flow and reduces uric acid. As a result, Lipitor is now being prescribed as an off-label treatment for maintaining kidney health and managing creatinine levels.

SUPPLEMENTS

The following nutritional supplements support kidney health and, therefore, balanced creatinine levels. Ask your doctor about proper dosing before taking any of these substances.

SUPPLEMENTS FOR HIGH CREATININE		
Supplements	**Dosage**	**Considerations**
Cordyceps	525 mg two to three times a day.	Helps with lung function by increasing oxygen to the cells, and has shown to improve BUN and creatinine levels in laboratory studies. It is especially recommended for people who have conditions like diabetes and high blood pressure, which increase the risk of kidney failure. Also reported to support liver function. While some medical literature suggests that cordyceps rebalances immune activity, it should be used with caution if you have an autoimmune disease, such as lupus or multiple sclerosis, as it may cause the immune system to become more active.
Glutamine (L-glutamine)	2,000 mg three times a day.	Studies have shown that glutamine helps protect the kidneys against oxidative stress damage, as well as improve creatinine levels. Avoid if you suffer from severe liver disease, seizures, monosodium glutamate sensitivity, or mania. Do not take if you are pregnant or breastfeeding.
Goldenrod	15 to 20 drops two to three times a day.	Helps the kidneys remove wastes and excess fluid. People who have high blood pressure or fluid retention (edema) related to heart or kidney disease should not use goldenrod. The supplement should not be taken with diuretics, as this may cause the loss of too much fluid. Women who are pregnant or breastfeeding should avoid using.
N-acetyl cysteine (NAC)	500 to 750 mg twice a day.	NAC is an antioxidant that is reported to help protect against blood vessel damage and clots due to insulin resistance, diabetes, and other blood sugar regulation problems. It also helps improve the body's capacity to decrease the harmful effects of toxins. NAC has been reported to improve kidney function in laboratory and human studies, and support glutathione production in the kidneys. It is generally well tolerated when taken in recommended dosages.

LIFESTYLE CHANGES

Diet is one of the primary contributing factors to raised creatinine levels. People whose diets are abundant in protein-rich foods typically lean towards the higher end of the normal creatinine range; in fact, levels can increase by as much as 10 to 30 percent due to excessive protein intake. Many times, people who are trying to build muscle increase their protein intake dramatically, which, along with intense workouts, can contribute to elevated creatinine levels because the body cannot adequately get rid of protein byproducts. If protein consumption is the cause of your high level, cut back on animal proteins, protein powders, dairy products, and other high-protein foods. Do not severely restrict your intake, however, as it's just as unhealthy to be protein deficient. Unless kidney failure is already present, you should also eat more garlic, fruits, vegetables, and other fiber-rich foods, which can help prevent the most common causes of renal failure. Fruits and vegetables are high in potassium, which aids in managing blood pressure; fiber improves diabetes management and intestinal health, which is often involved in autoimmunity; and garlic helps rid the body of heavy metals and reduce the risk of toxicity.

When high creatinine levels are caused by dehydration, the long-term solution is to maintain adequate hydration. Drinking about two to three liters of water per day is essential for keeping your body well-hydrated and maintaining proper kidney function. If you regularly exercise or perform manual labor, be sure to drink more than the required amount to compensate for the water lost through perspiration. In addition, swap your morning coffee for a cup of green tea, and limit the amount of alcohol you drink, though eliminating alcoholic beverages altogether is ideal. After implementing the needed lifestyle changes, wait a few weeks and then have your level retested.

WHAT CAUSES LOW CREATININE LEVELS?

Low creatinine levels are usually not a cause for concern. The amount of creatinine in the blood depends partly on the amount of muscle tissue, so women tend to have lower levels than men. Low and slightly low levels are very common in pregnant women, as well as people—including many vegetarians—who follow a diet low in protein. Levels are also lower among the elderly, since muscle mass decreases as part of the natural aging process. While the vast majority of cases are caused by one of these three reasons, there are some medical conditions that may result in reduced levels, including:

- Advanced liver disease
- Cancer
- Drastic weight loss
- Malnutrition
- Muscular disorders, such as muscular dystrophy and myasthenia gravis
- Overhydration

An abnormal creatinine blood test is usually not the first indication of these conditions, but in some cases, it may help gauge their severity.

WHAT ARE THE SYMPTOMS OF LOW CREATININE?

There are no specific symptoms caused by low blood creatinine. Very low levels that are induced by other conditions, however, may result in symptoms like increased thirst and kidney pain, which are associated with a number of disorders. Elderly people whose muscle mass has deteriorated may fall more easily, resulting in potentially life-threatening bone fractures.

HOW CAN LOW CREATININE BE TREATED?

If your low level is due to severe weight loss or malnutrition, it is imperative that you increase your nutritional intake. This should be medically supervised. For low levels stemming from other conditions, you should make changes to your overall lifestyle and diet, preferably with the help of a nutrition specialist.

SUPPLEMENTS

Nutritional supplements may help raise creatinine levels, but this is a decision that is best made with your doctor. Some supplements that may be effective for normalizing levels are presented in the table below. Speak to a healthcare professional before deciding to use any of these supplements, especially creatine. Supplements can cause side effects and interact with certain medications, so it's important to have all the information available to you before taking any substance.

SUPPLEMENTS FOR LOW CREATININE

Supplements	Dosage	Considerations
Creatine	5 g twice a day for one week, continuing with 5 g a day.	Creatine is typically used to enhance athletic performance and increase muscle mass, which can raise BUN and creatinine levels. It may also be useful for treating congestive heart failure, hyperlipidemia, and neuromuscular disease. Supplements are safe when taken in recommended dosages, but may cause stomach cramps, muscle cramps, or muscle breakdown, which can lead to muscle tears and discomfort. Weight gain, increased body mass, heat intolerance, fever, dehydration, and electrolyte imbalances may also occur. Consult your medical provider before using.

Supplements	Dosage	Considerations
Whey protein	20 to 30 g (1 to 2 scoops added to a beverage) one to two times a day.	Studies have shown that whey protein is a form of protein that is both easily digested and superior to other proteins for muscle building. It has also been reported to improve immunity and work as an antioxidant in the body. However, high doses can cause increased bowel movements, nausea, thirst, bloating, cramps, reduced appetite, fatigue, and headaches. Avoid use if you are pregnant or breastfeeding.

LIFESTYLE CHANGES

If muscle mass is low, animal proteins should be consumed for some time because they are more bioavailable than other proteins. Eggs, whey protein, and fish can be incorporated into your diet as well. These foods, particularly eggs, are especially beneficial if you are also low in iron. Keep track of how much protein you consume on a daily basis to ensure you are taking in the amount needed to raise your creatinine level.

Did You Know?

You need to eat protein because it contains amino acids that help your bodies produce new cells and synthesize proteins that allow you to function properly. Animal-based proteins—meat, poultry, fish, dairy, and eggs—are called complete or high-quality proteins because they contain all of the essential amino acids that the body can't make for itself. If you have low BUN or creatinine levels, it may help to increase your intake of animal-based proteins.

13. BUN/CREATININE RATIO

The blood urea nitrogen (BUN) and creatinine blood tests are used to find the ratio of BUN to creatinine. This ratio, which provides a more accurate picture of kidney health, is usually not included on blood test results unless the BUN and/or creatinine values are abnormal. A normal BUN/creatinine ratio is between 10 to 1 and 20 to 1, with the target range between 12 to 1 and 16 to 1. High and low ratios can be indicative of kidney dysfunction and other medical conditions, so if your test results are abnormal, your doctor will order more comprehensive testing to determine the source of the problem.

WHAT ARE THE CAUSES OF HIGH AND LOW BUN/CREATININE RATIOS?

The most common cause of a high BUN/creatinine ratio is dehydration, as BUN rises more than creatinine when you are not adequately hydrated. Additional causes of a high ratio include:

- Congestive heart failure
- Dehydration
- Gastrointestinal bleeding
- Kidney disease or kidney stones
- Urinary tract obstruction

A low BUN/creatinine ratio can be caused by:

- Liver diseases, such as cirrhosis
- Low-protein diet
- Malnutrition
- Muscle disorders or muscle injury
- Pituitary dysfunction or pituitary hormone imbalance
- Pregnancy

Because both BUN and creatinine levels increase when the kidneys begin to fail, this ratio is not an important factor in detecting and diagnosing kidney failure.

WHAT ARE THE SYMPTOMS OF HIGH AND LOW BUN/CREATININE RATIOS?

Symptoms of an abnormal BUN/creatinine ratio, whether high or low, are always related to the underlying condition causing it. Physical indicators may include confusion, edema, fatigue, irregular heartbeat, and shortness of breath.

HOW CAN HIGH AND LOW BUN/CREATININE RATIOS BE TREATED?

If your BUN/creatinine ratio is abnormal, your physician will examine your individual counts of BUN and creatinine to get a better understanding of the abnormality. These individual readings determine how the imbalance should be treated. Once the problem has been identified, consult the appropriate sections of the BUN and creatinine chapters (see pages 123 and 130) to find out how it may be remedied with medical treatments, lifestyle changes, or both.

SUPPLEMENTS

There are several nutritional supplements you can take to help stabilize your ratio depending on the cause of the imbalance. The supplements in the table below have a variety of functions, such as supporting blood pressure, improving gastrointestinal function, promoting kidney health, and detoxifying the body. Before taking a supplement, check with your doctor to make sure it is appropriate for your needs. Your doctor may also be able to provide you with important information about the product, as well as recommend a dose that is safe and effective for your particular problem.

SUPPLEMENTS FOR ABNORMAL BUN/CREATININE RATIOS

Supplement	Dosage	Considerations
Coenzyme Q_{10} (CoQ_{10})	30 mg three times a day or 50 mg twice a day, depending on dose per capsule.	CoQ_{10} is important for energy production, oxygen use, high blood pressure, and heart health, especially in people with kidney disorders. It can also boost endurance, improve insulin sensitivity, and lower triglycerides and blood glucose levels. This supplement is especially recommended if you are taking statin drugs, red yeast rice, and certain diabetes medications, which may result in a CoQ_{10} deficiency.
Cordyceps	525 mg two to three times a day.	Helps with lung function by increasing oxygen to the cells, and has shown to improve BUN and creatinine levels in laboratory studies. It is especially recommended for people who have conditions like diabetes and high blood pressure, which increase the risk of kidney failure. Also reported to support liver function. While some medical literature suggests that cordyceps rebalances immune activity, it should be used with caution if you have an autoimmune disease, such as lupus or multiple sclerosis, as it may cause the immune system to become more active.

Supplement	Dosage	Considerations
Goldenrod	15 to 20 drops two to three times a day.	Helps the kidneys remove wastes and excess fluid. People who have high blood pressure or fluid retention (edema) related to heart or kidney disease should not use goldenrod. The supplement should not be taken with diuretics, as this may cause the loss of too much fluid. Women who are pregnant or breastfeeding should avoid using.
Green tea or green tea extract	3 to 6 cups (tea) or 250 mg one to two times a day (extract).	Helps improve antioxidant and lipid levels. When taken with other supplements and diet/lifestyle changes, green tea extract is reported to assist in weight loss. It can also help regulate glucose levels, lower triglycerides, and prevent kidney stones, which may result from high calcium. If taking an extract, use a form standardized to 90-percent polyphenols (specifically EGCG). Tell your doctor if you are currently taking aspirin or anticoagulant drugs like warfarin (Coumadin), as green tea extract may increase the risk of bleeding.
L-arginine (HCl sustained release)	1,000 mg (two 500-mg capsules) three times a day.	L-arginine helps regulate blood pressure and may be effective for lowering mildly elevated levels. The substance has also been found to boost endurance and improve exercise ability in people with heart failure. There is some evidence that it may indirectly help metabolism problems resulting from kidney failure. People with low blood pressure or heart problems should avoid using this supplement. Talk to your doctor before taking if you have asthma.
Nettle	If using a liquid extract, take 15 to 30 drops two to three times a day. If using the capsule form, take 50 to 100 mg two to three times a day.	Used to improve kidney function and relieve allergy symptoms such as runny nose. They are also known to be effective in preventing urinary problems, such as urinary tract infections. May cause sweating and upset stomach. Consult your physician before taking if you have diabetes, kidney or liver disease, or urinary or prostate problems. Women who are pregnant or breastfeeding should not use before speaking to their doctor.
Selenium	200 mcg once a day.	Has been reported to help protect the kidneys. Selenium also helps protect the body against mercury toxicity, which can damage the liver and kidneys. Never take more than the recommended dose. Symptoms of selenium toxicity include vomiting, stomach pain, hair loss, brittle nails, and fatigue.

14. GLOMERULAR FILTRATION RATE (GFR)

BUN and creatinine levels by themselves are sometimes insufficient measures of kidney health, especially if kidney disease is suspected or has already developed. The best way to measure kidney function is by calculating the *glomerular filtration rate*, or GFR, which reflects the amount of blood that is filtered per minute and generally correlates with urinary output. *Glomeruli* are tiny filters inside your kidneys that remove waste products from the blood while preventing the loss of important blood components, such as proteins and blood cells. When GFR falls below a certain level, it indicates kidney dysfunction. Doctors calculate GFRs of people who have chronic kidney disease (CKD), diabetes, heart disease, high blood pressure, or a family history of CKD. Frequent urinary tract infections and urinary blockages are also situations that may prompt a doctor to find a person's GFR.

GFR is not measured with a separate blood test; it is calculated by plugging a person's blood creatinine value, age, sex, height, and weight into an equation. Race is also taken into consideration, since the genetics of African Americans affect how their kidneys process and filter wastes. GFR values are measured in milliliters per minute (mL/min) and categorized according to the stage of kidney damage reflected. Therefore, there is no target or optimal range. Please note that "evidence of kidney damage" refers to elevated BUN and creatinine levels, as well as protein in the urine.

REFERENCE RANGES FOR GLOMERULAR FILTRATION RATE (GFR)

GFR (mL/min)	Severity of Kidney Damage
90 to 120 with no evidence of kidney damage	Normal
Greater than 90 with evidence of kidney damage	Stage 1 (Beginning of kidney damage)
60 to 89	Stage 2 (Mild kidney damage)
30 to 59	Stage 3 (Moderate kidney damage)
15 to 29	Stage 4 (Severe kidney damage)
Less than 15	Stage 5 (Kidney failure)

Young adults usually have a GFR of 120 to 130 mL/min, and this number gradually declines—usually by 0.5 to 1.0 mL/min—as a normal part of the aging process. Some conditions can cause temporary decreases in GFR, including infections, cysts, and urinary tract obstructions, which can occur with kidney stones. When GFR is low, physicians look for additional signs of kidney damage, such as protein in the urine, to determine if kidney failure is, in fact, occurring. Chronically low GFR—a low reading that lasts for three months or more—is a sign of chronic kidney disease with an increased chance of cardiovascular disease and other medical complications. GFR under 15 mL/min requires dialysis, an artificial process of removing wastes from the blood. Although GFR may slightly increase during pregnancy, high values are rare; GFR tests are almost always intended for spotting and reversing low rates. Keeping track of changes in GFR over time is crucial for detecting chronic kidney disease and related conditions, as well as for making decisions about treatment.

WHAT CAUSES LOW GFR?

The main reason for chronically low GFR is chronic kidney disease, or CKD. In the United States, the most common cause of CKD is diabetes, followed closely by high blood pressure. More specifically, the hallmarks of insulin resistance—high blood sugar, high insulin, and high triglycerides, for example—are associated with low GFR. This actually makes insulin resistance the most important factor, as it leads to both diabetes and high blood pressure. Polycystic kidney disease—a condition characterized by cysts in the kidneys that permanently damage the glomeruli—can also cause CKD and lead to chronic kidney failure. There is also an increasingly high rate of kidney damage and kidney failure due to the overuse of over-the-counter painkillers like aspirin, acetaminophen, ibuprofen, and naproxen. Additional causes of low GFR include:

- Diet low in animal proteins, such as vegetarian and vegan diets
- Heavy metal toxicity
- Kidney stones
- Medications
- Tumors
- Urinary tract infection or urinary blockage

Further testing may be needed to determine the cause of your low rate if none of the factors above apply to you.

WHAT ARE THE SYMPTOMS OF LOW GFR?

While GFR alone does not produce physical symptoms, the underlying cause often does. Warning signs of chronic kidney disease include fatigue, edema (water retention), poor appetite, dry itchy skin, muscle cramps, poor concentration, and an increased need to urinate. Although not common, some people also experience pain near the kidneys. As the disease progresses, anemia, nausea, and numbness of the hands and feet can also occur. If low GFR is a concern for you, familiarize yourself with the symptoms of CKD and other associated conditions. Consult your doctor if you have experienced any of the possible symptoms.

HOW CAN LOW GFR BE TREATED?

When low GFRs are due to chronic kidney disease, treatment depends on the condition's level of severity. Although it is not a cure, dialysis is a life-saving procedure for people with kidney failure. In cases of acute (sudden) kidney failure, dialysis can be used until proper kidney function is restored. Chronic cases call for long-term dialysis or temporary use of the therapy until a kidney transplant can be performed, if such a measure is necessary.

For long-term disease management, patients with chronic kidney disease must follow a renal diet. This entails decreasing intake of foods containing phosphorus and potassium, which build up in the body when the kidneys are unable to remove them. Phosphorus buildup can result in calcium loss in the bones, and high potassium may disrupt normal heartbeat and cause cardiac arrest. Protein intake should also be considered when implementing a renal diet. Some doctors may recommend decreasing protein intake in cases of early-stage kidney failure, as some past studies have shown that reducing protein consumption can slow the progression of the disease. Protein should not be cut out of the diet entirely, since it is needed for certain physiological functions. CKD patients who are on dialysis are generally put back on higher-protein diets to maintain muscle mass and overall health. If you have kidney disease, your doctor will determine if a renal diet is necessary and then, depending on the stage of your disease, decide on an appropriate nutritional regimen.

People who do not have chronic kidney disease may choose to take supplements or modify their lifestyle to promote optimal GFR. This should be done with the assistance of a healthcare professional.

SUPPLEMENTS

You can protect your kidneys and enhance their function by taking one or more of the supplements below. Choose reputable products and always ask your doctor about potential side effects and proper dosage amounts before supplementing with any substance.

SUPPLEMENTS FOR LOW GFR		
Supplement	**Dosage**	**Considerations**
Alpha-lipoic acid	600 mg one to two times a day.	Reported to help with blood sugar uptake and use in the body. Also helps detoxify the body, protect the kidneys, and improve cholesterol levels. Make sure that the raw material provider for the product is from Europe to guarantee effectiveness.
Bonito fish peptides	500 mg three times a day.	This supplement has been found to help reduce blood pressure that is elevated. Fish peptides are reported to be safe when taken in the recommended dosage. Take with food to avoid minor stomach irritation.
Cordyceps	525 mg two to three times a day.	Helps with lung function by increasing oxygen to the cells, and has shown to improve BUN and creatinine levels in laboratory studies. It is especially recommended for people who have conditions like diabetes and high blood pressure, which increase the risk of kidney failure. Also reported to support liver function. While some medical literature suggests that cordyceps rebalances immune activity, it should be used with caution if you have an autoimmune disease, such as lupus or multiple sclerosis, as it may cause the immune system to become more active.
GTF (Glucose Tolerance Factor) chromium	200 to 400 mcg once a day.	Chromium is important for blood sugar and insulin regulation. Additionally, people who have a diet high in refined carbohydrates like sugar may also be low in chromium. Use under a doctor's supervision if you are diabetic, as it may affect medication dosage. Do not use if you have kidney or liver problems, chromate or leather contact allergy, or a behavioral psychiatric condition such as schizophrenia or depression.
Goldenrod	15 to 20 drops two to three times a day.	Helps the kidneys remove wastes and excess fluid. People who have high blood pressure or fluid retention (edema) related to heart or kidney disease should not use goldenrod. The supplement should not be taken with diuretics, as this may cause the loss of too much fluid. Women who are pregnant or breastfeeding should avoid using.

Supplement	Dosage	Considerations
Green tea or green tea extract	3 to 6 cups (tea) or 250 mg one to two times a day (extract).	Helps improve antioxidant and lipid levels. When taken with other supplements and diet/lifestyle changes, green tea extract is reported to assist in weight loss. It can also help regulate glucose levels, lower triglycerides, and prevent kidney stones. If taking an extract, use a form standardized to 90-percent polyphenols (specifically EGCG). Tell your doctor if you are currently taking aspirin or anticoagulant drugs like warfarin (Coumadin), as green tea extract may increase the risk of bleeding.
Magnesium	250 to 500 mg twice a day.	Use magnesium aspartate, citrate, taurate, glycinate, or any amino acid chelate. Supports bone building and balances calcium intake. The ratio of calcium-to-magnesium intake should be between 1 to 1 and 2 to 1. This supplement is reported to improve blood vessel function and insulin resistance, in addition to decreasing LDL cholesterol, total cholesterol, and triglycerides. Also essential for phase-I liver detoxification. If you experience loose stools after taking magnesium, cut your dose in half and gradually increase over the course of a few months. Consult your health-care provider for dosage advice.
N-acetyl cysteine (NAC)	500 to 750 mg twice a day.	NAC is an antioxidant that is reported to help protect against blood vessel damage and clots due to insulin resistance, diabetes, and other blood sugar regulation problems. It also helps improve the body's capacity to decrease the harmful effects of toxins. NAC has been reported to improve kidney function in laboratory and human studies, and support glutathione production in the kidneys. It is generally well tolerated when taken in recommended dosages.
Nettle	If using a liquid extract, take 15 to 30 drops two to three times a day. If using the capsule form, take 50 to 100 mg two to three times a day.	Used to improve kidney function and relieve allergy symptoms such as runny nose. They are also known to be effective in preventing urinary problems, such as urinary tract infections. May cause sweating and upset stomach. Consult your physician before taking if you have diabetes, kidney or liver disease, or urinary or prostate problems. Women who are pregnant or breastfeeding should not use before speaking to their doctor.

Supplement	Dosage	Considerations
Probiotics	20 billion CFUs twice a day.	Probiotics help normalize beneficial flora in the gastro intestinal tract, and are reported to decrease triglyceride and cholesterol levels. They are also reported to improve BUN levels and quality of life in people with kidney disease. It's best to use heat-stable products that do not require refrigeration. If using an antibiotic, wait three hours before taking probiotics. If diarrhea occurs, decrease your dosage. If this side effect persists for longer than 48 hours, stop taking the supplement and contact your doctor. Live cultures should be guaranteed through the date of expiration on label. For optimal results, take probiotics with meals, as food improves the survivability of the cultures.
Selenium	200 mcg once a day.	Has been reported to help protect the kidneys. Selenium also helps protect the body against mercury toxicity, which can damage the liver and kidneys. Never take more than the recommended dose. Symptoms of selenium toxicity include vomiting, stomach pain, hair loss, brittle nails, and fatigue.
Zinc	25 to 50 mg once a day.	Zinc is important in immunity and acts as an anti-oxidant. It is also reported to help regulate blood sugar. May also be used by men to treat low testosterone and support prostate health. Take zinc in the form of an amino acid chelate or citrate. Check with your doctor before using.

LIFESTYLE CHANGES

Diet is crucial when it comes to preventing low GFR, as well as managing or avoiding the conditions that may cause it. If you are insulin resistant or at high risk for developing the condition, the dietary guidelines below will help you better control your blood glucose, blood pressure, and triglycerides and cholesterol levels. Managing these levels will prevent the decline in kidney function that leads to low GFR.

- Avoid excess salt. Sodium can be harmful to people whose kidneys are impaired. When the kidneys cannot rid the body of sodium properly, it builds up in the bloodstream and can cause high blood pressure and edema. For this reason, limit your total daily intake to 2,400 mg. Studies on the famous DASH (Dietary Approaches to Stop Hypertension) diet found that reduced intake of sodium—one of the diet's hallmarks—is effective for lowering blood pressure.

• Avoid refined sugars and carbohydrates. Eating a diet high in sugar and refined carbohydrates leads to increased blood levels of insulin and glucose, which can damage your cells, including kidney cells. Impaired kidney cells may result in restricted blood flow in the kidneys and affect their ability to balance electrolytes. Over time, this process leads to kidney damage. In addition, more and more medical research is validating low-carbohydrate diets as effective ways to manage body weight, diabetes, and high blood pressure. The goal is to allow for a moderate intake of complex carbohydrates like whole grains, while still maintaining a normal weight and healthy blood sugar level. Most people can get about 50 percent of their calories from carbohydrates, but if you take in this amount and still cannot stabilize your blood sugar, you may have to further reduce your consumption. A registered dietitian can help you learn how to decrease your intake and eat healthier versions of carbohydrates, such as low-starch fruits and vegetables.

• Eliminate trans fats. These man-made fats, which are added to cookies, doughnuts, potato chips, margarine, fast food items, and other processed foods, are hazardous to your health. Trans fats trigger inflammatory processes in the body, paving the way for conditions like high blood pressure and insulin resistance that ultimately lead to heart disease and diabetes. Trans fats also weaken circulation because they contribute to the hardening of arteries, which places an added burden on the kidneys. It's important to avoid foods containing partially hydrogenated oils, which continue to be widely used in the food industry. Check labels on packaged crackers, cookies, chips, and other snacks, that are high in both trans fats and sugars—a double whammy for your health. Replace these harmful foods with healthy fats, which are needed to maintain cell membranes and nerve cells. Healthy fats are found in nuts, seeds, avocados, lean meats, fish, olive oil, organic butter, and coconut oil. Flax seeds and flax oil are also healthy fats, but do not use them in cooking, and be sure to keep them refrigerated.

• Stay hydrated. Studies have shown that drinking adequate water may help reduce appetite and facilitate weight loss, both of which can help you better manage high blood sugar. Additionally, meeting your daily water requirement helps the kidneys filter blood and flush toxins out of the body. One study found that, when done over a long period of time, regularly drinking a sufficient amount of water is correlated with lower rates of chronic kidney disease. Experts generally recommend drinking 2 to 3 liters of water per day depending on your size, climate, physical activity, and health. In weight-loss studies, people were successful in shedding pounds when they drank two 8-ounce glasses of water before meals. However, if you have kidney disease, be careful not to drink too much water, as this may lead to overhydration.

- Stock your kitchen with organic foods. Whenever possible, buy foods that are certified organic products. Pesticides, heavy metals, and other toxins that are often found in nonorganic foods have been linked to insulin resistance. Additionally, heavy metals are known to be very hard on the kidneys.

- Take in adequate minerals. Chromium, magnesium, and zinc are essential minerals that support the balance and regulation of both blood sugar and insulin. While it's possible to get the required amounts in supplement form (see the table on page 11), it's ideal to take in mineral-rich foods. Chromium is not found in large amounts in any type of food, but more concentrated sources include onions, tomatoes, and brewer's yeast. Magnesium is contained in pumpkin seeds, spinach, Swiss chard, and soybeans, and zinc is abundant in venison, beef, and lamb. Remember to buy organic meats from grass-fed animal sources.

In addition to modifying your diet, you should exercise regularly and try to lose excess weight—measures that will help improve or prevent insulin resistance. Having your blood pressure and GFR tested regularly is also a good idea, especially if you are at an increased risk of developing kidney disease. If you are a smoker, you should seek help from your physician to quit the habit. Smoking is a known cause of high blood pressure and directly leads to kidney damage. However, this damage is reversible if smoking is stopped. Finally, it is best to limit or eliminate alcohol. While one or two drinks per day—depending on whether you are male or female—can lower certain health risks, excessive alcohol intake can raise your blood pressure and cause kidney damage. People who drink excessively have been found to have thickened glomeruli and enlarged kidneys.

CONCLUSION

Whether it's used to check for a condition, to test the effectiveness of medication, or simply as part of a routine medical exam, the results of a basic metabolic panel test can be invaluable when it comes to matters of your health. This panel looks at values that determine your body's internal maintenance and how well certain physiological processes, from glucose absorption to removal of wastes, are being carried out. When these basic functions cannot be properly executed, your body is thrown out of balance, paving the way for serious health problems. While many of these conditions are treatable with diet and lifestyle modifications, others, such as diabetes and kidney disease, are usually lifelong ailments that require careful management. Detecting an abnormality before it turns into an acute or chronic medical issue is potentially life saving, and regular BMP tests play a key role in this.

When reading the results of your blood test, it's important to remember that a normal value is not necessarily an optimal value. If your results are on either the high or low end of the normal range, you should ask your doctor about the implications for your health and what you can do to reach the target range. In general, it's a good idea to make positive lifestyle changes regardless of whether your test results are normal or abnormal. Adjusting your diet, adopting healthy habits, and quitting unhealthy ones are fundamental to disease prevention and have a powerful influence on your overall health. Nutritional supplements can also be used to reinforce the benefits of a healthy lifestyle, so ask your physician to recommend high-quality products. Finally, keep in mind that the best thing you can do for your well-being is to be proactive. A simple blood test can be the first step to becoming an advocate for yourself and your health.

PART 3

The Hepatic Function Panel

The liver plays a number of essential roles in the body and is responsible for hundreds of vital chemical reactions. From one blood draw, a lab assesses your total protein level, as well as the specific levels of two classes of proteins called albumin and globulin; the presence of a natural orange-yellow pigment called bilirubin; and the levels of liver enzymes found in the blood, including alanine aminotransferase (ALT), alkaline phosphatase (ALP), aspartate aminotransferase (AST), and gamma-glutamyltransferase (GGT). For example, it synthesizes glycogen from excess glucose in the blood, which it stores and metabolizes back into glucose when blood sugar levels are low. In addition to glycogen, it stores fat-soluble vitamins such as D and A, as well as the chemical elements iron and copper. The liver also produces bile, which is required for fat digestion, and amino acids, which are used for numerous purposes throughout the body. Finally, it detoxifies the body and removes waste, filtering the blood several times a day and breaking down substances such as environmental chemicals, hormones, alcohol, and drugs for elimination. Perhaps one of its most important functions is the removal of nitrogen, a waste product of protein metabolism, which it coverts into a compound called *urea* for ultimate excretion via urination. As you can see, virtually anything that goes through your mouth will end up getting processed by the liver, especially if the lining of the gut has been compromised, so monitoring liver function is important.

The hepatic function panel focuses on the primary indicators of liver function and can be used to detect liver damage. From one blood draw, a lab assesses your total protein level, as well as the amounts of *bilirubin* (both the direct and indirect forms) and the enzymes *alanine aminotransferase* (ALT), *alkaline phosphatase* (ALP), and *aspartate aminotransferase* (AST) in your system. While the most common things that can go wrong with the liver are cell injury or death, which most generally occurs from either excessive alcohol consumption or an accumulation of fat in the liver, this organ can also be damaged by hepatitis viruses A, B, or C, which cause inflammation. Additionally, an overload of toxic substances can result in significant problems. Not only are these substances harmful in and of themselves, but the degree of detoxification activity they cause the liver to undergo can be harmful, creating high levels of dangerous unstable molecules known as *free radicals*.

Did You Know?

The liver is the largest of the body's internal organs and is vital to proper physical functioning. As illustrated by the Greek myth of Prometheus—a trickster who was chained to a rock and made to have an eagle eat his liver each day, only to have it grow back in time for the eagle to feast again the next—the liver is the only organ capable of regenerating lost tissue. It can actually repair or regenerate up to 50 percent of damaged or destroyed matter!

15. TOTAL PROTEIN

The total protein count of the hepatic panel is the sum of two classes of proteins called *albumin* and *globulin*. This measurement can determine your nutritional status, diagnose kidney or liver disease, and evaluate the strength of your immune system. It is also used to investigate the cause of *edema*, which refers to a buildup of fluid that leads to swelling somewhere in the body, generally the ankles. Calculated in grams per deciliter of blood (g/dL), total protein levels fall into the following ranges.

REFERENCE RANGES FOR TOTAL PROTEIN

Total Protein (g/dL)	Category
Greater than 8.0	High
6.5 to 8.0	Normal
Less than 6.5	Low
Target Range: 7.2 to 7.5 g/dL	

Both high and low readings warrant further investigation into individual albumin and globulin levels, as well as the ratio between the two.

WHAT CAUSES HIGH TOTAL PROTEIN?

Total protein will be high when albumin or globulin production is elevated due to any number of reasons. While a temporary high protein count may point to acute infection, consistently high total protein levels can suggest a problem such as:

- Adrenal cortical hypofunction
- Alcoholism
- Chronic bacterial infection, such as tuberculosis
- Chronic viral infection, such as hepatitis
- Collagen vascular disease, such as rheumatoid arthritis, systemic lupus, or scleroderma
- Cryoglobulinemia
- Dehydration (often associated with such conditions as diabetic acidosis and chronic diarrhea)
- Diabetes
- Elevated cortisol due to chronic stress
- Heavy metal toxicity

- Hemolysis
- Hypersensitivity states
- Kidney dysfunction
- Leukemia
- Liver dysfunction
- Medications, including nonsteroidal anti-inflammatory drugs (NSAIDs), gold sodium thiomalate, penicillamine, and angiotensin-converting enzyme (ACE) inhibitors
- Nutritional deficiency
- Respiratory distress
- Sarcoidosis

If a lab test reveals high total protein levels, your doctor will seek to narrow down the cause of the problem by identifying exactly which protein is raised. While conditions such as dehydration typically result in high albumin, other issues, including leukemia and other diseases of the immune system, can cause high globulin.

WHAT ARE THE SYMPTOMS OF HIGH TOTAL PROTEIN?

Physical indicators of elevated protein include confusion, dehydration, edema, fatigue, frothy urine, and joint aches and pains. While these are serious problems that may be linked to serious health conditions, there are ways to lessen their impact and lower protein counts.

HOW CAN HIGH TOTAL PROTEIN BE TREATED?

Typically, the underlying cause of the imbalance must be treated in order to normalize protein levels. Once the condition has been determined, a few lifestyle adjustments may be able to treat the problem.

LIFESTYLE CHANGES

The most obvious step you can take is to decrease your protein intake, particularly avoiding foods that are high in albumin protein, which include fish, shellfish, chicken, turkey, and eggs. Any additional steps that should be taken will be determined by your physician after a comprehensive examination of your symptoms and blood test results.

WHAT CAUSES LOW TOTAL PROTEIN?

A low total protein level is usually the result of poor nutritional intake, but it may occur in spite of proper eating habits when protein is not adequately absorbed by the intestines. It may also happen if the body is damaged by an injury such as a severe burn, which would necessitate a significantly high amount of protein to keep up with the demands of the healing process. In fact, any type of healing or convalescence will sap protein from the body. Other causes of a low protein count include:

- Diarrhea
- Duodenal resections due to cancer
- Essential hypertension (high blood pressure with no known cause)
- Gastric bypass surgery
- Kidney disease
- Liver disease
- Pregnancy

Lastly, anti-ulcer medications such as proton-pump inhibitors (PPIs) and H_2 blockers make up the second-largest category of drugs currently being prescribed in the United States. They lower the production of stomach acid, thereby decreasing the body's absorption of protein. Although these substances are meant to be used for nine to twelve weeks, some people take them for years, which can considerably deplete their protein level.

WHAT ARE THE SYMPTOMS OF LOW TOTAL PROTEIN?

If you are not taking in or absorbing enough protein, the resulting low total protein level can have a significant impact on your health. It compromises immune function, leaving you more susceptible to infection, and makes it difficult to maintain lean muscle mass.

HOW CAN LOW TOTAL PROTEIN BE TREATED?

Low total protein is a serious issue, as it is associated with medical conditions like liver disease. While medically supervised treatment may be necessary, lifestyle modifications are also crucial.

LIFESTYLE CHANGES

One of the best ways to prevent a low level is to change your diet, which must include decreasing or eliminating alcohol consumption. You might also try increasing your intake of high-quality lean proteins, including fish, turkey, and, if you can find it, bison. Whenever possible, buy organic free-range meat, meaning it has been raised without chemical additives, hormones, or antibiotics. Additionally, cutting out refined sugars and carbohydrates from your diet will decrease inflammation and improve insulin function, which should enhance albumin synthesis in the liver. A reduction in dietary fat intake and soft drink consumption (due to the high-fructose corn syrup these beverages contain) is also recommended. Eating foods that help detoxify the kidneys, including asparagus, garlic, onions, and cruciferous vegetables such as cabbage and broccoli, can also be beneficial to your protein level. Maintaining healthy kidneys will help prevent protein from leaking into the urine.

If you have liver disease or another disorder causing low protein, your diet should be managed by a dietitian or a healthcare professional specializing in this area. People with liver or kidney disease must manage their protein levels on an individual basis. If your protein levels are on the low end of normal, you may want to take a digestive enzyme capsule. This can help your body break down proteins more effectively, thereby aiding in protein absorption. If you have had some type of abdominal surgery that has limited your ability to absorb protein, there are whey, rice, pea, and egg protein replacements available. These are generally sold in the form of a powder or beverage, which may be more readily absorbed.

A Helpful Tip

For a healthy liver, National Liver Foundation recommends the following sources of lean protein:

- Three ounces of meat, poultry (chicken), or fish (21 g protein)
- One cup of milk or yogurt (8 g)
- One large egg (7 g)
- Two tablespoons of peanut or other nut butters (7 g)
- One-half cup of tofu (7 g)
- One-fourth cup of cottage cheese (7 g)
- One ounce cheese (7 g)
- One-half cup of cooked, dried, pinto, kidney or navy beans (3 g)

16. ALBUMIN

Using amino acids derived from dietary protein, the liver produces about 9 to 12 g of albumin per day. Once produced, albumin in the blood makes up about 60 percent of the total protein level and is responsible for keeping the fluid portion of the blood contained within blood vessels. It also binds to key substances, including bilirubin, free fatty acids, hormones such as thyroxin and cortisol, nutrients like calcium and magnesium, as well as drugs, allowing them to travel throughout the body via the bloodstream. Albumin is also known to scavenge free radicals. Measured in grams per deciliter, albumin level ranges are detailed in the following table.

REFERENCE RANGES FOR ALBUMIN

Albumin (g/dL)	Category
Greater than 5.0	High
3.7 to 5.0	Normal
Less than 3.7	Low
Target Range: 4.0 to 4.5 g/dL	

The categories apply for everyone except children under three years of age, for whom the normal range is broader, measuring 2.9 to 5.5 g/dL. Because albumin constitutes such a large part of the total protein count, reasons for abnormal albumin readings are often the same as those associated with abnormal total protein levels, such as kidney or liver disease, infection, and dehydration.

WHAT CAUSES HIGH ALBUMIN?

High albumin levels, also called *hyperalbuminemia,* are almost always related to dehydration, which can be caused by something as simple as a lack of fluid intake or something as serious as the increased urination that occurs at the onset of diabetes. Other reasons for high albumin include:

- Hypochlorhydria (low stomach acid content)
- Inflammation of the digestive tract (generally caused by a condition such as irritable bowel syndrome or colitis)
- Kidney or liver disease

- Malnutrition
- Medications, including anabolic steroids, glucocorticoids, estrogen, growth hormone, and insulin
- Pregnancy eclampsia (seizures and coma during pregnancy)
- Protein supplements
- Retinol (vitamin A) deficiency

Although the reports of people developing excessively high albumin from using protein supplements are very rare, the possibility should be considered if you take protein pills as part of an exercise regimen.

WHAT ARE THE SYMPTOMS OF HIGH ALBUMIN?

Even before high albumin is detected by a blood test, symptoms of the problem may arise, which include bleeding from the gastrointestinal tract, bone aches and pains, confusion, dark urine, diarrhea, dizziness, edema in the abdomen or belly, fatigue, fever and chills, increased thirst, itchiness, jaundice (yellowing of the eyes and skin), loss of appetite, pale or light-colored stool, and profuse sweating.

Because these symptoms may be indicative of a number of health conditions, it would be wise to consult your doctor if you experience any of them.

HOW CAN HIGH ALBUMIN BE TREATED?

Once you have addressed the underlying issue with your doctor, you can remedy high albumin with a few essential adjustments to your lifestyle, as well as supplements.

SUPPLEMENTS

As high albumin has been linked to kidney and liver problems, you may consider dietary supplements that are protective of these organs, such as the substances listed below. While these substances can be helpful, never take any supplement without the guidance of your doctor, as your situation may prohibit its use or call for a reduced dosage. You should also ask your doctor about L-glutamine, curcumin, and melatonin, which have been shown to support the kidneys as well.

SUPPLEMENTS FOR HIGH ALBUMIN		
Supplement	**Dosage**	**Considerations**
Cordyceps	1,100 mg twice a day.	Helps with lung function by increasing oxygen to the cells, and has shown to improve BUN and creatinine levels in laboratory studies. It is especially recommended for people who have conditions like diabetes and high blood pressure, which increase the risk of kidney failure. Also reported to support liver function. While some medical literature suggests that cordyceps rebalances immune activity, it should be used with caution if you have an autoimmune disease, such as lupus or multiple sclerosis, as it may cause the immune system to become more active.
Milk thistle extract (standardized to 80-percent silymarins)	300 mg once or twice a day.	Milk thistle is reported to support liver function. May have a laxative effect and cause nausea, diarrhea, indigestion, gas, bloating, fullness or pain, and loss of appetite. Avoid if you have an allergy to ragweed and related plants, a hormone-sensitive condition such as breast cancer or uterine fibroids, or are pregnant or breastfeeding.
N-acetyl cysteine (NAC)	400 mg twice a day.	NAC is an antioxidant that is reported to help protect against blood vessel damage and clots due to insulin resistance, diabetes, and other blood sugar regulation problems. It also helps improve the body's capacity to decrease the harmful effects of toxins. NAC has been reported to improve kidney function in laboratory and human studies, and support glutathione production in the kidneys. It is generally well tolerated when taken in recommended dosages.

LIFESTYLE CHANGES

First, it's important to stay hydrated. Aim to drink approximately 2 to 3 liters of water that has been purified through reverse osmosis (RO) or filtration per day. In addition, try to adopt a diet that will protect your liver and kidneys, and consider the recommended dietary supplements.

If high albumin levels are associated with kidney disease, your doctor will likely put you on what is known as a *renal diet* in order to protect your kidneys from further damage. It consists of low-phosphorus and low-potassium foods and strictly regulates protein intake. You should also discontinue the use of any protein supplements and limit foods high in albumin protein, such as fish, fowl, shellfish, and eggs, until your albumin level returns to normal. Once albumin has been lowered, discuss your regular protein consumption with your doctor. While protein consumption should likely remain at a minimum, recent studies suggest that the generous consumption of vegetables, which contain nephroprotective antioxidants and potassium, may safeguard kidney function from elevated protein in the diet, even in diabetics with compromised kidney function. Vegetable consumption has an alkalizing effect on the urine and spares mineral loss. Finally, if high albumin has been associated with liver disease, alcohol consumption should be stopped altogether.

WHAT CAUSES LOW ALBUMIN?

Low albumin levels, or *hypoalbuminemia,* can arise when your body is fighting an infection, healing a burn, or simply malnourished. It may even occur when a person experiences *polydipsian,* or excessive thirst; whenever a person takes in too much water, either by drinking large volumes or by intravenous (IV) fluid therapy, proteins in the blood are diluted. The following conditions are also connected to low albumin.

- Chronic debilitating disease, such as rheumatoid arthritis
- Dehydration
- Gastrointestinal conditions that cause protein loss, such as diarrhea
- Gastrointestinal dysbiosis (microbial imbalance within the gastrointestinal tract)
- Hemorrhage
- Hypocalcemia (low calcium level)
- Hypothyroidism (underactive thyroid gland)
- Inflammatory bowel disease, such as Crohn's disease, which causes malabsorption
- Liver dysfunction
- Medication interactions or side effects of certain pharmaceuticals, including chemotherapy or weight-loss drugs such as phentermine (Adipex) and sibutramine (Meridia)
- Neoplastic disease, such as leukemia and Hodgkin's lymphoma
- Nephrotic syndrome (kidney damage)
- Peptic ulcer
- Shock and trauma

Because low albumin may be the result of a variety of serious health conditions, it is important to get your blood checked if you notice any of the symptoms of this problem.

WHAT ARE THE SYMPTOMS OF LOW ALBUMIN?

Low albumin can manifest itself many ways. It can cause edema in the abdomen or belly, fatigue, increased perspiration, elevated risk of bone fracture, jaundice, and confusion.

HOW CAN LOW ALBUMIN BE TREATED?

As is the case with high albumin, treatment should focus on the cause of the problem. The guidelines highlighted below may be beneficial.

SUPPLEMENTS

Certain supplements may be directly or indirectly helpful. While alpha-lipoic acid and arginine promote kidney health, and L-glutamine is good for your digestive tract and supports glutathione production in the kidneys, a handful of other substances can also help low albumin issues. The fact that these products can be acquired without a prescription does not mean they are harmless. Always consult your doctor to discuss the possible side effects of any supplement you are considering.

SUPPLEMENTS FOR HIGH ALBUMIN		
Supplement	**Dosage**	**Considerations**
Alpha-lipoic acid	300 mg twice a day.	Reported to help with blood sugar uptake and use in the body. Also helps detoxify the body, protect the kidneys, and improve cholesterol levels. Make sure that the raw material provider for the product is from Europe to guarantee effectiveness.
Glutamine (L-glutamine)	3,000 to 5,000 mg twice a day.	Studies have shown that glutamine helps protect the kidneys against oxidative stress damage, as well as improve creatinine levels. Avoid if you suffer from severe liver disease, seizures, monosodium glutamate sensitivity, or mania. Do not take if you are pregnant or breastfeeding.
L-arginine (HCl sustained release)	1,000 to 2,000 mg twice a day.	L-arginine helps regulate blood pressure and may be effective for lowering mildly elevated levels. The substance has also been found to boost endurance and improve exercise ability in people with heart failure. There is some evidence that it may indirectly help metabolism problems resulting from kidney failure. People with low blood pressure or heart problems should avoid using this supplement. Talk to your doctor before taking if you have asthma.
Whey protein	20 g (1 to 2 scoops added to a beverage) one to three times a day.	Studies have shown that whey protein is a form of protein that is both easily digested and superior to other proteins for muscle building. It has also been reported to improve immunity and work as an antioxidant in the body. However, high doses can cause

Supplement	Dosage	Considerations
Whey protein *(continued)*		increased bowel movements, nausea, thirst, bloating, cramps, reduced appetite, fatigue, and headaches. Avoid use if you are pregnant or breastfeeding.

LIFESTYLE CHANGES

While exogenous albumin, or albumin that has been artificially synthesized outside the body, is not used to raise levels of this protein, your doctor may recommend an increase in dietary protein intake. Before you increase the protein level of your diet, however, your overall health will need to be evaluated. If the underlying cause of low albumin is an infection, it is a good idea to take in plenty of high quality proteins to support immune function and restore normal albumin levels. If you have existing kidney disease, however, you should not increase your protein intake. Patients with liver disease should also not consume more protein despite low albumin levels, as the liver can no longer remove nitrogen waste. If nitrogen were to build up along with other toxins, it would cause a type of brain dysfunction called *hepatic encephalopathy,* symptoms of which include confusion, disorientation, personality changes, and erratic behavior. As a rule, patients with kidney illnesses follow the renal diet, which is designed to control dietary intake of phosphorus, sodium, potassium, protein, and fluids according to each patient's individual needs.

Other suggested food-related measures involve practices that may restore gut health and improve protein absorption in the digestive system, such as:

- Lowering sugar and refined carbohydrate intake
- Limiting bread, rice, cereal, and pasta, especially in the morning
- Eliminating high-fructose corn syrup and fruit juice, and minimizing high-glycemic fruit, such as pineapple, bananas, and dried fruit
- Increasing consumption of low-glycemic foods, such as beans, peas, zucchini, squash, and low-starch vegetables, including asparagus, cabbage, green beans, and sprouts, to five to nine servings per day
- Eating more sources of soluble fiber, such as flaxseed and guar gum, and drinking at least eight glasses of water per day
- Minimizing or eliminating fast food. If this is not possible, opt for a salad when eating at a fast food restaurant.

17. GLOBULIN

Together with albumin, globulin forms the total protein level on a blood test lab report. It includes carrier proteins, enzymes, clotting factors, and, predominantly, antibodies. Globulin is categorized into three main groups: alpha globulins, beta globulins, and gamma globulins. While alpha globulins and beta globulins are primarily transport proteins, gamma globulins are mainly comprised of *immunoglobulins* (Igs), also known as antibodies. These proteins are produced by the immune system in response to an infection or allergic reaction, and after organ transplantation. Globulin ranges are as follows:

REFERENCE RANGES FOR GLOBULIN	
Globulin (g/dL)	**Category**
Greater than 3.5	High
2.0 to 3.5	Normal
Less than 2.0	Low
Target Range: 2.8 to 3.2 g/dL	

Individual alpha and beta globulin levels also have target ranges, but unlike the total globulin count, which is measured in grams per deciliter, they are measured in grams per liter. Alpha globulin has a target range of 0.2 to 0.3 g/L, and beta globulin has a target range of 0.7 to 1.0 g/L. There a few different types of gamma globulins, each of which has its own target range. These are not typically included in a regular lab panel.

WHAT CAUSES HIGH GLOBULIN?

Because gamma globulins account for a majority of the globulin level, a high globulin count, also known as *hypergammaglobulinemia,* most commonly suggests that antibodies have been elevated to fight off an infection, which may be acute or chronic, or as a result of an allergic reaction. Other causes include:

- Autoimmune disease, such as rheumatoid arthritis or systemic lupus erythematosus (SLE)
- Blood coagulation disorders
- Cancer
- Inflammatory bowel disease, such as ulcerative colitis or Crohn's disease
- Leukemia
- Liver disease, including biliary cirrhosis and obstructive jaundice

- Medication interaction or side effect
- Nephrosis (kidney dysfunction)
- Peptic ulcer

While many of these conditions are quite serious, try not to be alarmed by a high globulin level. Remember, it is typically a sign of your body doing what it is supposed to do in the face of an infection or allergy.

WHAT ARE THE SYMPTOMS OF HIGH GLOBULIN?

Physical indicators of high globulin include confusion, edema, fatigue, increased perspiration, and pain due to inflammation. These symptoms, of course, should not be ignored. If connected to high globulin levels, they may be associated with one of the previously listed causative conditions, signaling liver toxicity, kidney damage, cancer, chronic inflammatory disease, or gastrointestinal dysbiosis, also known as an imbalance of bacteria in the gut. (See the inset below.)

HOW CAN HIGH GLOBULIN BE TREATED?

Once the primary cause of high globulin has been identified, focused treatment should be able to normalize this protein. If globulin levels are elevated due to an allergy, locate and eliminate the allergen. If infection is present, your doctor will take steps to clear it from your system. If a peptic ulceration is

The Importance of Balanced Gut Flora

Elevated globulins are almost always due to allergies or infection, both of which are related to the digestive tract's balance of gut flora and integrity of intestinal tissue. Antibiotics, unfortunately, which are used to help fight infection, destroy the beneficial bacteria in the gut. Modern society's dependence on antibiotics has resulted in a large number of people with a depleted amount of good flora, and this problem is still not fully recognized for the significant role it is playing in gut-related diseases and conditions. While you may be able to improve your level of healthful gut flora by eating fermented foods like yogurt and kefir, which include these bacteria, it is probably more effective to use probiotic supplements, which contain high doses of friendly bacteria, in an effort to regain balance. (See page 168.)

spotted, your doctor will seek to heal it. Finally, if globulin is high because of chronic inflammation or an autoimmune disease, therapy for these conditions should help bring globulin levels down. Additional treatments are highlighted in the sections that follow.

DRUGS

As high globulin levels are most often the result of infection, antibiotics may be prescribed to fight the problem. Unfortunately, antibiotics wipe out not only the infection but also the healthful bacteria, leaving the gut flora compromised and the stage set other conditions that might lead to elevated globulin again. Antibiotics are necessary for active infections, but sometimes, natural alternatives can be used for cold or flu-like symptoms (see the table on page 164). If antibiotics are absolutely necessary, you can restore gut health with probiotic supplements, which contain beneficial bacteria. Certain formulations of probiotics are designed improve kidney function by helping remove the waste product urea from the body. This action relieves some of the burden placed on these organs, which are normally responsible for the elimination of the nitrogen-containing substance. You can find guidelines for probiotics supplements in many of the supplement tables provided throughout this book.

SUPPLEMENTS

While there are dietary supplements recommended to lower globulin, they depend upon the underlying condition associated with the issue. Once your doctor has determined the cause of your high globulin reading, you will be able to consider the supplements best suited to your situation. For example, if high globulin is linked to autoimmune disease or chronic inflammation, the following substances may be helpful.

SUPPLEMENTS FOR HIGH GLOBULIN ASSOCIATED WITH AUTOIMMUNE DISEASE OR CHRONIC INFLAMMATION

Supplement	Dosage	Considerations
IgG powder	15 to 20 g mixed in a favorite sugar-free non-dairy beverage each day.	Used to reduce inflammatory signaling in the gastrointestinal tract.

Supplement	Dosage	Considerations
Omega-3 essential fatty acids DHA and EPA (fish oil)	1,000 mg up to four times a day.	Fish oil acts as an antioxidant and decreases inflammation in the body, in addition to supporting heart and blood vessel health. Speak to your doctor before taking if you are on blood-thinning medication, as fish oil may increase the risk of bleeding. Be sure to use only high-quality oils that have been tested for contaminants.
Peppermint oil (with enteric coating)	Take as directed on the label or as directed by your healthcare provider.	Used to treat inflammatory bowel disease. May cause heartburn or an allergic reaction such as flushing, headache, or mouth sores.
Turmeric phytosome	300 to 500 mg three times a day with meals.	This is a type of turmeric extract that contains phosphatidylcholine, a beneficial phosolipid that has significantly higher absorbability.

The nutritional supplements below may be effective for fighting off the flu or common cold, especially if they are used as soon as symptoms are experienced.

SUPPLEMENTS AS AN ALTERNATIVE TO ANTIBIOTICS

Supplement	Dosage	Considerations
Andrographis paniculata (standardized to 50 percent andrographolides)	150 mg once a day for preventive purposes; 300 to 600 mg once a day if symptoms are present.	May be effective for treating the common cold, as well as reducing fever and sore throat. Avoid use if you have an autoimmune disorder.
Esberitox (Echinacea)	3 tablets three times a day while symptoms are present.	Do not use if you are allergic to the daisy (Echinacea) plant family.
Oscillococcinum	1 tube (1 g) every 6 hours up to three times a day.	Do not use for colds, as it is not indicated. Take at the first sign of flu symptoms for the best results.

Finally, if an erosion of the lining of the stomach or small intestine, also known as a *peptic ulcer,* is causing your high globulin count, the following supplements may be recommended. Keep in mind that these substances should not be used as treatment for ulcers, but considered supportive nutrition.

SUPPLEMENTS FOR HIGH GLOBULIN ASSOCIATED WITH PEPTIC ULCER		
Supplement	**Dosage**	**Considerations**
Colostrum	1,000 to 2,000 mg one to three times a day, taken on an empty stomach, either one hour before or two hours after a meal.	Use a product made from the pre-milk of New Zealand cattle. Avoid use if you are pregnant, breastfeeding, or allergic to cow's milk or milk products.
Deglycyrrhizinated licorice (DGL)	400 to 800 mg three times a day, chewed either one hour before or two hours after a meal, and at bedtime.	Do not use if you are scheduled to undergo surgery.
Zinc carnosine	1 capsule (containing 8 mg zinc and 29.5 mg L-carnosine) up to four times a day for one month, and 1 to 2 capsules two times a day thereafter.	Has been shown to enhance healing of the stomach lining, among other gastrointestinal benefits. It may also help protect the liver.

In addition, probiotics and L-glutamine have been reported to protect the gastric mucosa, so speak to your physician to determine if these supplements can fulfill your health needs. Remember, although supplements may be used to treat the underlying causes of high globulin, potential side effects may prohibit you from taking advantage of such treatment. Talk to your doctor to see which substance might be right for you.

LIFESTYLE CHANGES

While the solution lies in addressing the issue with your physician, there are a few lifestyle modifications you can make that may be beneficial. The dietary practices used to treat high globulin are the same as those used to remedy low albumin, as both problems are related to gut health. The main goal is to cut down or eliminate sugar from your daily meals. Sugar promotes the overgrowth of the intestinal yeast known as *candida albicans.* While candida is a normal part of gut flora, too much of it can result in a number of health problems that would raise globulin levels. Other related dietary advice includes:

- Lowering refined carbohydrate intake
- Limiting bread, rice, cereal, and pasta, especially in the morning
- Eliminating high-fructose corn syrup and fruit juice, and minimizing high-glycemic fruit, such as pineapple, bananas, and dried fruit

- Eating more sources of soluble fiber, such as flaxseed and guar gum, and drinking at least eight glasses of water per day
- Increasing consumption of low-glycemic foods, such as beans, peas, zucchini, squash, and low-starch vegetables, including asparagus, cabbage, green beans, and sprouts, to five to nine servings per day
- Minimizing or eliminating your consumption of fast food, or opting for healthier choices at restaurants, such as salad

In addition to watching what you eat, getting adequate sleep can help balance and restore the immune system, which will normalize your globulin count. Get at least six to eight hours of quality sleep nightly. Learning how to cope with stress is also very important. Stress raises levels of the hormone cortisol, which lowers the production of the immunoglobulin IgA, making you more prone to food allergies. Exercise, even a small daily amount, can reduce the effects of stress and help you sleep better. Incorporate thirty minutes of physical activity into your day, three to five times a week. The mere act of walking is beneficial, but a combination of aerobics and strength training is best.

If you use anti-inflammatory drugs to alleviate problems such as arthritis pain, try to cut down on the dose or use an alternative product, as these pharmaceuticals can break down the mucosal linings of the intestines, thereby weakening your gut flora and raising your globulin level. You might want to try glucosamine, which facilitates collagen hydration and improves mobility. Natural anti-inflammatory agents, like Boswellia and curcumin, are also helpful, as they inhibit the production of inflammatory cytokines. Finally, get tested for food intolerances and allergies. You might be able to return your globulin count to a normal range by simply eliminating a certain food from your diet.

WHAT CAUSES LOW GLOBULIN?

Health conditions that compromise the immune system are generally associated with a low globulin count, or *hypogammaglobulinemia*. These illnesses include:

- Acute hemolytic anemia
- Alpha-1 antitrypsin deficiency, which often leads to emphysema
- Immunodeficiency syndromes
- Liver dysfunction

- Lymphocytic leukemia
- Malignant lymphoproliferative disorder
- Malnutrition or protein loss
- Medication interactions or side effects of certain drug treatments, including immunosuppressive therapy, chemotherapy, and steroids
- Renal disease
- Viral hepatitis
- Plasma cell dyscrasias

As many of the health conditions that cause low globulin are quite serious, it is important to see your doctor if you experience any symptoms of the problem.

WHAT ARE THE SYMPTOMS OF LOW GLOBULIN?

Low globulin levels are suspected when a person exhibits fatigue, pain, or an increased susceptibility to colds, flu, and other infections.

HOW CAN LOW GLOBULIN BE TREATED?

The easiest way to support globulin levels is to eat an overall healthful diet and take supplements, as detailed in the sections below.

SUPPLEMENTS

There are a number of supplements that can help you boost your immune system and raise your globulin count. Common examples are included in the table below. It's important to note, however, that while these substances can be beneficial to someone with a low globulin level, in severe cases, gamma globulin may need to be administered intravenously.

SUPPLEMENTS FOR LOW GLOBULIN

Supplement	Dosage	Considerations
Alfalfa herb	5 to 10 g three times a day.	Do not use this supplement if you have an autoimmune disease, such as lupus or multiple sclerosis, a hormone-sensitive condition, such as breast cancer, or have had a kidney transplant. Diabetics use with caution, as it may lower blood sugar. Avoid use if you are pregnant or breastfeeding.

Supplement	Dosage	Considerations
Chlorella	3 to 6 tablets (500 mg each) a day.	Do not use if you have an iodine sensitivity, weak immune system, or autoimmune disease, such as lupus. Avoid use if you are pregnant or breastfeeding.
Glutamine (L-glutamine)	5,000 mg once or twice a day.	Studies have shown that glutamine helps protect the kidneys against oxidative stress damage, as well as improve creatinine levels. Avoid if you suffer from severe liver disease, seizures, monosodium glutamate sensitivity, or mania. Do not take if you are pregnant or breastfeeding.
Immpower (AHCC)	6 capsules (500 mg each) a day, 2 with each meal for the first three to four weeks. Decrease to 2 capsules a day, one in the morning and one in the evening, thereafter.	Consider taking if viral hepatitis is present. Do not use if you have kidney disease due to its high phosphorus content.
N-acetyl cysteine (NAC)	400 mg twice a day.	NAC is an antioxidant that is reported to help protect against blood vessel damage and clots due to insulin resistance, diabetes, and other blood sugar regulation problems. It also helps improve the body's capacity to decrease the harmful effects of toxins. NAC has been reported to improve kidney function in laboratory and human studies, and support glutathione production in the kidneys. It is generally well tolerated when taken in recommended dosages.
Phyllanthus niruri (standardized to 3-percent bitter principles)	200 mg two to four times a day.	Taken if viral hepatitis is present. Use with caution if you are diabetic, as it may affect blood glucose levels. Do not use if you are pregnant, breastfeeding, or scheduled for surgery.
Probiotics	3 to 25 billion CFUs one to three times a day.	Probiotics help normalize beneficial flora in the gastrointestinal tract, which reduces production of acetaldehydes—a known cause of elevated liver enzymes. Probiotics are also reported to decrease triglyceride and cholesterol levels, and to improve BUN levels and quality of life in people with kidney disease. It's best to use heat-stable products

Supplement	Dosage	Considerations
Probiotics *(continued)*		that do not require refrigeration. If using an antibiotic, wait three hours before taking probiotics. If diarrhea occurs, decrease your dosage. If this side effect persists for longer than 48 hours, stop taking the supplement and contact your doctor. Live cultures should be guaranteed through the date of expiration on label. For optimal results, take probiotics with meals, as food improves the survivability of the cultures.
Reishi mushroom (standardized to 4 percent triterpenes and 10 percent polysaccharides, or beta-1,3-glucans)	150 to 300 mg three to four times a day.	If you take blood thinners, use only under a doctor's supervision. Avoid use if you have low blood pressure, thrombocytopenia, or are pregnant or breastfeeding.
Whey protein	20 to 30 g (1 to 2 scoops added to a beverage) two to three times a day.	Studies have shown that whey protein is a form of protein that is both easily digested and superior to other proteins for muscle building. It has also been reported to improve immunity and work as an antioxidant in the body. However, high doses can cause increased bowel movements, nausea, thirst, bloating, cramps, reduced appetite, fatigue, and headaches. Avoid use if you are pregnant or breastfeeding.

LIFESTYLE CHANGES

As low globulin is most often the result of disease, the most appropriate diet would be determined by the specific illness. As low globulin is directly related to a weakened immune system, treatment of the deficiency involves supporting immune integrity. If globulin levels are extremely low, you may be advised to eat low-bacteria foods because the immune system may not be strong enough to fight regular or even low levels of daily exposure to these microbes. Aside from dietary considerations, globulin improvement requires plenty of rest—at least seven to eight hours a night. Physical activity is also recommended, but nothing too strenuous. Yoga would be a good choice.

18. ALBUMIN/GLOBULIN (A/G) RATIO

In addition to total protein, a blood test will display the ratio of albumin to globulin, or A/G ratio, to determine whether or not your protein count is out of the normal range. Typically, the body will have a little more albumin than globulin, yielding an A/G ratio just over 1.0. Therefore, if you have an albumin count of 4.0 g/dL and a globulin count of 2.8 g/dL, your A/G ratio would be 1.4. An A/G ratio of 1.1 to 2.4 is considered normal. An overproduction of globulin or underproduction of albumin will result in a low A/G ratio, while a high A/G ratio may mean a deficiency of globulin. If your A/G ratio is high or low, your doctor will want to do a few follow-up tests to understand why it is outside the normal range.

REFERENCE RANGES FOR ALBUMIN/GLOBULIN

Albumin/Globulin	Normal Range
A/G Ratio	1.1 to 2.4

WHAT CAUSES A HIGH A/G RATIO?

A high A/G ratio is generally the result of a lack of gamma globulins, which suggests a compromised immune system. It is commonly associated with immune disorders, most of which are hereditary. In addition, an excess of *glucocorticoids,* which are a class of steroids that suppress the immune system, will result in a high A/G ratio. This problem may be found in people with chronic stress or adrenal tumors. An elevated A/G ratio may also be seen in cases of viral hepatitis and certain forms of leukemia, including lymphocytic leukemia. Other factors behind this issue include a high-protein, high-carbohydrate diet in connection with poor nitrogen retention, as well as hypothyroidism.

WHAT ARE THE SYMPTOMS OF A HIGH A/G RATIO?

Low globulin levels result in a weakened immune system, which causes fatigue, inflammation, and pain, and increases your risk of catching a cold, flu, or other infection.

HOW CAN A HIGH A/G RATIO BE TREATED?

If your A/G ratio is high, your doctor will want to look at your individual

albumin and globulin counts to get a better understanding of the abnormality. Treatment will be based on these individual protein readings. Once the problem has been identified, consult the appropriate sections of the previous chapters to find out how it may be remedied. (See pages 155 and 161.)

WHAT CAUSES A LOW A/G RATIO?

A low A/G ratio is the result of either an overproduction of globulin or an underproduction of albumin. Globulin levels usually rise in the face of chronic inflammation or infection. High globulin may also point to a type of cancer known as myeloma or an autoimmune disease such as lupus. Albumin levels are typically low due to liver problems such as cirrhosis, which reduces albumin production, or kidney problems, which result in a loss of this protein.

WHAT ARE THE SYMPTOMS OF A LOW A/G RATIO?

Individuals with a low A/G ratio may exhibit confusion, increased perspiration, fatigue, edema, and pain due to inflammation.

HOW CAN A LOW A/G RATIO BE TREATED?

If your A/G ratio is low, your doctor will want to look at your individual albumin and globulin counts to get a better understanding of the abnormality. Treatment will be based on these individual protein readings. Once the problem has been identified, consult the appropriate sections of the previous chapters to find out how it may be remedied.

19. BILIRUBIN

When aging red blood cells are broken down by the spleen, the normal byproduct is a natural orange-yellow pigment called *bilirubin*. This substance occurs in two forms. Before it reaches the liver, it is called *indirect* or *unconjugated bilirbuin*. Once it enters the liver, it attaches to certain sugars and becomes *direct* or *conjugated bilirubin*. A water-soluble substance, direct bilirubin is released into a digestive fluid called bile and stored in the gallbladder. Eventually, it is excreted from the body in stools. If the liver is damaged or diseased, it will not be able to process bilirubin as usual, causing the fluid to accumulate in the blood.

A blood test generally measures total bilirubin and direct bilirubin, and derives the indirect bilirubin level by subtracting direct bilirubin from the total amount. Normal ranges of both total and direct bilirubin appear below.

REFERENCE RANGES FOR BILIRUBIN

Bilirubin Type	Normal Range (mg/dL)
Total Bilirubin	0.2 to 1.4
Direct Bilirubin	0.0 to 0.4

When total bilirubin is high, your doctor will take a closer look at the direct measurement. If direct bilirubin is normal, indirect bilirubin will be calculated.

WHAT CAUSES HIGH BILIRUBIN?

More than half of newborn babies have a higher than normal bilirubin level, which results in a condition called *neonatal jaundice*, or *neonatal hyperbilirubinemia*. It occurs when the infant's liver begins to process bilirubin, which had formerly been managed by the mother's system. It is typically temporary and does not require treatment. If the bilirubin level is particularly high, the baby may be given *phototherapy*—artificial daylight that is known to break down bilirubin.

While the cause of high bilirubin in a newborn is relatively easy to identify, it may be a little more difficult to determine in an adult. Other reasons behind an elevated bilirubin level include:

- Biliary stricture (abnormal narrowing of the common bile duct)
- Gallbladder infection
- Gilbert's syndrome
- Healing of large hematomas (bruises)
- Hemolysis
- Hepatitis
- Liver failure
- Mononucleosis
- Pernicious anemia
- Sickle cell disease
- Significant bile duct obstruction, such as a stone or tumor
- Transfusion reaction

In addition to the medical conditions just mentioned, the medications on the list below may also increase bilirubin levels.

- Allopurinol (Lopurin)
- Anabolic steroids
- Antibiotics, including isoniazid (Tubizid), rifampin (Rifadin), and sulfonamides
- Antimalarial drugs
- Azathioprine (Imuran)
- Chlorpropamide (Diabinese)
- Cholinergics
- Epinephrine
- MAO inhibitors
- Methotrexate (Rheumatrex)
- Methyldopa (Aldomet)
- Nicotinic acid
- Opiates, including codeine, morphine, meperidine, and oxycodone
- Oral contraceptives
- Quinidine
- Theophylline (Aerolate III)

Depending on which form of bilirubin is elevated, a high measurement can indicate different causes. High direct bilirubin suggests such problems as gallbladder dysfunction or cancer. If indirect bilirubin is raised, it may be the result of a health condition such as cirrhosis or viral hepatitis.

WHAT ARE THE SYMPTOMS OF HIGH BILIRUBIN?

Due to the color of bilirubin, a buildup of this substance will eventually result in the yellowing of the skin and the whites of the eyes known as jaundice. Other symptoms that point to an elevation of bilirubin include bone aches and pains, confusion, dark urine, dehydration, diarrhea, dizziness, edema in the abdomen or belly, fatigue, fever or chills, gastrointestinal bleeding, increased perspiration, itchiness, loss of appetite, and pale or light-colored stools.

HOW CAN HIGH BILIRUBIN BE TREATED?

High bilirubin may be lowered through medical methods such as a blood transfusion or the previously mentioned use of phototherapy, while lifestyle habits and dietary supplements may help maintain a healthy immune system, as well as proper liver and gallbladder function.

Drugs

The symptoms of high bilirubin can be frustrating and uncomfortable. This is especially true of the itchiness associated with this problem, as it cannot be reduced with the use of topical ointments, like corticosteroids, or antihistamines. If you experience itchiness due to high bilirubin, your doctor can prescribe the drug cholestyramine, which lowers bile acid, thereby reducing bilirubin and alleviating the itchy feeling. Exercising and losing weight may improve the effectiveness of this drug. If you are considering this medication, talk to your doctor to see what type of fitness program might be right for your situation.

DRUGS FOR HIGH BILIRUBIN	
Drug	**Considerations**
Cholestyramine resin (bile acid sequestrant) *Questran*	Potential side effects include blurred vision, diarrhea, fatigue, headache, liver problems, loss of appetite, memory loss, nausea, and vomiting. Bile acid sequestrants can also increase your risk of bleeding and deplete the body of essential nutrients, such as beta-carotene, calcium, folic acid, iron, magnesium, phosphorus, vitamin B_{12}, vitamin D, vitamin E, and vitamin K. Therefore, it is recommended that you take a daily multivitamin or mineral supplement while using bile acid sequestrants.

SUPPLEMENTS

Additionally, dietary supplements may help maintain the health of your liver and the strength of your immune system, which are often weakened in cases of high bilirubin. Some options are listed in the table below. Not every supplement is appropriate for every health situation, however, so talk to your healthcare provider before taking any substance to treat high bilirubin.

SUPPLEMENTS FOR HIGH BILIRUBIN		
Supplement	**Dosage**	**Considerations**
Alpha-lipoic acid	300 mg two to three times a day.	Reported to help with blood sugar uptake and use in the body. Also helps detoxify the body, protect the kidneys, and improve cholesterol levels. Make sure that the raw material provider for the product is from Europe to guarantee effectiveness.
Immpower (AHCC)	6 capsules (500 mg each) a day, 2 with each meal for the first three to four weeks. Decrease to 2 capsules a day, one in the morning and one in the evening, thereafter.	Consider taking if viral hepatitis is present. Do not use if you have kidney disease due to its high phosphorus content.
Milk thistle extract (standardized to 80-percent silymarins)	80 to 160 mg one to three times a day.	Milk thistle is reported to support liver function. May have a laxative effect and cause nausea, diarrhea, indigestion, gas, bloating, fullness or pain, and loss of appetite. Avoid if you have an allergy to ragweed and related plants, a hormone-sensitive condition, such as breast cancer or uterine fibroids, or are pregnant or breastfeeding.
N-actetyl cysteine (NAC)	400 mg twice a day.	NAC is an antioxidant that is reported to help protect against blood vessel damage and clots due to insulin resistance, diabetes, and other blood sugar regulation problems. It also helps improve the body's capacity to decrease the harmful effects of toxins. NAC has been reported to improve kidney function in laboratory and human studies, and support glutathione production in the kidneys. It is generally well tolerated when taken in recommended dosages.
Sulforaphane	50 mg one to two times a day.	Helps support liver detoxification.
Turmeric phytosome	300 to 500 mg three times a day with meals.	This is a type of turmeric extract that contains phosphatidylcholine, a beneficial phosolipid that has significantly higher absorbability.

LIFESTYLE CHANGES

If you have high bilirubin, any recommended changes to your diet will be based on the cause of the elevation. For example, if bilirubin is raised because of a bile duct obstruction, you may be advised to go on a low-fat diet. If the problem is due to liver damage, you will be told to avoid alcohol completely. A low-protein diet should also be followed if the damage is severe.

Aside from dietary changes, other lifestyle changes may also be helpful, such as decreasing your stress level and getting an adequate amount of sleep every night. Yoga or meditation can help alleviate anxiety, while a minimum of seven hours of sleep should provide adequate rest. In addition, exercise, even if it is only a small amount daily, is a good idea, as it promotes immune health, glucose regulation, and blood circulation. Finally, getting some sun will reduce bilirubin. Exposure to sunlight actually helps break down this substance in the blood.

WHAT CAUSES LOW BILIRUBIN?

Low bilirubin can be a side effect of certain drugs, including barbiturates, penicillin, caffeine, and high doses of salicylates such as aspirin. It is rare and not typically cause for alarm. It can, however, be associated with spleen dysfunction, the hardening of medium and large arteries known as *arteriosclerosis,* and the depressive mood condition called *seasonal affective disorder,* so your doctor may want to have a closer look at a low reading.

WHAT ARE THE SYMPTOMS OF LOW BILIRUBIN?

Symptoms of this problem do not result from the low bilirubin itself, but rather from the conditions to which it may be linked. For example, you may experience sudden numbness or chest pain if low bilirubin is connected to arteriosclerosis, while an underactive spleen can cause fatigue.

HOW CAN LOW BILIRUBIN BE TREATED?

If low bilirubin is a side effect of medications or other chemicals, levels should return to normal once the use of these substances is discontinued. If the issue is associated with the health conditions mentioned in the previous section, your doctor will seek to treat these underlying conditions appropriately. Low bilirubin, however, is not generally seen as a concern, and will likely not require treatment.

20. ALANINE AMINOTRANSFERASE (ALT)

Alanine aminotransferase (ALT) is an enzyme that is found in the liver and, to a lesser extent, in the muscles, heart, kidneys, and pancreas. Along with the measurement of aspartate aminotransferase (see page 186), the ALT reading is one of the most important tests used to determine liver damage or disease. Normally, blood levels of ALT are low. When the liver is diseased or damaged, however, it releases ALT into the bloodstream, causing levels of this enzyme to rise.

In healthy individuals, ALT levels can vary 10 to 30 percent from day to day, and may fluctuate by as much as 45 percent during a single day. The highest ALT levels generally occur in the afternoon and the lowest levels are typically found at night. Measured in international units per liter (IU/L), normal ranges for ALT differ slightly between men and women, and are as follows:

REFERENCE RANGES FOR ALANINE AMINOTRANSFERASE (ALT)

Category	ALT Normal Range (IU/L)
Men	0 to 55
Women	0 to 40

As the normal range for both men and women begins at 0 IU/L, there really isn't a problem with low levels of this enzyme. In fact, low levels are expected in a healthy person.

WHAT CAUSES HIGH ALT?

High ALT may occur for a wide variety of reasons. The list below includes the most common causes of this problem.

- Alcohol abuse
- Autoimmune hepatitis
- Biliary obstruction
- Chemical intoxication by heavy metals or pesticides
- Cirrhosis
- Congestive heart failure
- Diabetes or insulin resistance
- High body mass index (BMI), also known as obesity
- Influenza
- Kidney disease
- Liver disease
- Mononucleosis

- Muscular dystrophy
- Myocardial infarction
- Pancreatic dysfunction
- Strenuous exercise
- Viral hepatitis
- Vitamin B_6 deficiency

Additionally, elevated ALT may be a side effect of certain medications, including:

- Acetaminophen (Tylenol)
- Antibiotics such as tetracycline (Ala-Tet), sulfonamide (Bactrim), isoniazid (Tubizid), sulfamethoxazole (Gantanol), trimethoprim (Proloprim), and nitrofurantoin (Furadantin)
- Anticonvulsants such as phenobarbital (Solfoton), phenytoin (Dilantin), primidone (Mysoline), zonisamide (Zonegran)
- Antifungal drugs
- Cardiovascular drugs such as amiodarone (Cordarone), hydralazine (Apresoline), and quinidine (Quinidex)
- Heparin
- HMG-CoA reductase inhibitors such as atorvastatin (Lipitor), lovastatin (Mevacor), fluvastatin (Lescol), pravastatin (Pravachol), and simvastatin (Zocor)
- Methotrexate (Rheumex)
- Nonsteroidal anti-inflammatory drugs (NSAIDs), including ibuprofen (Advil) and naproxen (Aleve)
- Salicylates (aspirin)
- Tricyclic antidepressants such as amitriptyline (Elavil)
- Zileuton (Zyflo)

Finally, a few dietary supplements, including kava and red yeast rice, may also spike ALT measurements. Black cohosh is also suspected to raise ALT, though this has not been conclusively proven. Because high ALT levels are suggestive of liver disease, it is important to find out the exact reason behind such readings.

WHAT ARE THE SYMPTOMS OF HIGH ALT?

The symptoms of elevated ALT should never be ignored. See your doctor if you notice any of indicators of raised ALT, such as bone aches and pains, confusion, dark urine, dehydration, diarrhea, dizziness, edema in the abdomen or belly, fatigue, fever or chills, gastrointestinal bleeding, increased perspiration, itchiness, jaundice, loss of appetite, or pale or light-colored stool. If any of these symptoms are related to high ALT, treatment methods should be undertaken to protect the health of your liver.

HOW CAN HIGH ALT BE TREATED?

Treatment of high ALT involves supporting liver function and detoxification. If you are on medication that is metabolized in the liver, your doctor may tell you to stop or reduce the dosage, or take nutrients that can reduce ALT in spite of your drug therapy. Additional measures are provided in the following sections.

If your blood test shows a high ALT count, consult your physician to determine which supplements might be right for your situation.

SUPPLEMENTS FOR HIGH ALT

Supplement	Dosage	Considerations
Aged garlic extract	600 mg twice a day.	Aged garlic extract is used to protect the heart and blood vessels, and is reported to help decrease oxidative stress markers, including those related to blood sugar regulation problems. Aged garlic has also been reported to reduce liver enzymes and fatty liver, as well as decrease the formation of advanced glycation end-products (AGEs), which are implicated in various health problems, such as heart disease, kidney problems, and cancer. Aged garlic is not reported to interfere with blood thinners.
B-complex vitamins (containing at least 50 mg B_6)	1 tablet or capsule once a day, or as directed on the product label.	Typically listed as a B-25, B-50, or 5-100 supplement. Quality B-complex vitamins generally contain vitamins B_1 (thamin), B_2 (riboflavin), B_3 (niacin), B_5 (pantothenic acid), B_6 (pyridoxine), folic acid, and B_{12} (cyanocobalamin). Betaine (TMG) should also be added for increased protection. B vitamins can be found in quality multivitamins and mineral supplements as well. Speak to your health-care provider before taking if you have a medical condition, including anemia, diabetes, and liver problems.

Supplement	Dosage	Considerations
Magnesium	200 to 300 mg three times a day.	Use magnesium aspartate, citrate, taurate, glycinate, or any amino acid chelate. Supports bone building and balances calcium intake. The ratio of calcium-to-magnesium intake should be between 1 to 1 and 2 to 1. This supplement is reported to improve blood vessel function and insulin resistance, in addition to decreasing LDL cholesterol, total cholesterol, and triglycerides. Also essential for phase-I liver detoxification. If you experience loose stools after taking magnesium, cut your dose in half and gradually increase over the course of a few months. Consult your health-care provider for dosage advice.
Milk thistle extract (standardized to 80-percent silymarins)	160 mg two to three times a day. If phytosome is used, take 100 mg two to three times a day.	Milk thistle is reported to support liver function. May have a laxative effect and cause nausea, diarrhea, indigestion, gas, bloating, fullness or pain, and loss of appetite. Avoid if you have an allergy to ragweed and related plants, a hormone-sensitive condition such as breast cancer or uterine fibroids, or are pregnant or breastfeeding.
Probiotics	3 to 25 billion CFUs one to three times a day.	Probiotics help normalize beneficial flora in the gastrointestinal tract, which reduces production of acetaldehydes—a known cause of elevated liver enzymes. Probiotics are also reported to decrease triglyceride and cholesterol levels, and to improve BUN levels and quality of life in people with kidney disease. It's best to use heat-stable products that do not require refrigeration. If using an antibiotic, wait three hours before taking probiotics. If diarrhea occurs, decrease your dosage. If this side effect persists for longer than 48 hours, stop taking the supplement and contact your doctor. Live cultures should be guaranteed through the date of expiration on label. For optimal results, take probiotics with meals, as food improves the survivability of the cultures.

LIFESTYLE CHANGES

Dietary suggestions include limiting fatty foods, refined sugars, and carbohydrates, and refraining from alcohol consumption completely. If elevated ALT is the result of a vitamin B_6 deficiency, increase your intake of foods that contain this vitamin, such as peanuts, legumes, potatoes, and bananas. Quitting smoking is also helpful, as the habit decreases vitamin B_6 in the body.

21. ALKALINE PHOSPHATASE (ALP)

Alkaline phosphatase (ALP) is an enzyme that is produced mainly in the liver and bone, with a small amount coming from the kidneys, intestines, and, if you are pregnant, the placenta. On a blood test, elevated ALP values are used extensively as tumor markers and to diagnose liver disease, although they may also be seen in connection with bone injury, pregnancy, or skeletal growth. Normal ranges vary slightly according to gender and age, and are listed below.

REFERENCE RANGES FOR ALKALINE PHOSPHATASE (ALP)	
Category	**ALP Normal Range (IU/L)**
Men 15 to 20 years old	45 to 400
Men 20 to 60 years old	25 to 150
Men 60 to 100 years old	25 to 160
Women 15 to 20 years old	45 to 400
Women 20 to 60 years old	25 to 150
Women 60 to 100 years old	25 to 165
Target Range for Both Men and Women: 72.5 IU/L	

ALP levels should always be measured after fasting, as food ingestion can raise them by as much as 30 international units per liter (IU/L). Because an elevated ALP level can be linked to a variety of serious health conditions, your doctor will want to determine the reason behind a high reading.

WHAT CAUSES HIGH ALP?

In the case of natural bone growth, bone healing, or pregnancy, elevated ALP is expected and not a concern. On many occasions, however, a serious health condition, such as any one of the disorders or diseases listed below, is responsible for a rise in this enzyme.

- Autoimmune disorders
- Biliary obstruction
- Bone cancer
- Celiac disease
- Chemical intoxication by heavy metals or pesticides
- Cirrhosis
- Congestive heart failure

- Diabetes
- Extrahepatic and intrahepatic cholestasis
- Hyperparathyroidism
- Hypervitaminosis D
- Leukemia
- Liver cancer
- Liver disease
- Osteoblastic bone disease
- Paget's disease
- Pancreatic cancer
- Parasites
- Primary biliary cirrhosis
- Primary sclerosing cholangitis
- Pulmonary infarction
- Sepsis
- Shingles
- Viruses such as cytomegalovirus (CMV), hepatitis, and mononucleosis

In addition to high ALP levels resulting from health problems, side effects of certain drugs may also increase ALP. These substances include:

- Acetaminophen (Tylenol)
- Allopurinol (Zyloprim)
- Antibiotics
- Anticonvulsants
- Anti-inflammatories, such as ibuprofen (Advil)
- Birth control pills
- Oral hypoglycemic medications, such as metformin (Glucophage) and chlorpropamide (Diabinese)
- HMG-CoA reductase inhibitors
- Corticosteroids, such as cortisone (Prednisone)
- Phenothiazines, such as chlorpromazine (Thorazine)
- Methyltestosterone (Android)
- Methyldopa (Aldomet)
- Narcotic pain medicines (Lortab, Vicodin, Percocet)
- Propranolol (Inderal)
- Tricyclic antidepressants, such as amitriptyline (Elavil)

Even if you suspect that high ALP is the result of a medication, never stop taking a drug without talking first to your doctor.

WHAT ARE THE SYMPTOMS OF HIGH ALP?

Symptoms of high ALP include bone pain and fractures, confusion, dehydration, dark urine, diarrhea, dizziness, edema in the abdomen or belly, fatigue, fever or chills, gastrointestinal bleeding, increased perspiration, itchiness, jaundice, loss of appetite, pale or light-colored stools, and vitamin D deficiency.

HOW CAN HIGH ALP BE TREATED?

While your doctor will want to treat any underlying condition associated with elevated ALP, such as a parathyroid disorder or diabetes, you can modify your diet and lifestyle to maintain liver and bone health. Below are some helpful suggestions for improving your diet and lifestyle to support balanced ALP levels.

SUPPLEMENTS

Dietary supplements may be recommended when elevated amounts of ALP are present. The following table details the wide variety of helpful substances at your disposal. Before beginning a supplement regimen, check with your doctor to verify that the recommended dosages are appropriate for your situation.

SUPPLEMENTS FOR HIGH ALP

Supplement	Dosage	Considerations
Aged garlic extract	600 mg one to three times a day.	Aged garlic extract is used to protect the heart and blood vessels, and is reported to help decrease oxidative stress markers, including those related to blood sugar regulation problems. Aged garlic has also been reported to reduce liver enzymes and fatty liver, as well as decrease the formation of advanced glycation end-products (AGEs), which are implicated in various health problems, such as heart disease, kidney problems, and cancer. Aged garlic is not reported to interfere with blood thinners.
Immpower (AHCC)	6 capsules (500 mg each) a day, 2 with each meal for the first three to weeks. Decrease to 2 capsules a day, one in the morning and one in the evening, thereafter.	Consider taking if viral hepatitis is present. Do not use if you have kidney disease due to its high phosphorus content.
Magnesium	400 mg twice a day.	Use magnesium aspartate, citrate, taurate, glycinate, or any amino acid chelate. Supports bone building and balances calcium intake. The ratio of calcium-to-magnesium intake should be between 1 to 1 and 2 to 1. This supplement is reported to improve blood vessel function and insulin resistance, in addition to decreasing LDL cholesterol, total cholesterol, and triglycerides. Also essential for phase-I liver detoxification. If you experience loose stools after taking

Supplement	Dosage	Considerations
Magnesium *(continued)*		magnesium, cut your dose in half and gradually increase over the course of a few months. Consult your health-care provider for dosage advice.
Milk thistle extract (standardized to 80-percent silymarins)	140 to 200 mg two to three times a day.	Milk thistle is reported to support liver function. May have a laxative effect and cause nausea, diarrhea, indigestion, gas, bloating, fullness or pain, and loss of appetite. Avoid if you have an allergy to ragweed and related plants, a hormone-sensitive condition, such as breast cancer or uterine fibroids, or are pregnant or breastfeeding.

LIFESTYLE CHANGES

You may increase your intake of phytoestrogen-rich foods such as flax seed, sesame seeds, pomegranates, and soy, as phytoestrogens protect your bones. To care for your liver, cut down on the consumption of refined sugar and carbohydrates, as well as fatty foods such as fried edibles and full-fat dairy products. Doing so will reduce stress placed on the liver. In addition, the weight lost by following such a diet will improve the functioning of this organ. Opt for salads with grilled lean meats like chicken and fish. Eat more calcium-containing foods, such as green leafy vegetables and low-fat dairy products. Finally, get thirty minutes of exercise a day at least three times a week. Physical activity may help reduce risk of osteoporosis and bone fractures.

WHAT CAUSES LOW ALP?

A number of medical conditions may result in a low ALP reading, including:

- Achondroplasia
- Cardiopulmonary bypass pump use
- Congenital hypophosphatasia
- Hypothyroidism
- Magnesium deficiency
- Malnutrition
- Milk-alkali syndrome (Burnett's syndrome)
- Pernicious anemia
- Scurvy (vitamin C deficiency)
- Zinc deficiency

WHAT ARE THE SYMPTOMS OF LOW ALP?

Symptoms of low ALP include premature loss of teeth, bone fractures, and bone pain.

HOW CAN LOW ALP BE TREATED?

Low ALP should be addressed by taking action to support bone, liver, and kidney health. Specific substances that may help this goal are highlighted below.

SUPPLEMENTS

Consider the following supplements to promote healthy ALP levels. Once your doctor has determined the underlying cause of low ALP, you will be better able to identify the supplements that might be helpful. Discuss all your options with your physician.

SUPPLEMENTS FOR LOW ALP

Supplement	Dosage	Considerations
Magnesium	250 to 500 mg twice a day.	Use magnesium aspartate, citrate, taurate, glycinate, or any amino acid chelate. Supports bone building and balances calcium intake. The ratio of calcium-to-magnesium intake should be between 1 to 1 and 2 to 1. This supplement is reported to improve blood vessel function and insulin resistance, in addition to decreasing LDL cholesterol, total cholesterol, and triglycerides. Also essential for phase-I liver detoxification. If you experience loose stools after taking magnesium, cut your dose in half and gradually increase over the course of a few months. Consult your health-care provider for dosage advice.
Milk thistle extract (standardized to 80-percent silymarins)	140 to 200 mg two to three times a day.	Milk thistle is reported to support liver function. May have a laxative effect and cause nausea, diarrhea, indigestion, gas, bloating, fullness or pain, and loss of appetite. Avoid if you have an allergy to ragweed and related plants, a hormone-sensitive condition, such as breast cancer or uterine fibroids, or are pregnant or breastfeeding.
Vitamin B_{12} (cyanocobalamin)	100 to 1,000 mcg once a day.	There are no known toxicities associated with vitamin B_{12} consumption.
Zinc carnosine	1 capsule (containing 8 mg zinc and 29.5 mg L-carnosine) up to four times a day for one month, and 1 to 2 capsules two times a day thereafter.	Has been shown to enhance healing of the stomach lining, among other gastrointestinal benefits. It may also help protect the liver.

22. ASPARTATE AMINOTRANSFERASE (AST)

Aspartate aminotransferase (AST) is an enzyme mainly present in the liver, although it is found to a lesser degree in the heart, muscles, kidneys, and pancreas. AST readings are typically low unless one of these tissues are damaged and then releases this enzyme into the bloodstream. Low AST readings are generally a sign of good health and not cause for concern.

In combination with the ALT count (see page 177), AST is predominantly used to identify liver damage and disease. AST readings can fluctuate between 5 and 10 percent from one day to the next in the same individual. In addition, AST levels are generally 15 percent higher in African American men than Caucasian men, while obese men often display mildly elevated AST. Finally, moderate exercise can increase AST to almost three times the normal limit for up to twenty-four hours. AST ranges are listed below.

REFERENCE RANGES FOR ASPARTATE AMINOTRANSFERASE (AST)

AST (IU/L)	Category
Less than 5	Low
5 to 40	Normal
Greater than 40	High

The ranges can vary between laboratories, so be sure to check the reference range on your lab report.

WHAT CAUSES HIGH AST?

Elevated AST levels may occur for a number of reasons, all of which are linked by their ability to damage the liver and other tissues that contain this enzyme. They are as follows:

- Alcohol abuse
- Autoimmune hepatitis
- Biliary obstruction
- Chemical intoxication by heavy metals or pesticides
- Cirrhosis
- Congestive heart failure
- Diabetes and/or insulin resistance
- High BMI (obesity)
- Hyperthyroidism
- Influenza

- Kidney disease
- Liver disease
- Mononucleosis
- Muscular dystrophy
- Myocardial infarction (heart attack)
- Nonalcoholic steatosis
- Pancreatic dysfunction
- Strenuous exercise
- Vitamin B_6 deficiency
- Viral hepatitis

Several medications may also increase AST, including the following:

- Acetaminophen (Tylenol)
- Antibiotics such as tetracycline (Ala-tet), sulfonamide (Bactrim), isoniazid (Tubizid), sulfamethoxazole (Gantanol), trimethoprim (Proloprim), and nitrofurantoin (Furadantin)
- Anticonvulsants such as phenobarbital (Solfoton), phenytoin (Dilantin), primidone (Mysoline), and zonisamide (Zonegran)
- Antifungal drugs
- Cardiovascular drugs such as amiodarone (Cordarone), hydralazine (Apresoline), and quinidine (Quinidex)
- Heparin
- HMG-CoA reductase inhibitors such as atorvastatin (Lipitor), lovastatin (Mevacor), fluvastatin (Lescol), pravastatin (Pravachol), and simvastatin (Zocor)
- Methotrexate (Rheumex)
- Nonsteroidal anti-inflammatory drugs (NSAIDs), including ibuprofen (Advil) and naproxen (Aleve)
- Progesterone
- Salicylates (aspirin)
- Tricyclic antidepressants such as amitriptyline (Elavil)
- Zileuton (Zyflo)

Your healthcare provider will be able to identify the reason for a raised AST reading and recommend the appropriate steps to take to bring the level back to normal.

WHAT ARE THE SYMPTOMS OF HIGH AST?

See your doctor if you notice any symptoms of raised AST, including bone aches and pains, confusion, dark urine, dehydration, diarrhea, dizziness, edema in the abdomen or belly, fatigue, fever or chills, gastrointestinal bleeding, increased perspiration, itchiness, jaundice, loss of appetite, or pale or light-colored stools.

HOW CAN HIGH AST BE TREATED?

Treatment usually depends on supporting healthy liver function, which may be achieved by adopting the following lifestyle and dietary habits.

SUPPLEMENTS

Dietary supplements may also combat the health conditions that lead to high AST. The table below lists a variety of natural compounds that may be helpful.

SUPPLEMENTS FOR HIGH AST

Supplement	Dosage	Considerations
Aged garlic extract	600 mg twice a day.	Aged garlic extract is used to protect the heart and blood vessels, and is reported to help decrease oxidative stress markers, including those related to blood sugar regulation problems. Aged garlic has also been reported to reduce liver enzymes and fatty liver, as well as decrease the formation of advanced glycation end-products (AGEs), which are implicated in various health problems, such as heart disease, kidney problems, and cancer. Aged garlic is not reported to interfere with blood thinners.
Andrographis paniculata extract (standardized to 50-percent andrographolides)	150 to 500 mg once a day.	May be effective for treating the common cold, as well as reducing fever and sore throat. Avoid use if you have an autoimmune disease, such as multiple sclerosis or lupus, or are trying to father a child or become pregnant. Avoid use if you are pregnant or breastfeeding.
B-complex vitamins (containing at least 50 mg B_6)	1 tablet or capsule once a day, or as directed on the product label.	Typically listed as a B-25, B-50, or 5-100 supplement. Quality B-complex vitamins generally contain vitamins B_1 (thamin), B_2 (riboflavin), B_3 (niacin), B_5 (pantothenic acid), B_6 (pyridoxine), folic acid, and B_{12} (cyanocobalamin). Betaine (TMG)

Supplement	Dosage	Considerations
B-complex *(continued)*		should also be added for increased protection. B vitamins can be found in quality multivitamins and mineral supplements as well. Speak to your health-care provider before taking if you have a medical condition, including anemia, diabetes, and liver problems.
Cordyceps	1,100 mg twice a day.	Helps with lung function by increasing oxygen to the cells, and has shown to improve BUN and creatinine levels in laboratory studies. It is especially recommended for people who have conditions like diabetes and high blood pressure, which increase the risk of kidney failure. Also reported to support liver function. While some medical literature suggests that cordyceps rebalances immune activity, it should be used with caution if you have an autoimmune disease, such as lupus or multiple sclerosis, as it may cause the immune system to become more active.
Immpower (AHCC)	6 capsules (500 mg each) a day, 2 with each meal for the first three to four weeks. Decrease to 2 capsules a day, one in the morning and one in the evening, thereafter.	Consider taking if viral hepatitis is present. Do not use if you have kidney disease due to its high phosphorus content.
Magnesium	200 to 400 mg twice a day.	Use magnesium aspartate, citrate, taurate, glycinate, or any amino acid chelate. Supports bone building and balances calcium intake. The ratio of calcium-to-magnesium intake should be between 1 to 1 and 2 to 1. This supplement is reported to improve blood vessel function and insulin resistance, in addition to decreasing LDL cholesterol, total cholesterol, and triglycerides. Also essential for phase-I liver detoxification. If you experience loose stools after taking magnesium, cut your dose in half and gradually increase over the course of a few months. Consult your health-care provider for dosage advice.

Supplement	Dosage	Considerations
Milk thistle extract (standardized to 80-percent silymarins)	160 mg two to three times a day. If phytosome is used, take 100 mg two to three times a day.	Milk thistle is reported to support liver function. May have a laxative effect and cause nausea, diarrhea, indigestion, gas, bloating, fullness or pain, and loss of appetite. Avoid if you have an allergy to ragweed and related plants, a hormone-sensitive condition, such as breast cancer or uterine fibroids, or are pregnant or breastfeeding.
Probiotics	3 to 25 billion CFUs one to three times a day.	Probiotics help normalize beneficial flora in the gastrointestinal tract, which reduces production of acetaldehydes—a known cause of elevated liver enzymes. Probiotics are also reported to decrease triglyceride and cholesterol levels, and to improve BUN levels and quality of life in people with kidney disease. It's best to use heat-stable products that do not require refrigeration. If using an antibiotic, wait three hours before taking probiotics. If diarrhea occurs, decrease your dosage. If this side effect persists for longer than 48 hours, stop taking the supplement and contact your doctor. Live cultures should be guaranteed through the date of expiration on label. For optimal results, take probiotics with meals, as food improves the survivability of the cultures.

LIFESTYLE CHANGES

Your first step should be to eliminate alcohol consumption completely. In addition, if you smoke, quit the habit. If you are overweight, it is important that you lose the extra pounds, as obesity is associated with non-alcoholic fatty liver. Exercise three to four times a week for approximately thirty to sixty minutes, and limit fatty foods, processed foods, high-glycemic foods, and dairy in your diet. Incorporate salads into your daily meals and opt for lean meats like chicken and fish. Protecting your liver is one of the most important steps you can take when abnormal hepatic panel readings such as high AST are found on a blood test, so take the time with your doctor to discuss the all the ways by which you might boost liver function.

23. GAMMA-GLUTAMYL TRANSFERASE (GGT)

Gamma-glutamyl transferase (GGT) is an enzyme found in numerous tissues throughout the body, including the kidneys, pancreas, spleen, heart, and, most significantly, the liver. While an elevated GGT reading suggests liver damage, it cannot reveal the cause of that damage on its own. GGT levels are analyzed in conjunction with ALP levels (see page 181) to help determine the illness of a patient. If both ALP and GGT are high, bile duct disease or liver disease is suspected. If ALP is raised but GGT is not, bone disease is likely. GGT is also very sensitive to alcohol use, so its elevation may simply be caused by alcohol consumption.

GGT levels can vary 10 to 15 percent from day to day. GGT activity decreases immediately after eating, and normal ranges differ slightly according to gender, as shown in the table below.

REFERENCE RANGES FOR GAMMA-GLUTAMYL TRANSFERASE (GGT)

Category	GGT Normal Range (IU/L)	GGT Target Range (IU/L)
Men	0 to 65	32.5
Women	0 to 45	22.5

The GGT levels of healthy African Americans are typically twice as high as those of Caucasians. Additionally, GGT may be 25 to 50 percent higher in obese individuals, and 10 percent higher in one-pack-a-day smokers.

WHAT CAUSES HIGH GGT?

The cause of an abnormal GGT reading is typically determined by comparing it to other measurements of the hepatic panel. High GGT counts may be associated with the following conditions.

- Alcohol abuse
- Autoimmune hepatitis
- Biliary obstruction
- Cancer
- Chronic obstructive pulmonary disease (COPD)
- Cirrhosis
- Congestive heart failure
- Diabetes
- Excessive magnesium consumption
- Hyperthyroidism

- Influenza
- Kidney disease
- Liver disease, particularly non-alcoholic fatty liver disease (See the inset on page 193)
- Myocardial infarction (heart attack)
- Obesity
- Pancreatic dysfunction
- Rheumatoid arthritis
- Strenuous exercise
- Viral hepatitis

Dietary supplements, including kava and red yeast rice, can also raise GGT levels. Black cohosh has also been reported to elevate GGT, but this is still in question. Finally, the wide variety of medications listed below may increase GGT as well:

- Acetaminophen (Tylenol)
- Anabolic steroids
- Antibiotics such as tetracycline (Ala-tet), sulfonamide (Bactrim), isoniazid (Tubizid), sulfamethoxazole (Gantanol), trimethoprim (Proloprim), and nitrofurantoin (Furadantin)
- Anticonvulsants such as phenobarbital (Solfoton), phenytoin (Dilantin), primidone (Mysoline), and zonisamide (Zonegran)
- Antifungal drugs
- Cardiovascular drugs such as amiodarone (Cordarone), hydralazine (Apresoline), and quinidine (Quinidex)
- Heparin
- HMG-CoA reductase inhibitors such as atorvastatin (Lipitor), lovastatin (Mevacor), fluvastatin (Lescol), pravastatin (Pravachol), and simvastatin (Zocor)
- Methotrexate (Rheumex)
- Nonsteroidal anti-inflammatory drugs (NSAIDs), including ibuprofen (Advil) and naproxen (Aleve)
- Salicylates (aspirin)
- Synthetic progesterone
- Tricyclic antidepressants such as amitriptyline (Elavil)
- Zileuton (Zyflo)

Your doctor will let you know if you need to adjust the dosage of your medication or discontinue its use. Never change your medication regimen without talking to your physician.

Insulin Resistance and Nonalcoholic Fatty Liver Disease

As you now know, elevated liver enzymes usually occur as an early indication that the liver is sustaining damage. In addition to hepatitis, the most common cause of injury to the liver is fatty liver disease. Until recently, fatty liver disease was primarily associated with chronic alcohol abuse. The truth, however, is that nonalcoholic fatty liver disease is now the leading cause of elevated liver enzymes.

A diet high in refined carbohydrates and sugar can tax the body's ability to process glucose, which can lead to insulin resistance. When insulin resistance is present, the body cannot shuttle glucose out of the bloodstream properly. The liver turns the excess glucose into triglycerides, which it then attempts to expel into the body as fat. When carbohydrate and sugar intake is consistently too high, the liver cannot rid itself of these triglycerides, causing them to build up in the liver as fat. This nonalcoholic fatty liver then elevates liver enzymes.

The liver has a tremendous ability to restore damaged cells, so if the source of the fatty liver is eliminated and the damage is not too extensive, the liver can repair itself. A low-carb, low-sugar diet has been shown to reverse the conditions that lead to nonalcoholic fatty liver disease, which some predict will be the number one cause of liver transplants over the next decade. Currently, the disease affects 22 percent of those who are obese, which means the healthcare system will be facing a serious problem if people do not change their lifestyle and lose excess weight.

WHAT ARE THE SYMPTOMS OF HIGH GGT?

Symptoms of high GGT include bone aches and pains, confusion, dark urine, dehydration, diarrhea, dizziness, edema in the abdomen or belly, fatigue, fever or chills, gastrointestinal bleeding, increased perspiration, itchiness, jaundice, loss of appetite, or pale or light-colored stool.

HOW CAN HIGH GGT BE TREATED?

As stated, if high GGT is being caused by medication, you may be asked to reduce the dosage or stop the medication all together. Provided below are some lifestyle and dietary measures you can take to normalize GGT.

SUPPLEMENTS

Dietary supplements can be effective in the treatment of high GGT and as a protective measure for overall liver health. Helpful substances are listed below, but your choice of supplement will depend upon the underlying cause of elevated GGT.

SUPPLEMENTS FOR HIGH GGT		
Supplement	**Dosage**	**Considerations**
Aged garlic extract	600 mg twice a day.	Aged garlic extract is used to protect the heart and blood vessels, and is reported to help decrease oxidative stress markers, including those related to blood sugar regulation problems. Aged garlic has also been reported to reduce liver enzymes and fatty liver, as well as decrease the formation of advanced glycation end-products (AGEs), which are implicated in various health problems, such as heart disease, kidney problems, and cancer. Aged garlic is not reported to interfere with blood thinners.
GTF (Glucose Tolerance Factor) chromium	400 to 800 mcg twice a day.	Chromium is important for blood sugar and insulin regulation. Additionally, people who have a diet high in refined carbohydrates like sugar may also be low in chromium. Use under a doctor's supervision if you are diabetic, as it may affect medication dosage. Do not use if you have kidney or liver problems, chromate or leather contact allergy, or a behavioral psychiatric condition such as schizophrenia or depression.
Magnesium	400 mg twice a day.	Use magnesium aspartate, citrate, taurate, glycinate, or any amino acid chelate. Supports bone building and balances calcium intake. The ratio of calcium-to-magnesium intake should be between 1 to 1 and 2 to 1. This supplement is reported to improve blood vessel function and insulin resistance, in addition to decreasing LDL cholesterol, total cholesterol, and triglycerides. Also essential for phase-I liver detoxification. If you experience loose stools after taking magnesium, cut your dose in half and gradually increase over the course of a few months. Consult your health-care provider for dosage advice.

Supplement	Dosage	Considerations
Phosphatidyl-choline (at least 35-percent choline)	500 to 1,000 mg up to two times a day.	Low choline in the diet can result in the inability to package and transport fat out of the liver. Side effects may include upset stomach and loose stools. Theoretically, it may interact with anticholinergic or acetylcholinesterase-inhibiting drugs, since taking in choline may increase acetylcholine production.
Probiotics	5 to 10 billion CFUs two to three times a day.	Probiotics help normalize beneficial flora in the gastrointestinal tract, which reduces production of acetaldehydes—a known cause of elevated liver enzymes. Probiotics are also reported to decrease triglyceride and cholesterol levels, and to improve BUN levels and quality of life in people with kidney disease. It's best to use heat-stable products that do not require refrigeration. If using an antibiotic, wait three hours before taking probiotics. If diarrhea occurs, decrease your dosage. If this side effect persists for longer than 48 hours, stop taking the supplement and contact your doctor. Live cultures should be guaranteed through the date of expiration on label. For optimal results, take probiotics with meals, as food improves the survivability of the cultures.

LIFESTYLE CHANGES

Quitting smoking and losing weight may be recommended. You should limit high-glycemic foods and foods containing refined sugars and carbohydrates. If your gall bladder is involved, limit fatty foods as well. Vegetables, fruits, legumes, and lean meats such as chicken should be staples of your diet. You should also increase your intake of omega-3 fatty acids by eating more cold-water fish like salmon, halibut, and haddock.

WHAT CAUSES LOW GGT?

If GGT levels are consistently on the lower end of the spectrum, your doctor may suspect health conditions such as hypothalamic malfunction or hypothyroidism. Decreased GGT may also result from low amounts of magnesium in the bloodstream, or even pregnancy. Lastly, certain drugs may lower GGT. These medications include:

- Antibiotics and antifungal agents
- Antiretroviral drugs
- Birth control pills
- Cholestyramine (Questran)

- Corticosteroids
- Digoxin (Lanoxin)
- Diuretics
- Hormonal replacement therapy
- Proton-pump inhibitors such as lansoprazole (Prevacid), omeprazole (Prilosec), pantoprazole (Protonix), rabeprazole (Aciphex), and esomeprazole (Nexium)
- Salicylates such as aspirin

While low GGT levels are not as alarming as high readings, your doctor will still want to know the cause and treat the issue accordingly.

WHAT ARE THE SYMPTOMS OF LOW GGT?

Low GGT may cause symptoms that include anxiety, dry skin, fatigue, heart palpitations or arrhythmias, insomnia, muscle weakness and cramps, restless leg syndrome, and tremors, which are also signs of low magnesium and hypothyroidism.

HOW CAN LOW GGT BE TREATED?

If the underlying reason for low GGT is a health condition such as hypothalamic malfunction or hypothyroidism, your doctor will treat it with the necessary medical therapy. If low GGT is the result of low magnesium, the following supplements and dietary changes may help.

SUPPLEMENTS

The supplements below may be effective for normalizing GGT due to magnesium deficiency. However, if the cause of your low level is hypothyroidism, refer to the section on thyroid hormones (see page 268) for guidance on choosing supplements to support thyroid function.

SUPPLEMENTS FOR LOW GGT

Supplement	Dosage	Considerations
Magnesium	300 mg two to three times a day.	Use magnesium aspartate, citrate, taurate, glycinate, or any amino acid chelate. Supports bone building and balances calcium intake. The ratio of calcium-to-magnesium intake should be between 1 to 1 and 2 to 1. This supplement is reported to improve blood vessel function and insulin resistance, in addition to decreasing LDL cholesterol, total cholesterol, and triglycerides. Also essential for phase-I

Supplement	Dosage	Considerations
Magnesium *(continued)*		liver detoxification. Use magnesium aspartate, citrate, malate, taurate, threonate, or amino acid chelate. If you experience loose stools after taking magnesium, cut your dose in half and gradually increase over the course of a few months. Consult your health-care provider for dosage advice.

LIFESTYLE CHANGES

Increase your consumption of magnesium-containing foods, which include seeds, nuts, legumes, cereal grains, and dark leafy greens and vegetables. Magnesium capsules may also be recommended.

CONCLUSION

The liver is an integral part of many vital functions in the body. The health of this organ is tremendously important to monitor, which makes the hepatic panel a big component of the average blood test. While certain liver problems may seem beyond your control, there are, nevertheless, many steps you can take to lessen or avoid liver damage. They all have to do with alleviating the burden placed on this organ, as most of the recommendations in this section explain. While there are numerous helpful dietary supplements to consider, adjusting your diet can also offer significant benefits. By eating organic foods, you reduce your exposure to chemicals that would normally increase the detoxification workload of the liver. By incorporating healthful vegetables, fruits, whole grains, and lean proteins into your diet, you ensure that your body gets all the nutrients, fiber, antioxidants, and amino acids it requires to promote the liver's detoxification process. Similarly, drinking an adequate amount of water each day will help flush out toxins. Additionally, a high-antioxidant, low-sugar meal plan will protect the liver from free radical damage and even reduce the creation of these destructive substances.

While you are watching what you eat, you should also exercise and learn to control stress, as doing so will reduce your risk of insulin resistance-related fatty liver disease. And by addressing underlying causes of liver problems and easing the burden on this organ, you may be able to reduce your reliance on medications such as aspirin or ibuprofen, which are hard on the liver. The truth is that there is a lot you can do to support healthy liver function, and making these lifestyle adjustments is a good idea whether or not a blood test shows abnormal readings on your hepatic panel. Be proactive with your overall well-being and you will be amazed at the results.

PART 4

Complete Blood Count

A complete blood count, or CBC, is one of the most commonly administered lab tests. It is usually done as part of a routine physical examination, but can also be used to evaluate the effectiveness of medical treatments, as well as to identify the cause of symptoms like fatigue, weakness, and bruising. In addition, the CBC helps health-care professionals diagnose conditions such as anemia, bone marrow disorders, nutritional deficiency, and various types of infection.

Complete blood counts calculate the different types of blood cells—red blood cells (RBCs), platelets, and white blood cells (WBCs)—as well as their characteristics, such as the average concentration of hemoglobin in a red blood cell. Also included are measurements of the different kinds of white blood cells, which can change daily depending on occurrences in the body. More specifically, the complete blood count consists of the following lab values:

- **The number of red blood cells,** which carry oxygen to the cells and carbon dioxide back to the lungs to be removed from the body. A decrease in red blood cells can cause an oxygen deficit and lead to *anemia*—a low count of RBCs—while an increase may raise the risk of clotting.

- **The concentration of hemoglobin,** iron-containing molecules in red blood cells that act as the vehicle for oxygen and carbon dioxide transport.

- **Hematocrit,** the proportion of blood volume that contains red blood cells, which should be significantly greater than the proportions of white blood cells and platelets.

- **Mean corpuscular volume (MCV),** which is a calculation of the average size of a red blood cell. This measurement is also used to determine red cell distribution width (RDW), a number that represents the variation in size among red blood cells.

- **Mean corpuscular hemoglobin (MCH),** or the average amount of hemoglobin contained in a single red blood cell.

- **Mean corpuscular hemoglobin concentration (MCHC),** a measurement of the amount of hemoglobin found in a group of red blood cells rather than only one.

- **The number of platelets,** which are tiny cell fragments essential for clotting. Too few platelets can cause abnormal bleeding, while an excess contributes to unnecessary clot formation, increasing the risk of heart attack, stroke, and pulmonary embolism.

- **The number of white blood cells,** which serve as a vital part of the immune system by protecting the body from foreign bacteria, viruses, and other pathogens. The five basic white blood cell types are neutrophils, lymphocytes, monocytes, eosinophils, and basophils, all of which play distinct roles in maintaining immunity. They also exist in different amounts that fluctuate depending on whether an infection or illness is present.

Abnormal readings of these values frequently, but do not necessarily, indicate a medical problem. As you learn about the various causes, symptoms, and treatment methods for high and low counts in this section, remember that this information is not intended to replace the advice of your physician.

Consider This

Blood has three basic components: 55 percent is plasma, the fluid in which the red and white blood cells are suspended; 45 percent is made up of red blood cells, which carry oxygen to your body's cells and remove carbon dioxide from them; and less than 1 percent is composed of white blood cells, which fight infection and disease. In addition, plasma also contains cells called platelets, which help the blood clot in the event of an injury.

24. RED BLOOD CELLS

Red blood cells (RBCs) are the most plentiful type of cell in the blood, accounting for approximately 40 to 45 percent of the body's blood supply. These cells are responsible for carrying oxygen to the tissues and organs, as well as for bringing carbon dioxide back to the lungs so that it can be removed (exhaled) from the body. Red blood cells derive their color from the protein *hemoglobin* (see page 210), which is contained in each cell and serves as the vehicle of oxygen and carbon dioxide transport. With an average lifespan of 120 days, RBCs are constantly being replenished. A hormone known as *erythropoietin* (EPO), which is secreted mainly by the kidneys, plays a vital role in RBC production by stimulating stem cells in the bone marrow to produce more red blood cells when oxygen levels decrease. EPO also helps boost the rate at which red blood cells reach maturity. Iron, folate (also known as folic acid or vitamin B_9), and vitamin B_{12} are required for the manufacture of RBCs as well.

Normal ranges for red blood cell counts, which are expressed as cells per microliter (cells/mcL), vary according to age and sex.

REFERENCE RANGES FOR RED BLOOD CELL COUNTS

Category	Normal RBC Count (cells/mcL)
Men	4.7 to 6.1 million
Women	4.2 to 5.4 million
Children and Adolescents (under 18 years of age)	4.0 to 5.5 million
Infants	4.8 to 7.1 million

A red blood cell count is usually performed during a routine physical and is used to help diagnose *polycythemia* (high red blood cell count), *anemia* (low blood cell count), and various blood disorders. If an abnormality is detected, other values in the complete blood count, or CBC, are examined to identify the cause of the imbalance.

WHAT CAUSES A HIGH RED BLOOD CELL COUNT?

There are numerous reasons for a high red blood cell count, or polycythemia. RBC production increases when the body's oxygen levels are low because of a medical condition or because the external oxygen supply is limited, such as at high-altitude locations. The number of red blood cells also rises when the kidneys release too much erythropoietin, causing the bone marrow's stem cells to produce more RBCs. Moreover, a decrease in blood plasma, the liquid part of the blood, can also lead to higher levels of red blood cells. Each of these processes can be triggered by a number of factors, including:

- Bone marrow disorders, including *polycythemia vera* (primary polycythemia)
- Chronic obstructive pulmonary disease (COPD)
- Congenital heart disease
- Dehydration
- Heart failure
- Hemoglobinopathies, genetic defects that impair the ability of RBCs to transport oxygen efficiently
- Kidney cancer
- Kidney transplant
- Living at high altitudes, where oxygen levels are lower
- Medications such as anabolic steroids, erythropoietin (EPO), gentamicin (Gentamicin), and methyldopa (Aldomet)
- Pulmonary fibrosis
- Smoking
- Various types of heart and lung disease

The complications of high RBC counts vary depending on the type of polycythemia present. In primary polycythemia, which is an inherent (rather than acquired) disorder of the bone marrow, the high number of RBCs increases the thickness of the blood and, therefore, slows down the rate at which it flows through the body. This raises the risk of blood clot formation, which can cause a heart attack, stroke, or pulmonary embolism. Primary polycythemia can also create additional clotting problems and kidney dysfunction. Very rarely, the condition can turn into leukemia. The complications of secondary polycythemia—an elevated RBC count caused by other health conditions—are usually related to the underlying illness or disorder, and thus vary widely.

WHAT ARE THE SYMPTOMS OF A HIGH RED BLOOD CELL COUNT?

In some people, an elevated red blood cell count may not produce any symptoms, while others may have nonspecific symptoms such as abdominal bloating, dizziness, fatigue, and headache. For reasons that have not yet been determined, people who have primary polycythemia may experience itchiness, usually right after showering or bathing. Physical indicators such as chest pain and shortness of breath are also possible, particularly in those who have heart or respiratory problems due to their high red blood cell count.

HOW CAN A HIGH RED BLOOD CELL COUNT BE TREATED?

Treatment for elevated red blood cells depends on the cause. Treatments with drugs, supplements, and lifestyle modification are detailed below.

DRUGS

The main therapy for primary polycythemia is phlebotomy, or the drawing of blood, but medications such as hydroxyurea (Hydrea) and antiplatelet drugs may also be used to prevent the formation of blood clots. These medications are potentially unsafe for those who have clotting problems, however, and should be avoided by these patients. High RBC counts due to other medical conditions (secondary polycythemia) can be managed by treating the underlying problem, such as dehydration, heart disease, or lung disease.

LIFESTYLE CHANGES

In general, people who have an excess of red blood cells should limit their intake of foods that are high in iron, folate, and vitamin B_{12}, which are essential nutrients for RBC production. People who do a great deal of aerobic exercise generally have higher RBC and hemoglobin counts, since their bodies require more oxygen—which is delivered via hemoglobin (see page 210). Your doctor will design a treatment plan and provide appropriate recommendations based on the specifics of your condition.

WHAT CAUSES A LOW RED BLOOD CELL COUNT?

Anemia, the most common blood disorder among the US population, is the name given to any deficiency of healthy red blood cells. There are more than 400 types of anemia, which can be grouped into three main categories: (1) Anemia caused by bleeding, (2) anemia caused by the reduction of red blood cells or the production of defective red blood cells, and (3) anemia caused by the premature destruction of red blood cells. The types of anemia that fall into these three categories, as well as their common causes, are discussed in this section.

ANEMIA CAUSED BY BLEEDING

Loss of blood over time, which is known as chronic bleeding, can lead to anemia. Common causes of this general type of anemia include gastrointestinal problems, like hemorrhoids and ulcers, as well as menstruation and prolonged use of NSAIDs, such as aspirin and ibuprofen.

ANEMIA CAUSED BY REDUCED OR DEFECTIVE RED BLOOD CELLS

There are a number of conditions that can cause a reduction in the body's level of red blood cells or, alternatively, result in the production of abnormal red blood cells that lack the ability to properly function. The kinds of anemia that fall into this category include:

- **Aplastic anemia.** This type of anemia is caused by problems with the bone marrow, which may either be inherited or induced by external factors such as medication (chloramphenicol), infection, or chemotherapy or radiation treatment. The bone marrow fails to produce stem cells, many of which eventually develop into red blood cells. The result is an absence of RBCs.

- **Anemia of chronic disease.** People who have chronic illnesses very often also have low red blood cell counts. Advanced kidney disease, cancer (especially blood cancers like leukemia and multiple myeloma), hypothyroidism, and autoimmune diseases such as lupus can all cause anemia.

- **Iron-deficiency anemia.** The body requires iron to make hemoglobin, the RBC component that acts as the vehicle for oxygen transport. Iron-deficiency anemia can be caused by breastfeeding or pregnancy, a diet lacking in iron-rich foods, endurance training, and menstruation. People who donate blood very frequently or suffer from digestive disorders like Crohn's disease may also develop iron-deficiency anemia.

- **Megaloblastic anemia.** This occurs due to a deficiency of folate (folic acid) or vitamin B_{12}, which are needed to manufacture red blood cells. A diet low or lacking in meat and/or vegetables can result in a deficiency of these nutrients. The drug phenytoin (Dilantin) can also lead to megaloblastic anemia, since it can reduce the amount of folate in the body.

- **Pernicious anemia.** When the body cannot absorb vitamin B_{12}, pernicious anemia develops. Possible causes include Crohn's disease, parasitic infections of the intestinal tract, and other medical conditions.

- **Sickle cell anemia.** A genetic disorder that mainly affects African Americans, sickle cell anemia is characterized by the production of abnormal red blood cells shaped like crescents, or sickles. These defective RBCs break down quickly, so the amount of oxygen able to reach tissues and organs is greatly diminished.

- **Thalassemia.** As an inherited condition, thalassemia—a disorder in which RBCs do not grow properly—mostly affects people of African, Mediterranean, Middle Eastern, and Southeast Asian descent. However, it can also develop as a result of lead exposure or poisoning.

Additional causes of anemias in this category include alcohol abuse, certain medications, and intestinal disorders such as celiac disease.

ANEMIA CAUSED BY RED BLOOD CELL DESTRUCTION

There are a number of reasons for the development of *hemolytic anemia*, or anemia caused by the premature destruction of RBCs. It may be inherited—as in the cases of sickle cell anemia and thalassemia, which also fall into this group—or occur as a result of infection, the use of certain medications like quinidine, or the presence of toxins in the body due to liver or kidney disease. Severe burns, chemical exposure, high blood pressure, and blood clotting disorders can also cause hemolytic anemia.

Regardless of the type, anemia tends to cause hypoxia, or low oxygen levels in the body, since there are not enough red blood cells to provide an adequate amount of oxygen to the cells. Insufficient oxygen can cause fatigue and lower your capacity for physical activity. Most cases of anemia are mild enough to be easily managed and do not cause major complications. However, if left untreated, severe anemia can damage organs and bring about heart arrhythmias or heart failure, especially in the elderly and people who suffer from other serious medical conditions.

WHAT ARE THE SYMPTOMS OF A LOW RED BLOOD CELL COUNT?

Symptoms of a low blood cell count are dependent on the severity of the condition. In cases of chronic anemia, the body may adjust to decreased oxygen levels and, in effect, no physical symptoms occur. When symptoms are present, however, they usually include weakness and fatigue, shortness of breath, pale skin, headache, heart palpitations, dizziness, mental confusion, and loss of sex drive.

HOW CAN A LOW RED BLOOD CELL COUNT BE TREATED?

Different types of anemia require different treatments. Depending on the specific cause of your low red blood cell count, as well as the severity of your symptoms, your doctor may treat you with fluids, oxygen therapy, or, if appropriate, injections of erythropoietin (EPO), iron, or vitamin B_{12}. Severe cases of anemia may call for a blood transfusion, bone marrow transplant, or other aggressive treatment. Low counts caused by mild nutritional deficiencies, however, can usually be treated as follows.

SUPPLEMENTS

Nutritional supplements may be helpful for raising your red blood cell count, but again, ask your doctor's advice before beginning use. The supplements below can increase red blood cells by improving nutrient absorption, correcting a nutritional deficiency, strengthening RBCs, or enhancing the body's use of oxygen. Keep in mind that the supplements listed here will not necessarily address your particular problem. Once you know the cause of your anemia, ask a healthcare professional if there is an appropriate supplement for you to take.

SUPPLEMENTS FOR LOW RBC COUNTS

Supplement	Dosage	Considerations
B-complex vitamins (containing at least 50 mg B_6)	1 tablet or capsule once a day, or as directed on the product label.	Typically listed as a B-25, B-50, or 5-100 supplement. Quality B-complex vitamins generally contain vitamins B_1 (thamin), B_2 (riboflavin), B_3 (niacin), B_5 (pantothenic acid), B_6 (pyridoxine), folic acid, and B_{12} (cyanocobalamin). Betaine (TMG) should also be added for increased protection. B vitamins can be found in quality multivitamins and mineral supplements as well. Speak to your health-care provider before taking if you have a medical condition, including anemia, diabetes, and liver problems.
Coenzyme Q_{10} (CoQ_{10})	30 mg three times a day or 50 mg twice a day, depending on dose per capsule.	CoQ_{10} is important for energy production, oxygen use, high blood pressure, and heart health, especially in people with kidney disorders. It can also boost endurance, improve insulin sensitivity, and lower triglycerides and blood glucose levels. This supplement is especially recommended if you are taking statin drugs, red yeast rice, and certain diabetes medications, which may result in a CoQ_{10} deficiency.

Supplement	Dosage	Considerations
Iron	325 mg (1 tablet) once a day.	May temporarily cause constipation or stomach cramps. Men should not use unless under a doctor's order.
Phosphatidyl-serine	100 mg three times a day.	Helps to build the cell walls of red blood cells. Do not take if you are on blood-thinning medication or drugs for depression, glaucoma, or Alzheimer's disease. Do not use if you are pregnant or breast-feeding. Side effects may include insomnia and upset stomach.
Probiotics	3 to 10 billion CFUs two to three times a day.	Probiotics help normalize beneficial flora in the gastrointestinal tract, and are reported to decrease triglyceride and cholesterol levels. They are also reported to improve BUN levels and quality of life in people with kidney disease. It's best to use heat-stable products that do not require refrigeration. If using an antibiotic, wait three hours before taking probiotics. If diarrhea occurs, decrease your dosage. If this side effect persists for longer than 48 hours, stop taking the supplement and contact your doctor. Live cultures should be guaranteed through the date of expiration on label. For optimal results, take probiotics with meals, as food improves the survivability of the cultures.
Rhodiola (standardized)	150 to 300 mg one to three times a day.	Improves cellular oxygen levels and energy production. Side effects are rare, but may include irritability and insomnia.
Vitamin C (ascorbic acid/ ascorbate)	1,000 mg once a day.	Vitamin C has been found to lower CRP by about 25 percent when levels are elevated and increase iron absorption. Doses higher than 5,000 mg per day may cause diarrhea. Mineral ascorbates and Ester-C are buffered forms of vitamin C that decrease the likelihood of diarrhea. Do not take in large doses if you are prone to gout or kidney stones.

LIFESTYLE CHANGES

A low RBC count caused by a folate, iron, or vitamin B_{12} deficiency, though, can usually be corrected by restoring these nutrients to normal levels. Unless you have a disorder that prevents absorption of these nutrients, increasing your intake of the foods in the table on the following page should help correct anemia tied to an iron, folate, or vitamin B_{12} deficiency.

FOODS CONTAINING KEY NUTRIENTS FOR RBC PRODUCTION		
Iron	**Folate**	**Vitamin B_{12}**
• Artichokes • Chickpeas (garbanzo beans) • Dried beans • Dried fruits, such as prunes and raisins • Egg yolks • Iron-fortified cereals and grains • Leafy green vegetables, including collards, kale, and spinach • Lentils • Liver • Nuts, especially almonds, Brazil nuts, and cashews • Red meat • Scallops • Shellfish, particularly clams and oysters • Turkey or chicken giblets	• Asparagus • Beets • Black beans • Broccoli • Brewer's yeast • Brussels sprouts • Cantaloupe • Cauliflower • Chickpeas • Eggs • Fortified cereals • Grapefruit • Kidney beans • Leafy green vegetables, including spinach, collards, mustard and turnip greens • Lentils • Lima beans • Liver • Oranges • Papaya • Pinto beans • Romaine lettuce • Sprouts • Squash • String beans • Sunflower seeds • Wheat germ • Whole grain breads and cereals	• Cheese, particularly Swiss, Gjetost, mozzarella, and parmesan • Crab • Eggs • Fish, especially mackerel, herring, salmon, tuna, sardines, and cod • Fortified cereals • Lamb (mutton) • Liver • Lobster • Meat and poultry (beef, bison, chicken, turkey) • Shellfish (clams, oysters, mussels)

Be sure to buy organic, grass-fed beef that is free of hormones, antibiotics, and other potentially harmful substances. Also, choose lean, skinless cuts of poultry from free-range sources. Do not buy processed, packaged, or deli meats, which are usually filled with chemical additives. Additionally, if you are trying to increase your iron stores, avoid tea, which can inhibit the body's absorption of iron due to the presence of a substance called tannins in the tea. Coffee should be consumed at least one hour before or after taking in iron-containing foods or supplements. Also keep in mind that a single boiled egg can reduce iron absorption by as much as 28 percent in a given meal, so limit your intake.

In addition to following a balanced, iron-rich diet, you should also limit the number of times you exercise per week if you are iron deficient. Too much exercise can cause deformities in red blood cells and make them clump together, hindering oxygen transport. This is why athletes are susceptible to iron loss and, therefore, low red blood cell counts. Exercise in moderation and choose low-impact activities such as swimming, yoga, dancing, and aerobics.

Finally, choose the substances that you put in your body wisely. If you regularly use antacids or over-the-counter ulcer medication, be aware that these drugs may be depleting your iron reserves. Low acid production in the body leads to low iron levels, so consult your physician before taking a medicine that may further reduce your iron.

Did You Know?

Blood gets its color from a protein in red blood cells called hemoglobin. When oxygen attaches to the iron in hemoglobin, light reflection makes the chemical bond that forms between them appear red. The exact shade of red thus depends on the volume of oxygen within; brighter red blood contains more oxygen, darker red blood, less. Contrary to popular belief, at no point is your blood actually blue; the effect is essentially an optical illusion.

25. HEMOGLOBIN

The main component of red blood cells, hemoglobin (Hgb) is a protein molecule that does the physical transporting of oxygen and carbon dioxide through the body: Molecules of oxygen and carbon dioxide attach themselves to the hemoglobin, which delivers oxygen to cells and tissues, and returns carbon dioxide to the lungs to be exhaled. The hemoglobin, which contains iron, is also what gives RBCs their red color and proper circular shape.

Hemoglobin and red blood cell counts are obviously interconnected, but they are not always directly proportional, as red blood cells may contain unequal amounts of hemoglobin. In other words, even if your RBC count is normal, you may still have a higher- or lower-than-normal concentration of hemoglobin in your blood. Hemoglobin tests are often used to determine the severity of polycythemia, anemia, and bleeding disorders, but are also performed as part of a routine physical examination. Measured in grams per deciliter (g/dL), normal ranges for hemoglobin counts differ depending on an individual's age and sex. It's important to note that hemoglobin counts of endurance athletes can be as much as 30 percent higher than that of the average adult, which is considered normal.

REFERENCE RANGES FOR HEMOGLOBIN COUNTS

Category	Normal Hemoglobin (g/dL)
Men	14 to 18
Women	12 to 16
Children and Adolescents (under eighteen years of age)	11 to 13

Like other blood values, slightly high or slightly low levels of hemoglobin may be normal for some people. Still, if your blood test shows that your hemoglobin count falls too far outside the normal range for your demographic, your doctor will probably order more comprehensive testing to determine the cause.

WHAT CAUSES HIGH HEMOGLOBIN?

The causes of elevated hemoglobin levels coincide with those of high red blood cell counts. When RBC production increases due to low blood oxygen levels, heart or lung problems, an excess of the hormone erythropoietin (EPO), or bone marrow dysfunction, hemoglobin levels will also rise. More specific causes of high hemoglobin include:

- Dehydration
- Heart problems, including congenital heart disease and heart failure
- Kidney cancer
- Liver cancer
- Living at high altitudes
- Medications such as anabolic steroids (including testosterone) and methyldopa (Aldomet), a drug used to treat high blood pressure
- Overuse of EPO injections, which may be used to enhance athletic performance (blood doping)
- Polycythemia
- Poor lung function due to chronic obstructive pulmonary disease (COPD), emphysema, pulmonary fibrosis, or other lung diseases
- Smoking

High levels of hemoglobin are associated with increased blood thickness, which can slow down the flow of blood and, in turn, hinder oxygen transport. Clot formation is another possible complication of elevated hemoglobin, raising the risk of heart attacks, strokes, pulmonary embolisms, and blood clots elsewhere in the body.

WHAT ARE THE SYMPTOMS OF HIGH HEMOGLOBIN?

Symptoms caused by elevated hemoglobin levels are often linked to decreased oxygen levels. Indicators of poor oxygen circulation include bluish toes and fingers, as well as impaired mental function. Nonspecific symptoms of elevated hemoglobin levels are abdominal bloating, fatigue, headache, and shortness of breath.

HOW CAN HIGH HEMOGLOBIN BE TREATED?

Elevated hemoglobin by itself is not considered a disorder, but rather a symptom or result of a medical condition. Therefore, treatment must target the underlying cause.

LIFESTYLE CHANGES

Depending on the reason for your high level, your doctor may recommend decreasing your consumption of red meat and other foods rich in iron, since an excess of the nutrient is connected to elevated concentrations of hemoglobin. While lifestyle and dietary adjustments may not be enough to lower hemoglobin in all cases, they are helpful for long-term management of the condition and may reduce complications. After a thorough evaluation of your condition and symptoms, your doctor will decide a course of treatment that is right for you.

WHAT CAUSES LOW HEMOGLOBIN?

While not always a sign of illness, low hemoglobin levels can also be caused by a number of diseases and disorders characterized by low red blood cell counts, premature destruction of red blood cells, or blood loss. These include:

- Acute or chronic blood loss due to wounds, frequent blood donation, heavy menstrual periods, or bleeding of the gastrointestinal or urinary tract
- Anemia (aplastic, iron-deficiency, sickle cell, thalassemia, vitamin-deficiency)
- Bone marrow disorders
- Cancer, including leukemia, lymphoma (Hodgkin's and non-Hodgkin's), and multiple myeloma
- Cirrhosis of the liver
- Hypothyroidism
- Inflammation of the blood vessels (vasculitis)
- Kidney dysfunction or kidney failure
- Overhydration
- Medications, including certain chemotherapy drugs, phenytoin (Dilantin), and quinidine (Quinidex)

Keep in mind, though, that low hemoglobin is not necessarily a cause for concern. Some young women may have naturally low hemoglobin counts due to menstruation, and it's normal for levels to decrease during pregnancy.

WHAT ARE THE SYMPTOMS OF LOW HEMOGLOBIN?

Mild cases of low hemoglobin are common and generally symptom free. When a low level is due to anemia or another medical condition, however, dizziness, general weakness and fatigue, headache, and heart palpitations may occur. Report any symptom that persists or worsens to your doctor.

HOW CAN LOW HEMOGLOBIN BE TREATED?

If a low hemoglobin count requires treatment, therapy is always directed at the cause. Treatments for various types of anemia (see pages 203 to 209) are often appropriate, since low hemoglobin and low red blood cell counts are interrelated.

SUPPLEMENTS

The following nutritional supplements—which are also recommended for low red blood cell counts—may be effective for normalizing hemoglobin levels. Before deciding to take one of the substances below, discuss the supplement with your doctor or another knowledgeable healthcare professional.

SUPPLEMENTS FOR LOW HEMOGLOBIN

Supplement	Dosage	Considerations
B-complex vitamins (containing at least 50 mg B_6)	1 tablet or capsule once a day, or as directed on the product label.	Typically listed as a B-25, B-50, or 5-100 supplement.Quality B-complex vitamins generally contain vitamins B_1 (thamin), B_2 (riboflavin), B_3 (niacin), B_5 (pantothenic acid), B_6 (pyridoxine), folic acid, and B_{12} (cyanocobalamin). Betaine (TMG) should also be added for increased protection. B vitamins can be found in quality multivitamins and mineral supplements as well. Speak to your health-care provider before taking if you have a medical condition, including anemia, diabetes, and liver problems.
Coenzyme Q_{10} (CoQ_{10})	30 mg three times a day or 50 mg twice a day, depending on dose per capsule.	CoQ_{10} is important for energy production, oxygen use, high blood pressure, and heart health, especially in people with kidney disorders. It can also boost endurance, improve insulin sensitivity, and lower triglycerides and blood glucose levels. This supplement is especially recommended if you are taking statin drugs, red yeast rice, and certain diabetes medications, which may result in a CoQ_{10} deficiency.

Supplement	Dosage	Considerations
Iron	325 mg (1 tablet) once a day.	May temporarily cause constipation or stomach cramps. Men should not use unless under a doctor's order.
Phosphatidyl-serine	100 mg three times a day.	Helps to build the cell walls of red blood cells. Do not take if you are on blood-thinning medication or drugs for depression, glaucoma, or Alzheimer's disease. Do not use if you are pregnant or breastfeeding. Side effects may include insomnia and upset stomach.
Probiotics	3 to 10 billion CFUs two to three times a day.	Probiotics help normalize beneficial flora in the gastro-intestinal tract, and are reported to decrease triglyceride and cholesterol levels. They are also reported to improve BUN levels and quality of life in people with kidney disease. It's best to use heat-stable products that do not require refrigeration. If using an antibiotic, wait three hours before taking probiotics. If diarrhea occurs, decrease your dosage. If this side effect persists for longer than 48 hours, stop taking the supplement and contact your doctor. Live cultures should be guaranteed through the date of expiration on label. For optimal results, take probiotics with meals, as food improves the survivability of the cultures.
Rhodiola (standardized)	150 to 300 mg one to three times a day.	Improves cellular oxygen levels and energy production. Side effects are rare but may include irritability and insomnia.
Vitamin C (ascorbic acid/ ascorbate)	1,000 mg once a day.	Vitamin C has been found to lower CRP by about 25 percent when levels are elevated and increase iron absorption. Doses higher than 5,000 mg per day may cause diarrhea. Mineral ascorbates and Ester-C are buffered forms of vitamin C that decrease the likelihood of diarrhea. Do not take in large doses if you are prone to gout or kidney stones.

LIFESTYLE CHANGES

Low hemoglobin levels linked to a nutritional deficiency can be easily remedied with dietary changes. Refer to the table on page 208 for lists of foods that are rich in iron, folate, and vitamin B_{12}. Increasing your intake of these foods will greatly help you raise your hemoglobin count. Be sure to also limit your intake of tea, which can inhibit your absorption of iron, and if you drink coffee, consume it at least one hour before or after eating iron-containing foods or taking iron supplements.

26. HEMATOCRIT

Hematocrit is the proportion of your total blood volume that contains red blood cells. This measurement is not the same as a red blood cell count; it is expressed as a percentage and depends on both the number and size of the red blood cells. A hematocrit value reflects the proportion of your red blood cells in relation to the proportions of other cells present in your blood, and indicates if you have too many or too few RBCs. This value is needed in order to carry out an accurate assessment of anemia, polycythemia, and other blood disorders. It is also useful to reference when determining if an individual is dehydrated, or has a chronic disease or underlying malignancy. Normal hematocrit ranges for the average adult male, adult female, and child are provided in the table.

REFERENCE RANGES FOR HEMATOCRIT	
Category	**Normal Hematocrit (%)**
Men	36 to 50
Women	34 to 44
Children and Adolescents (under 18 years of age)	29 to 40

If the results of your complete blood count show that your hematocrit value is slightly higher or slightly lower than normal, it does not necessarily mean that you have a disease. Your doctor will evaluate your hematocrit alongside other lab values, as well as any reported symptoms.

WHAT CAUSES HIGH HEMATOCRIT?

The causes of high hematocrit values are generally the same as the causes of elevated red blood cell and hemoglobin counts. Among the many reasons for a high proportion of red blood cells are:

- Bone marrow disorders resulting in the overproduction of RBCs, such as polycythemia vera
- Congenital heart disease
- Dehydration
- Kidney disease
- Living at high altitudes
- Lung diseases such as emphysema and pulmonary fibrosis
- Overuse of erythropoietin (EPO) injections for athletic performance enhancement (blood doping)
- Smoking

If your hematocrit value is consistently high for an extended period of time, the cause of the abnormality will be investigated by your doctor in order to prevent complications.

WHAT ARE THE SYMPTOMS OF HIGH HEMATOCRIT?

The physical signs of high hematocrit values vary and are linked to the cause of the high level. The symptoms that occur are often the same as those associated with elevated hemoglobin counts—abdominal bloating, fatigue, headache, and shortness of breath.

HOW CAN HIGH HEMATOCRIT BE TREATED?

A high proportion of red blood cells can be corrected only by first treating the underlying medical issue. Your healthcare provider will determine an appropriate treatment based on the specific details of the condition.

LIFESTYLE CHANGES

Taking the necessary steps to improve your health will make a significant difference in how you feel each day. Adjust your diet by eating meat and other iron-rich foods in sparing quantities, as excessive iron intake can cause an increase in red blood cell production. You should also exercise for thirty to sixty minutes about three to four times per week, and maintain adequate hydration, which dilutes the number of red blood cells per volume. Dehydration, on the other hand, concentrates red blood cells by volume.

WHAT CAUSES LOW HEMATOCRIT?

A lower-than-normal proportion of red blood cells is generally caused by blood disorders, such as anemia, that result in an inadequate supply of healthy RBCs. However, since hematocrit test results reflect a *proportion* rather than a number, a low value can also indicate a surplus of white blood cells (WBCs), which normally make up a comparatively small portion of the blood. An excess of WBCs is typically a sign of an illness or infection, but may also signify that a more serious disease like cancer is present in the body. (See page 240 for more about white blood cell counts.) Specific causes of low hematocrit values include:

- Acute or chronic blood loss due to wounds, frequent blood donation, heavy menstrual periods, or internal bleeding, for example

- Anemia, including anemia of chronic disease, sickle cell anemia, thalassemia, iron-deficiency anemia, and megaloblastic anemia (anemia caused by vitamin B_{12} or folate deficiency)
- Certain types of cancer, particularly bone cancers and colon cancer
- Chronic inflammation
- Cirrhosis of the liver
- Infection
- Kidney failure
- Malnutrition
- Medications, such as certain chemotherapy drugs
- Overhydration

Women who are pregnant may also experience a temporary decrease in their hematocrit value due to increased fluid in their blood. The condition usually corrects itself after childbirth.

WHAT ARE THE SYMPTOMS OF LOW HEMATOCRIT?

Since anemia is a common cause of low hematocrit, symptoms of the disorder may be experienced depending on the severity of the condition. These include weakness, fatigue, rapid heartbeat, and dizziness, among others. However, an array of symptoms may occur, as low hematocrit is associated with a wide range of disorders.

HOW CAN LOW HEMATOCRIT BE TREATED?

Treatment for low hematocrit values depend on the underlying condition causing them, as well as the severity of that condition. A blood transfusion is one of the most aggressive treatments available, but this is used only in critical cases when there are no other options. In many cases, supplements and lifestyle adjustments can help correct the problem.

SUPPLEMENTS

The following supplements promote nutritional well-being and proper blood cell counts. Talk to your doctor before taking any substance, and inquire about dosage and potential side effects.

SUPPLEMENTS FOR LOW HEMATOCRIT		
Supplement	**Dosage**	**Considerations**
B-complex vitamins (containing at least 50 mg B_6)	1 tablet or capsule once a day, or as directed on the product label.	Typically listed as a B-25, B-50, or 5-100 supplement. Quality B-complex vitamins generally contain vitamins B_1 (thamin), B_2 (riboflavin), B_3 (niacin), B_5 (pantothenic acid), B_6 (pyridoxine), folic acid, and B_{12} (cyanocobalamin). Betaine (TMG) should also be added for increased protection. B vitamins can be found in quality multivitamins and mineral supplements as well. Speak to your health-care provider before taking if you have a medical condition, including anemia, diabetes, and liver problems.
Coenzyme Q_{10} (CoQ_{10})	30 mg three times a day or 50 mg twice a day, depending on dose per capsule.	CoQ_{10} is important for energy production, oxygen use, high blood pressure, and heart health, especially in people with kidney disorders. It can also boost endurance, improve insulin sensitivity, and lower triglycerides and blood glucose levels. This supplement is especially recommended if you are taking statin drugs, red yeast rice, and certain diabetes medications, which may result in a CoQ_{10} deficiency.
Iron	325 mg (1 tablet) once a day.	May temporarily cause constipation or stomach cramps. Men should not use unless under a doctor's order.
Phosphatidylserine	100 mg three times a day.	Helps to build the cell walls of red blood cells. Do not take if you are on blood-thinning medication or drugs for depression, glaucoma, or Alzheimer's disease. Do not use if you are pregnant or breastfeeding. Side effects may include insomnia and upset stomach.
Vitamin C (ascorbic acid/ ascorbate)	1,000 mg once a day.	Vitamin C has been found to lower CRP by about 25 percent when levels are elevated and increase iron absorption. Doses higher than 5,000 mg per day may cause diarrhea. Mineral ascorbates and Ester-C are buffered forms of vitamin C that decrease the likelihood of diarrhea. Do not take in large doses if you are prone to gout or kidney stones.

LIFESTYLE CHANGES

Low hematocrit caused by nutritional deficiency, though, can be remedied by adding the appropriate foods to your diet. (See the table on page 208 for foods rich in iron, folate, and vitamin B_{12}.) If the deficiency is severe, your doctor may recommend vitamin B_{12} injections to restore normal levels quickly. Still, you should adjust your diet and lifestyle as well to ensure that you maintain sufficient levels of these nutrients and, therefore, prevent anemia.

27. MEAN CORPUSCULAR VOLUME (MCV)

Mean corpuscular volume (MCV) is a measurement of the average volume, or size, of your red blood cells. *Macrocytosis* is the term used to describe larger-than-normal red blood cells, or high MCV, and *microcytosis* is the name for abnormally small red blood cells, or low MCV. The reference ranges used by most labs for this calculation, which is expressed in femtoliters, are provided in the table.

REFERENCE RANGES FOR MEAN CORPUSCULAR VOLUME (MCV)

MCV (fL)	Category
Greater than 100	High (macrocytic)
80 to 100	Normal
Less than 80	Low (microcytic)

MCV values are generally used to differentiate and diagnose various types of anemia. Anemia that is characterized by high or low MCV is categorized as either macrocytic or microcytic. It's important to note, however, that most cases of anemia are *normocytic,* meaning that MCV is within the normal range. It is also possible to have high MCV (macrocytosis) or low MCV (microcytosis) even if you are not anemic.

Additionally, mean corpuscular volume values are needed to calculate *red cell distribution width* (RDW), which reflects the amount of variation in RBC size and is taken into account when diagnosing various blood disorders. The normal range for RDW is 11.7 to 15.0 percent. Abnormal MCV and RDW are evaluated alongside the other CBC values, as well as any symptoms you exhibit.

WHAT CAUSES HIGH MCV?

High MCV is frequently a sign of a type of macrocytic anemia, a group that includes hemolytic anemia and megaloblastic (vitamin-deficiency) anemia. High MCV values may also be due to a deficiency of vitamin B_{12} or folic acid. The factors listed below can also result in an increase in MCV.

- Alcohol abuse
- Certain medications, such as anticonvulsants, chemotherapy drugs, some diabetes medications, oral contraceptives, and others
- Hemolytic anemia

- Hereditary anemia
- Hypothyroidism
- Intestinal imbalance
- Liver disease
- Malnutrition
- Megaloblastic anemia, which is caused by deficiencies of vitamins like B_{12}

There may also be an increase in mean corpuscular volume during pregnancy, but this change is only temporary.

WHAT ARE THE SYMPTOMS OF HIGH MCV?

High MCV alone does not produce symptoms, but people may experience symptoms related to the condition causing the high value. Common signs of anemia, for example, include dizziness, fatigue, headache, pale complexion, rapid heartbeat, and shortness of breath. High MCV is also associated with elevated aspartate aminotransferase (AST) and alanine aminotransferase (ALT) values, which are components of the hepatic function panel. (See pages 186 and 177 for more information on AST and ALT.)

HOW CAN HIGH MCV BE TREATED?

Normalizing MCV can be achieved only by treating the underlying disease or disorder. Chronic diseases, such as liver disease and hypothyroidism, must be dealt with by a specialist. When high MCV stems from alcohol abuse, addiction counseling and rehabilitation is necessary. Many, if not most, cases of high MCV are due to vitamin-deficiency anemia, so dietary modification and supplements may be sufficient for returning MCV to the normal range.

SUPPLEMENTS

B-complex vitamins can be used to boost your nutritional health. Do not take any product until you have consulted your physician. In addition to a B-complex vitamins, you should also take a separate folic acid supplement. Speak to your doctor about appropriate dosing and take only under the supervision of a health professional. Depending on the severity and nature of your deficiency, prescribed injections of vitamin B_{12} is another treatment option. Again, your doctor will determine whether or not this measure is necessary.

SUPPLEMENTS FOR HIGH MCV		
Supplement	**Dosage**	**Considerations**
B-complex vitamins (containing at least 50 mg B_6)	1 tablet or capsule once a day, or as directed on the product label.	Typically listed as a B-25, B-50, or 5-100 supplement. Quality B-complex vitamins generally contain vitamins B_1 (thamin), B_2 (riboflavin), B_3 (niacin), B_5 (pantothenic acid), B_6 (pyridoxine), folic acid, and B_{12} (cyanocobalamin). Betaine (TMG) should also be added for increased protection. B vitamins can be found in quality multivitamins and mineral supplements as well. Speak to your health-care provider before taking if you have a medical condition, including anemia, diabetes, and liver problems.

LIFESTYLE CHANGES

In all likelihood, your doctor will recommend that you increase your dietary intake of vitamin B_{12} and folate. (See the table on page 11.) Also remember to stay away from processed and packaged meats, and whenever possible, buy meats that are lean, organic, and grass-fed or free-range. You should also avoid alcohol—especially if you have liver disease.

WHAT CAUSES LOW MCV?

The most common reason for low MCV is iron deficiency, which may be due to low dietary intake of iron, blood loss through menstruation, or internal blood loss caused by other factors. Low MCV is associated with microcytic anemias, which include iron-deficiency anemia, sickle cell anemia, and thalassemia. Additional reasons for low MCV include:

- Acute or chronic bleeding due to menstruation, physical trauma, surgery, or ulcers, for example
- Cancer
- Decreased oxygen availability
- Deficiency in copper or vitamin B_6 (pyridoxine)
- Hemolytic anemia
- Kidney failure
- Lead poisoning
- Removal of the spleen (splenectomy)
- Rheumatoid arthritis

If your MCV is abnormal, your doctor will look at the other results of your CBC in order to determine a cause. Additional blood work may be necessary.

WHAT ARE THE SYMPTOMS OF LOW MCV?

A person may experience symptoms not from low MCV itself, but from the conditions underlying it. Anemia frequently induces headaches, fatigue, dizziness, rapid heartbeat, and shortness of breath, so notify your doctor if one or more of these symptoms apply to you.

HOW CAN LOW MCV BE TREATED?

Low MCV is not considered a disorder on its own, but rather an indicator or symptom of a medical condition. Therefore, correcting a low MCV depends on treating the underlying disorder or disease. Extreme situations may call for a blood transfusion, but cases caused by nutritional deficiency can usually be resolved with dietary and lifestyle improvements along with the appropriate supplements.

SUPPLEMENTS

Consider taking one of the supplements listed in the table below, as they have shown to support healthy blood counts. Because side effects and drug interactions are possible, speak to your doctor before using any substance.

SUPPLEMENTS FOR LOW MCV

Supplement	Dosage	Considerations
Coenzyme Q_{10} (CoQ_{10})	30 mg three times a day or 50 mg twice a day, depending on dose per capsule.	CoQ_{10} is important for energy production, oxygen use, high blood pressure, and heart health, especially in people with kidney disorders. It can also boost endurance, improve insulin sensitivity, and lower triglycerides and blood glucose levels. This supplement is especially recommended if you are taking statin drugs, red yeast rice, and certain diabetes medications, which may result in a CoQ_{10} deficiency.
Copper	1 to 4 mg once a day.	Use caution when supplementing with copper, as it can be toxic. Do not take a separate copper supplement without the guidance and supervision of a healthcare practitioner.
Iron	325 mg (1 tablet) once a day.	May temporarily cause constipation or stomach cramps. Men should not use unless under a doctor's orders.
Vitamin B_6	50 to 100 mg once a day.	Doses of higher than 100 mg per day should be approved by your health-care provider.

Supplement	Dosage	Considerations
Vitamin C (ascorbic acid/ ascorbate)	1,000 mg once a day.	Vitamin C has been found to lower CRP by about 25 percent when levels are elevated and increase iron absorption. Doses higher than 5,000 mg per day may cause diarrhea. Mineral ascorbates and Ester-C are buffered forms of vitamin C that decrease the likelihood of diarrhea. Do not take in large doses if you are prone to gout or kidney stones.

LIFESTYLE CHANGES

If you suffer from iron-deficiency anemia, increase your consumption of red meat, fish, and poultry, as well as dried beans and fruits, leafy green vegetables, and whole grains. Liver is by far the most iron-rich food, so if you do not mind eating it, it's highly beneficial to add it to your diet. Eating iron-fortified bread, cereal, and flour can also help boost your iron intake. (See the table on page 208 for more dietary sources of iron.) Low copper levels, which are associated with iron-deficiency anemia, can be raised by eating foods such as crimini mushrooms, molasses, kale, summer squash, asparagus, eggplant, and liver. Cashews and sesame seeds are also good sources of copper. In addition, you should eat more foods containing vitamin B_6, a nutrient found in brewer's yeast, legumes, liver, peanuts, potatoes, and wheat germ.

In terms of lifestyle, you should stop using antacids and over-the-counter ulcer medication if you have low iron, as low stomach acid is directly correlated with low blood iron levels. Limit your physical activity as well, since rigorous exercise is associated with iron loss. Choose low-impact activities like aerobics, dancing, swimming, and yoga, and work out in moderation if your iron levels are low.

A Helpful Tip

If your MCV value is low as a result of iron-deficiency anemia (anemia caused by low intake or absorption of iron), you should increase your intake of iron-rich foods. Red meat, oysters and clams, dried beans, and some leafy green vegetables are good sources. Because vitamin C helps your body absorb iron, for maximum effectiveness, pair your iron-rich food with a substance high in vitamin C, such as bell peppers, broccoli, or citrus fruit. If you are taking an iron supplement prescribed by a health-care professional, make sure to take it with vitamin C in order to maximize absorption.

28. MEAN CORPUSCULAR HEMOGLOBIN (MCH)

Mean corpuscular hemoglobin (MCH) is a measure of the average amount of hemoglobin contained in a single red blood cell. High hemoglobin content is often referred to as *hyperchromia,* and low content, *hypochromia.* Ranges of MCH, which is measured in picograms, are grouped into the categories listed in the table below. Keep in mind that these are the generally accepted ranges; precise values may vary by lab.

REFERENCE RANGES FOR MEAN CORPUSCULAR HEMOGLOBIN (MCH)

Mean Corpuscular Hemoglobin (pg/cell)	Category
Greater than 43	High (hyperchromic)
26 to 43	Normal
Less than 26	Low (hypochromic)

When anemia is present, calculating a person's MCH can help to determine the type of anemia, as well as its level of severity.

WHAT CAUSES HIGH MCH?

Understandably, when MCH is high (hyperchromic), it usually indicates the presence of macrocytic anemia—anemia characterized by red blood cells that are larger than normal in size. As mentioned earlier, hereditary and hemolytic anemias, as well as megaloblastic anemia, are often macrocytic. The common causes of high MCH overlap with those of high MCV and include:

- Alcoholism
- Certain medications, such as anticonvulsant drugs, diabetic medications, and oral contraceptives
- Hemolytic anemia
- Hereditary anemia
- Hypothyroidism
- Intestinal malabsorption of nutrients due to surgery or an underlying medical condition
- Liver disease
- Megaloblastic anemia

Your high MCH may be due to a condition that is not listed above. Additional blood tests may be needed to determine the cause of an abnormality and make an accurate diagnosis.

WHAT ARE THE SYMPTOMS OF HIGH MCH?

Disorders that cause high MCH may produce symptoms. Anemia, for example, is associated with nonspecific symptoms like dizziness, fatigue, headache, rapid heartbeat, and shortness of breath. Like high MCV, high MCH values are associated with elevated aspartate aminotransferase (AST) and alanine aminotransferase (ALT), which are included on the hepatic function panel. (See pages 186 and 177 for more information on AST and ALT.)

HOW CAN HIGH MCH BE TREATED?

Treatment for this condition is the same as that recommended for high MCV (see page 219). When the cause of the high value is a disease—whether liver disease, hypothyroidism, or alcoholism—you will most likely be referred to a specialist who can better address your specific problem. If a certain medication is causing your MCH to increase, your doctor should change or discontinue the prescription. Anemia may also require specific medical treatments depending on its severity. Taking an appropriate supplement and modifying your lifestyle also supports normal MCH.

SUPPLEMENTS

B-complex vitamins can be used to enhance your nutritional health. Consult your doctor before beginning a supplement regimen.

SUPPLEMENTS FOR HIGH MCH

Supplement	Dosage	Considerations
B-complex vitamins (containing at least 50 mg B_6)	1 tablet or capsule once a day, or as directed on the product label.	Typically listed as a B-25, B-50, or 5-100 supplement. Quality B-complex vitamins generally contain vitamins B_1 (thamin), B_2 (riboflavin), B_3 (niacin), B_5 (pantothenic acid), B_6 (pyridoxine), folic acid, and B_{12} (cyanocobalamin). Betaine (TMG) should also be added for increased protection. B vitamins can be found in quality multivitamins and mineral supplements as well. Speak to your health-care provider before taking if you have a medical condition, including anemia, diabetes, and liver problems.

LIFESTYLE CHANGES

If your high MCH stems from anemia caused by a deficiency of folic acid or vitamin B_{12}, it is possible to normalize your value through natural means. By incorporating the right foods into your diet, you can raise your levels of folate and vitamin B_{12}; folic acid is abundant in leafy green vegetables and most types of meat contain vitamin B_{12}. (Refer to the table on page 208 for more dietary sources of these nutrients.)

WHAT CAUSES LOW MCH?

Low MCH is associated with microcytic anemia, which is characterized by smaller-than-normal RBCs, and normocytic anemia, when red blood cells are normal in size but do not contain sufficient hemoglobin. When low MCH is a feature of anemia, the condition is said to be *hypochromic*. Causes of low MCH include:

- Acute or chronic bleeding due to menstruation, physical trauma, surgery, or ulcers, among other types of blood loss
- Deficiency in copper, vitamin B_6 (pyridoxine) or vitamin C
- Gastrointestinal cancer
- Hemolytic anemia
- Iron-deficiency anemia
- Lead poisoning
- Kidney disorders
- Removal of the spleen (splenectomy)
- Rheumatoid arthritis
- Sickle cell anemia
- Thalassemia

It's also possible that another condition is the source of your low MCH value. If necessary, your physician will order additional testing to pinpoint the cause of the abnormality.

WHAT ARE THE SYMPTOMS OF LOW MCH?

Symptoms associated with low MCH are generally triggered by the underlying disease or disorder. Tell your doctor if you experience symptoms such as dizziness, fatigue, headache, and shortness of breath, as these are common signs of anemia.

HOW CAN LOW MCH BE TREATED?

There are no treatments that specifically target low MCH values. To increase MCH, the underlying condition must be treated. Severe anemia may require a blood transfusion, but most cases are mild enough to be treated sufficiently with supplements and lifestyle modifications.

SUPPLEMENTS

One way to normalize MCH is nutritional supplementation. The supplements below can help prevent and control anemic conditions related to diet and lifestyle factors. Although low MCH can be due to copper deficiency, taking separate copper supplements without the supervision of your doctor is not generally advised, as they can be toxic when taken in excess. Always notify your physician before using a supplement, and be sure to ask about potential side effects and proper dosing.

SUPPLEMENTS FOR LOW MCH

Supplement	Dosage	Considerations
Iron	325 mg (1 tablet) once a day.	May temporarily cause constipation or stomach cramps. Men should not use unless under a doctor's orders.
Vitamin B_6	50 to 100 mg once a day.	Doses of higher than 100 mg per day should be approved by your healthcare provider.
Vitamin C (ascorbic acid/ ascorbate)	1,000 mg once a day.	Vitamin C has been found to lower CRP by about 25 percent when levels are elevated and increase iron absorption. Doses higher than 5,000 mg per day may cause diarrhea. Mineral ascorbates and Ester-C are buffered forms of vitamin C that decrease the likelihood of diarrhea. Do not take in large doses if you are prone to gout or kidney stones.

LIFESTYLE CHANGES

If the cause of low MCH is a deficiency of iron, vitamin B_6, or vitamin C, focus on adding the appropriate foods to your diet. Iron-rich foods include red meat, poultry, liver, fish, and other types of seafood, as well as leafy green vegetables, whole grains, and dried beans and fruits. In addition, low copper levels, which are associated with iron-deficiency anemia, can be raised by eating foods such as crimini mushrooms, molasses, kale, summer squash, asparagus, eggplant, and once again, liver. Cashews and sesame seeds are also good sources of copper. Filling your diet with leafy greens will also boost your vitamin C intake, while eating more fish, legumes, and potatoes will increase B_6 levels. (See the table on page 296 for more foods high in vitamin B_6.)

The lifestyle guidelines discussed for low MCV can also be applied to low MCH. In particular, be sure not to overexercise, as this can negatively affect iron levels and, therefore, hemoglobin production. Work out in moderation and choose mild forms of physical activity, such as dancing, yoga, and Pilates. Also keep in mind that using certain medications like antacids can reduce your iron stores. Speak to your doctor about changing or discontinuing such drugs if you have an iron deficiency.

29. MEAN CORPUSCULAR HEMOGLOBIN CONCENTRATION (MCHC)

Although closely related, mean corpuscular hemoglobin concentration (MCHC) and mean corpuscular hemoglobin (MCH) are distinct measurements. While MCH represents the average amount of hemoglobin in a single red blood cell, MCHC reflects the hemoglobin concentration in a given unit of packed red blood cells. As with MCV and MCH, calculating the MCHC can help health-care professionals better assess anemia and other blood disorders. Reference ranges for this lab value, which is measured in grams per deciliter (g/dL), are:

REFERENCE RANGES FOR MEAN CORPUSCULAR HEMOGLOBIN CONCENTRATION (MCHC)

Mean Corpuscular Hemoglobin Concentration (g/dL)	Category
Greater than 37	High
31 to 37	Normal
Less than 31	Low

Remember that ranges may vary depending on the lab you use. Your physician will determine if an abnormality is present and, if so, take the steps necessary to find the cause.

WHAT CAUSES HIGH MCHC?

In general, the possible reasons for a high MCHC are consistent with those of high MCV and MCH. However, a type of hereditary hemolytic anemia called *spherocytosis* has been associated with high MCHC. Anemia caused by a deficiency of vitamin B_{12} or folic acid is also known to cause high values. Other causes of high MCHC with which you are already familiar include:

- Alcoholism
- Certain medications, such as anticonvulsant drugs
- Hemolytic anemia
- Hereditary anemia
- Hypothyroidism
- Intestinal disturbances and malabsorption issues
- Liver disease
- Malnutrition
- Megaloblastic anemia

MCHC may also be higher in pregnant women, but values usually return to normal after giving birth.

WHAT ARE THE SYMPTOMS OF HIGH MCHC?

Symptoms of anemia are typical with high MCHC. Common signs include dizziness, fatigue, headache, pale complexion, rapid heartbeat, and shortness of breath. If another condition is the cause of an elevated MCHC, you may experience symptoms associated with that particular disease. Blood tests on the hepatic function panel can also help in the detection and diagnosis of hemoglobin abnormalities—high MCHC is associated with elevated aspartate aminotransferase (AST) and alanine aminotransferase (ALT) values. (See pages 186 and 177 for more information on AST and ALT.)

HOW CAN HIGH MCHC BE TREATED?

Treatment for high MCHC varies according to the cause of the abnormal value. If necessary, your doctor will refer you to a specialist who can better assess certain medical problems, such as liver disease and hypothyroidism. Likewise, alcohol abuse requires the attention of an addictions counselor. Some types of anemia may also necessitate specific treatments beyond dietary and lifestyle changes. In most cases, however, vitamin-deficiency anemia can be corrected by making some health-promoting adjustments to your everyday life.

SUPPLEMENTS

The following supplements support normal MCHC. While many supplements are useful in managing and preventing vitamin deficiencies, you should practice caution and consult your doctor before taking any substance—including those listed in the table below.

SUPPLEMENTS FOR HIGH MCHC

Supplement	Dosage	Considerations
B-complex vitamins (containing at least 50 mg B_6)	1 tablet or capsule once a day, or as directed on the product label.	Typically listed as a B-25, B-50, or 5-100 supplement. Quality B-complex vitamins generally contain vitamins B_1 (thamin), B_2 (riboflavin), B_3 (niacin), B_5 (pantothenic acid), B_6 (pyridoxine), folic acid, and B_{12} (cyanocobalamin). Betaine (TMG) should also be added for increased protection. B vitamins can be found in quality multivitamins and mineral supplements as well. Speak to your health-care provider before taking if you have a medical condition, including anemia, diabetes, and liver problems.

LIFESTYLE CHANGES

Eating more B_{12}- and folate-containing foods—shellfish, meats, fish, beans, and leafy green vegetables, for example—will help remedy anemia caused by insufficient levels of these nutrients. (The table on page 208 lists excellent dietary sources of folate and vitamin B_{12}.) For the most health benefits, choose organic lean meats from grass-fed or free-range sources. Also, stay away from processed and packaged products (including meats), as well as foods that contain hormones, antibiotics, and chemical additives. As a general rule, always follow the advice of your doctor when it comes to making decisions about treatment and prevention.

WHAT CAUSES LOW MCHC?

Conditions that can lower MCHC are generally the same as those for low MCV and low MCH (see pages 219 and 224). These include:

- Acute or chronic bleeding due to menstruation, physical trauma, surgery, or ulcers, for example
- Cancer
- Decreased oxygen availability
- Deficiency in copper or vitamin B_6 (pyridoxine)
- Hemolytic anemia
- Iron-deficiency anemia
- Kidney failure
- Lead poisoning
- Removal of the spleen (splenectomy)
- Rheumatoid arthritis
- Sickle cell anemia
- Thalassemia

Low MCHC is not always a cause for concern. Your doctor will evaluate all of your CBC test results in order to make a clear determination about what is causing your abnormal value.

WHAT ARE THE SYMPTOMS OF LOW MCHC?

Low MCHC itself does not produce symptoms, but you may experience symptoms of the condition causing the low level. Anemia frequently induces headaches, fatigue, dizziness, rapid heartbeat, and shortness of breath, so notify your doctor if one or more of these symptoms apply to you.

HOW CAN LOW MCHC BE TREATED?

When it comes to normalizing MCHC, the first step is always to treat the condition causing the low value. Treatment decisions should be made with your physician or the specialist to whom you are referred. Diet and lifestyle play a key role in combating conditions that can lead to low MCHC, particularly nutritional deficiency.

SUPPLEMENTS

You may consider taking a nutritional supplement to help balance your blood counts. The supplements in the table below may be beneficial if you have low MCHC, but you should seek the advice of your physician to ensure safe usage of the products, especially if you have a copper deficiency that may require a separate supplement. Do not take copper without first consulting your healthcare provider.

SUPPLEMENTS FOR LOW MCHC

Supplement	Dosage	Considerations
Iron	325 mg (1 tablet) once a day.	May temporarily cause constipation or stomach cramps. Men should not use unless under a doctor's orders.
Vitamin B_6	50 to 100 mg once a day.	Doses of higher than 100 mg per day should be approved by your healthcare provider.
Vitamin C (ascorbic acid/ascorbate)	1,000 mg once a day.	Vitamin C has been found to lower CRP by about 25 percent when levels are elevated and increase iron absorption. Doses higher than 5,000 mg per day may cause diarrhea. Mineral ascorbates and Ester-C are buffered forms of vitamin C that decrease the likelihood of diarrhea. Do not take in large doses if you are prone to gout or kidney stones.

LIFESTYLE CHANGES

If you suffer from anemia caused by low iron, copper, or vitamin B_6, center your diet around foods rich in these nutrients. Foods with the highest iron concentrations include red meat, liver, poultry, fish, leafy green vegetables, whole grains, nuts, beans, and dried fruits, while copper is plentiful in crimini mushrooms, eggplant, kale, asparagus, liver, and molasses. And to increase your B_6 level, incorporate brewer's yeast, wheat germ, peanuts, legumes, and potatoes into your diet. (See the table on page 296 for more dietary sources of vitamin B_6.)

It's also important to limit how often you exercise if your iron stores are low. As mentioned already, overexercising can lead to iron loss, so choose non-intense forms of physical activity if you are trying to increase your iron. You can still get sufficient exercise by engaging in low-impact workouts such as dancing, yoga, Pilates, and swimming.

Last but not least, keep in mind that certain substances can affect MCHC. For example, antacid use is correlated with low iron, leading to low MCHC as well. If you take an antacid regularly, discuss alternatives with your doctor.

30. PLATELETS

Although they make up only a small portion of the blood, platelets are indispensable to your health. Their main function is to stop bleeding by swelling, clumping together, and forming a sticky plug, or clot. Platelets also transport other blood components, including inflammatory compounds called cytokines, as well as neurotransmitters, or brain chemicals. Approximately 2 percent of the neurotransmitter serotonin, a vital chemical that acts as a mood enhancer, is contained in the platelets. The reference ranges for platelet counts in adults, which are often measured using cubic millimeters (mm^3), are:

REFERENCE RANGES FOR PLATELET COUNTS

Platelets (mm^3)*	Category
Greater than 400,000	High
150,000 to 400,000	Normal
Less than 150,000	Low

*Depending on the testing laboratory, other units, such as microliters (μl , may be used to measure platelets.

The upper limit of the normal range is slightly higher for children, at around 450,000 mm^3. Keep in mind that ranges may differ from those above depending on the lab you use, so do not be alarmed if your number is slightly out of range. Still, if you have concerns, you should talk to your physician. Abnormal platelet counts are linked to a host of medical conditions ranging from infections to cancer. Autoimmune diseases, blood loss, chronic inflammation, and iron deficiency are also associated with both high and low levels.

WHAT CAUSES A HIGH PLATELET COUNT?

An elevated platelet count fall into one of two categories. It can be the result of a primary condition called *thrombocythemia,* in which the bone marrow overproduces the cells that form platelets. The cause of this disorder is unknown and in some cases may be triggered by a genetic mutation. Alternatively, a high count may be symptomatic of (secondary to) another condition. This is referred to as *secondary thrombocytosis*—the overproduction of platelets—and may be induced by:

- Autoimmune diseases, such as rheumatoid arthritis
- Blood loss
- Certain cancers, including colon cancer
- Chronic inflammation
- Elevated homocysteine and C-reactive protein (CRP) levels
- High red blood cell count (polycythemia)
- Infection
- Iron-deficiency anemia
- Living at high altitudes
- Medications, such as erythropoietin (EPO), estrogen, oral contraceptives, and steroids
- Spleen disorders or spleen removal
- Strenuous exercise
- Vitamin-B deficiency

Elevated platelet levels are dangerous and may cause abnormal bleeding, as well as unnecessary blood clotting. This can lead to heart attack, stroke, pulmonary embolism, or blockages in other parts of the body.

WHAT ARE THE SYMPTOMS OF A HIGH PLATELET COUNT?

Elevated platelet levels do not always produce specific symptoms, but general symptoms may include headache, numbness in the hands and feet, and weakness. If blood clotting occurs, confusion, difficulty breathing, dizziness, nausea, changes in speech, and pain in the abdomen, jaw, or neck may ensue. Seizures and momentary loss of consciousness are possible as well. Warning signs of abnormal bleeding include bruising or bleeding easily, bleeding in the mouth or gums, and frequent nosebleeds. These symptoms require immediate medical attention.

HOW CAN A HIGH PLATELET COUNT BE TREATED?

If an elevated platelet count is a temporary reaction to certain factors, such as an infection or surgery, treatment is not always necessary. In all other cases of secondary thrombocytosis, the underlying condition must be treated first in order to normalize the platelet count. If your physician deems it necessary, aspirin or another anticoagulant drug may be prescribed. Natural approaches to reducing platelet counts are described below.

SUPPLEMENTS

Nutritional supplementation should be considered as a complementary treatment. The supplements below have been shown to promote balanced platelet levels, but their effectiveness depends on the underlying cause of your condition. Speak to your doctor before beginning a regimen, and take any substance only as directed.

SUPPLEMENTS FOR HIGH PLATELET COUNTS		
Supplement	**Dosage**	**Considerations**
Green tea or green tea extract	3 to 6 cups of tea, or 250 to 500 mg of the extract a day.	Helps decrease platelet aggregation, as well as improve antioxidant and lipid levels. When used in combination with other supplements and a healthy diet and lifestyle, green tea extract may also aid in weight loss. Other reported benefits include glucose regulation and kidney stone prevention. If taking an extract, use a form standardized to 90-percent polyphenols (specifically EGCG). Tell your doctor if you are currently taking aspirin or anticoagulant drugs like warfarin (Coumadin), as green tea extract may increase the risk of bleeding.
Iron	325 mg (1 tablet) once a day.	May temporarily cause constipation or stomach cramps. Men should not use unless under a doctor's orders.
Resveratrol	30 to 100 mg up to three times a day.	Ask your doctor before using if you have a hormone-sensitive condition such as uterine fibroids or breast cancer.
Whey protein	20 to 30 g (1 to 2 scoops added to a beverage) twice a day.	Has been reported to minimize platelet aggregation. Studies have shown that whey protein is a form of protein that is both easily digested and superior to other proteins for muscle-building. It has also been reported to improve immunity and work as an antioxidant in the body. However, high doses can cause increased bowel movements, nausea, thirst, bloating, cramps, reduced appetite, fatigue, and headaches. Avoid use if you are pregnant or breastfeeding.

LIFESTYLE CHANGES

There are also some natural ways to prevent conditions leading to high platelet counts. Eating certain foods, especially those containing vitamin K and omega-3 fatty acids, can support platelet balance. Vitamin K, which is essential for clot formation, is abundant in dark leafy greens like kale, spinach, and collard and mustard greens. Omega-3s are important because they decrease production of thromboxane, a substance that helps platelets to function properly. These fatty acids are found in cold-water fish (particularly halibut, mackerel, and salmon), flax seeds, and walnuts. Increasing your intake of foods that enhance liver and kidney detoxification is also beneficial, so incorporate cruciferous vegetables such as cabbage, broccoli, and asparagus into your diet, as well as onions and garlic.

At the same time, there are several dietary and lifestyle habits that are best to avoid. Stay away from food that can promote inflammation, including processed meats, fried foods, baked goods, fast food, and any commercial product that contains artificial sweeteners, chemical additives, or saturated and trans fats. It's also important to minimize—and ideally, eliminate—your exposure to pesticides, plastics, and heavy metals, which are often found in nonorganic foods. To ensure your food is chemical-free, buy locally grown organic produce whenever possible. Finally, eliminate alcohol and smoking from your lifestyle, and be careful not to engage in an excessive amount of exercise. Over-exercising can increase clotting factors such as platelets, thereby encouraging clot formation.

WHAT CAUSES A LOW PLATELET COUNT?

A low platelet count may be due to factors inhibiting their production, causing them to break down, or confining them in the spleen, in turn decreasing the amount in the blood. Among these factors are:

- Anemia caused by bone marrow disorders or bone marrow suppression
- Autoimmune disorders, such as lupus and rheumatoid arthritis
- Bacterial infection in the blood (sepsis)
- Chemotherapy
- Deficiency of vitamin B_{12} or folic acid, which reduces ability of bone marrow to make platelets
- Enlarged spleen
- Excessive alcohol consumption
- Hemolytic uremic syndrome (HUS), a rare condition causing a severe decline in platelet count
- Idiopathic thrombocytopenic purpura (ITP), a disease in which the body mistakenly produces antibodies to attack and destroy platelets
- Leukemia

- Medications such as anticoagulants (notably heparin), anticonvulsants, anti-inflammatory drugs, aspirin, gold salts, quinidine, quinine, and sulfa antibiotics
- Thrombotic thrombocytopenic purpura (TTP), an uncommon disorder causing the formation of blood clots throughout the body
- Toxic chemical or heavy metal exposure
- Viral infections like HIV and hepatitis

Slightly low platelet counts are common in pregnant women, but the deficiency usually resolves itself shortly after giving birth. In general, a low platelet count is a concern because it typically leads to abnormal bleeding, which can make surgery and even some forms of physical activity dangerous. Severely low counts, though rare, can cause internal bleeding, which can be fatal when it affects the brain or intestines.

WHAT ARE THE SYMPTOMS OF A LOW PLATELET COUNT?

Low levels of platelets cause abnormal bleeding, which manifests as symptoms such as excessive or easy bruising, prolonged bleeding of cuts and wounds, bleeding mouth and gums, nosebleeds, and bleeding under the skin, or *petechiae*. Other physical indicators include heavy menstrual flow and blood in the urine and/or stools.

HOW CAN A LOW PLATELET COUNT BE TREATED?

Mild cases of low platelet counts do not always require treatment. However, very low levels and low counts caused by an underlying disorder call for therapy that is tailored to the particular condition. Common treatment methods—which may include drugs, supplements, and/or lifestyle change—are detailed in this section.

DRUGS

Depending on the cause and severity of your low count, your doctor may prescribe a drug therapy or medical procedure. For instance, there are a few different options for idiopathic thrombocytopenic purpura (ITP), including corticosteroids to block antibody production, the drug rituximab (a monoclonal antibody), and intravenous gamma globulin to boost the immune system. Spleen removal is also a treatment option, and in more serious situations, a blood transfusion.

SUPPLEMENTS

Nutritional supplements are helpful for keeping your platelet count within a normal range. Consult your physician before taking a supplement.

SUPPLEMENTS FOR LOW PLATELET COUNTS		
Supplement	**Dosage**	**Considerations**
Folic acid	1 mg once a day.	Doses greater than 1 mg per day should be taken only under the monitoring and supervision of a physician.
Iron	325 mg (1 tablet) once a day.	May temporarily cause constipation or stomach cramps. Men should not use unless under a doctor's orders.
Vitamin C (ascorbic acid/ ascorbate)	Up to 1,000 mg three times a day.	Vitamin C has been found to lower CRP by about 25 percent when levels are elevated and increase iron absorption. Doses higher than 5,000 mg per day may cause diarrhea. Mineral ascorbates and Ester-C are buffered forms of vitamin C that decrease the likelihood of diarrhea. Do not take in large doses if you are prone to gout or kidney stones.

LIFESTYLE CHANGES

It is also possible to manage the condition with certain lifestyle changes. Your doctor will probably recommend discontinuing the use of some medications, including antacids like Alka-Seltzer, acetaminophen (Anacin), ibuprofen (Advil), naproxen (Aleve) and various forms of aspirin such as ASA, Bufferin, Ecotrin, Excedrin, Fiorinal, and Percodan. Dietary adjustments are also in order. For example, increase your intake of foods rich in vitamin K, which helps stimulate platelet production. However, you should reduce (or eliminate) consumption of dairy products and alcohol, as they contain substances that inhibit the production of platelets. In addition, avoid activities that may lead to injury, including contact and high-risk sports like rugby, skiing, wrestling, and football, all of which can be dangerous for people prone to bleeding.

31. WHITE BLOOD CELLS

White blood cells (WBCs), also known as *leukocytes,* are an essential component of the immune system, serving to protect the body from harmful microorganisms. When an infection develops in the body, the number of white blood cells quickly increases, and the cells are transported to the infection site to attack and destroy the bacteria, virus, or other "bug" causing it. There are five types of WBCs that circulate in the blood—*neutrophils, lymphocytes, monocytes, eosinophils,* and *basophils*—and the concentrations of each can fluctuate on a day-to-day basis. The specific role and function of each type are described below.

- **Neutrophils.** This is the most common type of white blood cell, accounting for more than 50 percent of your body's supply. Neutrophils are the cells that engulf and destroy infection-causing bacteria and other harmful pathogens. Immature neutrophils are known as *band cells,* while fully developed neutrohpils are called *polys.*

- **Lymphocytes.** The two types of lymphocytes are B cells and T cells, which are produced in lymphoid tissue of the spleen, lymph nodes, and thymus gland. The B cells make antibodies that attack bacteria and toxins, and T cells target once-healthy cells in the body that have become cancerous or overtaken by a virus.

- **Monocytes.** These WBCs, which are distinguished by their large nucleus, develop into either *macrophages* or *dendritic cells.* Macrophages ingest microbes that the body recognizes as dangerous, while dendritic cells acquire *antigens*—foreign substances that trigger antibody production—so that T cells are able to identify them.

- **Eosinophils.** Found in the bloodstream as well as the lining of various tissues, eosinophils contain proteins that aid the body in fighting off parasitic infections. However, when these cells accumulate, they can actually contribute to the kind of inflammation that occurs in allergic disorders such as asthma. The medical term for an abnormally high number of eosinophils is *eosinophilia,* a condition that is considered to be a reaction to a certain disease, allergen, or parasite, rather than a disease itself.

- **Basophils.** Constituting less than 1 percent of the total white blood count, basophils are present in both the blood and tissues, and, like other WBCs, help to ward off foreign invaders. However, basophils are unique in their ability to kill parasites that are external to the body, including ticks. Additionally, basophils release heparin, an anticoagulant, and histamine, a blood-thinning substance. Basophils are similar to eosinophils in that when their number climbs too high, they can contribute to allergies and other inflammatory reactions in the body. In fact, histamine is the substance that causes allergy symptoms like itchy skin, runny nose, and watery eyes, which is why those who suffer from allergies usually take antihistamine medication for relief.

Measuring the number of the different white blood cells in the body is useful for diagnosing infections and other diseases. This blood test is called a *white blood cell differential test,* and it calculates the number of each WBC type as well as the total WBC count, all of which are measured in micrograms per liter (mcg/L). The normal ranges for the different kinds of white blood cells vary, but the generally accepted ranges for adults are provided in the table. Some labs may be at zero if the immune system is not under a specific type of stress.

REFERENCE RANGES FOR WHITE BLOOD CELL COUNTS

White Blood Cell Count	Normal Range (mcg/L)
Total white blood cells	4,500 to 11,000*
Neutrophils	1,800 to 7,800 (50 to 70 percent of total)
Lymphocytes	1,000 to 4,800 (15 to 45 percent of total)
Monocytes	0 to 800 (0 to 10 percent of total)
Eosinophils	0 to 450 (0 to 6 percent of total)
Basophils	0 to 200 (0 to 2 percent of total)

*For pregnant women, the normal range for total white blood cells is 5,900 to 17,000 mcg/L.

If one or more of your WBC counts is abnormal, your doctor will order further testing to determine the cause. It is important to realize, though, that an abnormality does not necessarily mean you have a serious medical condition. As you will see, both high and low WBC counts can be triggered by a wide range of factors, and not all of them are significant.

WHAT CAUSES A HIGH WHITE BLOOD CELL COUNT?

The medical term for a high white blood cell count is *leukocytosis.* An elevated level usually indicates that an infection is present in the body, but may also be caused by lifestyle factors such as strenuous exercise and eating too many refined carbohydrates and sugars. These foods increase insulin release, thereby driving up baseline WBC counts. In other cases, though, the underlying cause is more severe. The following conditions are associated with high WBC counts:

- Allergies, especially severe allergic reactions
- Bacterial or viral infections
- Bone marrow disorders such as myelofibrosis and polycythemia vera
- Certain medications, including allopurinol (Zyloprim), aspirin, corticosteroids, epinephrine, quinine (Qualaquin), and triamterene (Dyrenium)
- Chronic inflammatory conditions, like rheumatoid arthritis
- Eating a large meal
- Intense exercise
- Kidney failure
- Leukemia
- Malnutrition
- Removal of the spleen
- Severe physical or emotional stress
- Smoking
- Thyroid imbalance, particularly autoimmune thyroiditis
- Tissue damage due to injuries such as burns

Another condition may be the reason for your high count, so work with your doctor to find an accurate diagnosis.

WHAT ARE THE SYMPTOMS OF A HIGH WHITE BLOOD CELL COUNT?

Since an increased number of WBCs usually means that the body is trying to fight off an infection or illness, you may experience symptoms such as swollen lymph nodes, inflammation, or fever. General indicators of leukocytosis also include weight loss, poor appetite, bruising, and bleeding. Symptoms associated with specific medical conditions—like bone marrow disorders and thyroid imbalance—may occur as well. If any of these symptoms sound familiar to you, seek the advice of your physician.

HOW CAN A HIGH WHITE BLOOD CELL COUNT BE TREATED?

Treatment for elevated white blood cell counts must be directed at the cause. Antibiotics are usually prescribed for infections, while anti-inflammatory drugs, such as aspirin and acetaminophen (Tylenol), may be used to reduce inflammation and fever. However, if an abnormally high count does not have any apparent cause, additional blood testing may be needed to clarify the source of the problem. A serious illness, like leukemia or other bone marrow disease, requires specific and aggressive treatments such as medication, intravenous fluids, bone marrow transplants, blood transfusions, or *leukocytoreduction*—a medical procedure used for decreasing the number of WBCs in leukemic patients. Treatment for an elevated WBC count should be obtained as soon as possible to order to prevent complications.

Although less serious causes of high WBC counts, such as bacterial and viral infections, require medical treatment in many instances, it is also possible to prevent and treat them naturally with dietary and lifestyle change, as detailed below.

SUPPLEMENTS

There are a number of nutritional supplements you can take to help fortify your immune system and improve WBC function. Consult your physician before using any product.

SUPPLEMENTS FOR HIGH WHITE BLOOD CELL COUNTS

Supplement	Dosage	Considerations
Beta-1,3-glucan	100 to 200 mg once a day.	Improves the activation and function of WBCs. Women who are pregnant or breastfeeding should avoid use.
Moducare	40 mg (2 capsules) twice a day.	Taken if thyroid antibodies are present.
Omega-3 essential fatty acids DHA and EPA (fish oil)	1,000 mg up to four times a day.	Fish oil acts as an antioxidant and decreases inflammation in the body, in addition to supporting heart and blood vessel health. Speak to your doctor before taking if you are on blood-thinning medication, as fish oil may increase the risk of bleeding. Be sure to use only high-quality oils that have been tested for contaminants.

Supplement	Dosage	Considerations
Probiotics	5 to 10 billion CFUs one to two times a day.	Probiotics help normalize beneficial flora in the gastrointestinal tract, and are reported to decrease triglyceride and cholesterol levels. They are also reported to improve BUN levels and quality of life in people with kidney disease. It's best to use heat-stable products that do not require refrigeration. If using an antibiotic, wait three hours before taking probiotics. If diarrhea occurs, decrease your dosage. If this side effect persists for longer than 48 hours, stop taking the supplement and contact your doctor. Live cultures should be guaranteed through the date of expiration on label. For optimal results, take probiotics with meals, as food improves the survivability of the cultures.
Reishi mushroom (standardized to 4 percent triterpenes and 10 percent polysaccharides, or beta-1,3-glucans)	150 to 300 mg three to four times a day.	If you take blood thinners, use only under a doctor's supervision. Avoid use if you have low blood pressure, thrombocytopenia, or are pregnant or breastfeeding.
Zinc	25 to 50 mg once a day.	Zinc is important in immunity and acts as an antioxidant. It is also reported to help regulate blood sugar. May also be used by men to treat low testosterone and support prostate health. Take zinc in the form of an amino acid chelate or citrate. Check with your doctor before using.

LIFESTYLE CHANGES

The goal of your diet should be to decrease your consumption of foods that lead to inflammation—a primary cause of high WBCs—as you increase your intake of immunity-boosting foods. First, cut out commercial baked goods and processed foods containing artificial sweeteners and other chemical additives, which promote inflammatory conditions in the body. Any food containing saturated or trans fats, like fried and fast food, should also be avoided. Second, allergens like wheat, dairy products, and soy should be eliminated from your diet, since they can both cause inflammation and raise WBC levels, especially if you have an underlying allergy or sensitivity. And to counteract inflammation, incorporate omega-3s into your diet by eating cold-water fish (halibut, mackerel, and salmon in particular), walnuts, and flax seeds. Omega-3s are loaded with benefits, including anti-inflammatory properties.

At the same time, you can bolster your immune system by eating foods rich in zinc and selenium—minerals found in lean meats, liver, eggs, and seafood, especially oysters. Zinc is also plentiful in whole grains and pumpkin seeds. Additional sources of selenium include Brazil nuts, dairy products, garlic, and certain vegetables like cabbage, celery, cucumbers, and radishes. Minerals are often lost through food processing, so when possible, buy foods that are fresh and organic.

Your lifestyle is central to maintaining a strong immune system. Lessen your exposure to environmental contaminants, such as pesticides, heavy metals, and plastics, by purchasing products free of these ingredients, which can compromise your immunity. Additionally, strive to get at least seven hours of sleep per night, drink plenty of filtered water (approximately 2 to 3 liters per day), and exercise in moderation. If your white blood cell count is already high, you may want to consider restricting the amount you exercise until your number returns to normal. Remember, overexertion can cause a spike in WBCs.

WHAT CAUSES A LOW WHITE BLOOD CELL COUNT?

While a high WBC count is not always cause for concern, a lower-than-normal number of white blood cells, or *leukopenia,* usually suggests a medical problem—though some individuals are genetically predisposed to a below-normal WBC count. Autoimmune diseases, bone marrow disorders, cancer, viral infections that impair the bone marrow, and certain drugs can all cause a drop in white blood cell counts. Below is a list of specific causes of low counts, and many are similar to the causes of high WBCs. This is because if the immune system is activated and producing too many white blood cells, the body may wear out its ability to make WBCs. Neutrophil levels are most affected by this process, while other counts may remain within the normal range or become slightly elevated.

- Allergies
- Autoimmune diseases, such as rheumatoid arthritis and lupus
- Bone marrow dysfunction caused by conditions such as aplastic anemia, myelofibrosis, and other congenital disorders
- Chemotherapy and radiation therapy
- Chronic inflammation
- Hypersplenism (destruction of blood cells by the spleen)
- Hyperthyroidism
- Immune deficiency caused by diseases like HIV/AIDS
- Infectious diseases
- Leukemia
- Nutritional deficiency, especially in vitamins A, B, C, E, selenium, and zinc

In addition, the following medications may reduce the total number of white blood cells in the body:

- Anticonvulsants
- Antihistamines
- Anti-thyroid drugs
- Barbiturates
- Corticosteroids, such as cortisone, hydrocortisone, and prednisone
- Diuretics
- Sulfonamide antibiotics, including Bactrim (sulfameth-oxazole/trimethoprim)

The condition causing your low white blood cell count may not be included in the list above. Your doctor will evaluate your WBC differential test and any symptoms you may have in order to make a diagnosis.

WHAT ARE THE SYMPTOMS OF A LOW BLOOD CELL COUNT?

Physical indicators of a low blood cell count may include recurrent infections, slow-healing wounds, and fatigue. It is also possible that you will experience no symptoms at all. If you have a low number of WBCs, contact your doctor if you have signs of an infection, such as swollen lymph nodes, sore throat, fever, or skin lesions.

HOW CAN A LOW BLOOD CELL COUNT BE TREATED?

Depending on the cause, a low WBC count is treated with medication, lifestyle change, or both.

DRUGS

Infections can be treated with an appropriate antibiotic, but low counts associated with diseases may require drugs like pegfilgrastim (Neulasta) and filgrastim (Neupogen)—injections that stimulate the production of WBCs. Chemotherapy-induced leukopenia can also be treated with these medications. When a white blood cell level drops due to other medical therapies, such as pharmaceutical drugs, treatment may be delayed, adjusted, or discontinued until the WBC count normalizes.

SUPPLEMENTS

Nutritional supplements can also be potent immune-enhancers and help to normalize WBC counts. Speak to a healthcare professional before taking any substance below in order to ensure the safest and most effective use of the product.

SUPPLEMENTS FOR LOW WHITE BLOOD CELL COUNTS

Supplements	Dosage	Considerations
Beta-1,3-glucan	100 to 200 mg once a day.	Improves the activation and function of WBCs. Women who are pregnant or breastfeeding should avoid use.
Glutamine (L-glutamine)	3,000 to 5,000 mg twice a day.	Helps fuel WBC production, especially in individuals who regularly engage in strenuous exercise. Studies have shown that glutamine helps protect the kidneys against oxidative stress damage, as well as improve creatinine levels. Avoid if you suffer from severe liver disease, seizures, monosodium glutamate sensitivity, or mania. Do not take if you are pregnant or breastfeeding.
Multivitamin	Take as directed on the label.	A multivitamin/mineral supplement contains essential nutrients that help metabolism and blood sugar regulation. It also can be used to replace the nutrients that may be depleted due to blood sugar medications or a poor diet. Use only high-quality products. See page 11 for a list of essential nutrients to look for in a daily multivitamin.
Omega-3 essential fatty acids DHA and EPA (fish oil)	1,000 mg up to four times a day.	Fish oil acts as an antioxidant and decreases inflammation in the body, in addition to supporting heart and blood vessel health. Speak to your doctor before taking if you are on blood-thinning medication, as fish oil may increase the risk of bleeding. Be sure to use only high-quality oils that have been tested for contaminants.
Probiotics	5 to 10 billion CFUs one to two times a day.	Probiotics help normalize beneficial flora in the gastrointestinal tract, which improve immune function, and are reported to decrease triglyceride and cholesterol levels. They are also reported to improve BUN levels and quality of life in people with kidney disease. It's best to use heat-stable products that do not require refrigeration. If using an antibiotic, wait three hours before taking probiotics. If diarrhea occurs, decrease your dosage. If this side effect persists for longer than 48 hours, stop taking the supplement and contact your doctor. Live cultures should be guaranteed through the date of expiration on label. For optimal results, take probiotics with meals, as food improves the survivability of the cultures.

Supplements	Dosage	Considerations
Vitamin C (ascorbic acid/ ascorbate)	1,000 to 5,000 mg per day.	Vitamin C promotes the production of WBCs and has been found to lower CRP by about 25 percent when levels are elevated. Also shown to increase iron absorption. Doses higher than 5,000 mg per day may cause diarrhea. Mineral ascorbates and Ester-C are buffered forms of vitamin C that decrease the likelihood of diarrhea. Do not take in large doses if you are prone to gout or kidney stones.
Zinc	25 to 50 mg once a day.	Zinc is important in immunity and acts as an antioxidant. It is also reported to help regulate blood sugar. May also be used by men to treat low testosterone and support prostate health. Take zinc in the form of an amino acid chelate or citrate. Check with your doctor before using.

LIFESTYLE CHANGES

Minor illnesses, bacterial infections, and nutritional deficiency can also be the cause of a low white blood cell count. Self-care is essential when it comes to preventing and treating this type of leukopenia. As mentioned earlier, zinc and selenium, which are found in foods like lean meats, liver, eggs, and seafood, are vital minerals that help boost the immune system. Vitamin C, which is abundant in citrus fruits and dark leafy greens, is another important nutrient that you should be sure to work into your diet. Although it is not a cure for the common cold or flu, vitamin C activates WBCs to fight off infection, helping the immune system defend itself against invaders. The body uses up to six times more vitamin C when it's trying to fight off a bug. L-glutamine, an amino acid, is also used more by white blood cells when they need to become more active. For example, marathon runners and endurance athletes may experience a drop in L-glutamine after a major athletic event, making them more prone to illnesses like upper respiratory infections. Therefore, it may be helpful to take L-glutamine if you are training for a competition.

In addition, be careful about eating raw fish or undercooked meat, which can harbor bacteria and make you ill. This also goes for raw fruits and vegetables; while it's best to buy and eat them fresh, make sure you wash them before consuming. Adequate sleep—at least seven to restful hours per night—is also essential for maintaining a healthy immune system; studies show that getting five hours of sleep per night can cause a nine-fold increase in your risk of developing cold or flu. Moderate physical activity is important for stimulating WBC production, boosting your overall health, and lowering stress, which can make you more prone to illness and drive up your body's inflammatory response. And if your white blood cell count is currently low, be sure to avoid direct contact with people who are sick until your level returns to normal. This is especially important for those undergoing chemotherapy or another medical treatment that increases susceptibility to disease.

You should also follow the dietary and lifestyle guidelines for treating high white blood cell counts (see pages 243 to 245). Namely, avoid inflammation-causing foods, chemical additives, artificial sweeteners, and harmful chemicals found in many household and personal care products. All of these substances can trigger inflammatory conditions that wear down your body's immune response. For example, do not microwave food in plastic containers, drink out of plastic water bottles, or use products that contain phthalates. The presence of toxins and their negative impact on immunity is another good reason to buy your food organic when you can.

Of course, these lifestyle modifications will not necessarily raise your white blood cell count, but they do support overall wellness, as well as cut your risk of developing infections and other medical complications.

CONCLUSION

A complete blood count provides vital information about the status of your health, including bone marrow function, blood clotting, nutrition, oxygen transport, and immunity. Although some blood cell abnormalities are difficult—and in rare cases, impossible—to prevent, most are highly treatable, especially when they are caught early. If you experience one or more symptoms mentioned in this section, you should make an appointment with your physician. Even a symptom as general and seemingly harmless as fatigue can be a warning sign of something more serious that requires medication or other therapy.

Remember, there is plenty you can do in your everyday life to maintain normal CBC values. Your overall lifestyle—which includes sleep, exercise, and dietary patterns, as well as your use of certain products and drugs—is fundamental to keeping your blood healthy. If you don't already, eat foods rich in B vitamins, vitamin C, iron, selenium, and zinc to enhance blood cell production and bolster your immune system. Drinking water, getting adequate rest, quitting smoking, and regularly engaging in physical activity also promote general wellness and help prevent conditions that may lead to abnormal blood cell counts. You can also ask your health-care provider about specific nutritional supplements appropriate for your condition and needs. Supplements cannot replace a diet rich in whole foods, but in certain circumstances, you may not be able to get enough of a particular nutrient from the diet alone.

In sum, it is entirely possible to prevent, manage, and sometimes even reverse a blood cell abnormality. When you work with your physician, you can decide upon a course of action that is right for you and will put you on the road to better health.

Did You Know?

The first recorded human blood transfusion was performed in 1667 by French academic Jean-Baptiste Denis. Inspired by William Harvey's theory of blood circulation, Denis transferred sheep's blood to a feverish fifteen-year-old boy. The experiment seemed to be a success; the boy recovered and appeared to suffer no ill effects. The dangers of interspecies transfusion were not then understood, however; when subjects of subsequent transfusions died, the process was banned in France and England.

PART 5

Hormones

When most people hear the word hormones, they think of sexual development. The truth is, though, that hormones are responsible for so much more than just male and female sexual characteristics. They actually play a vital role in virtually every bodily process. Hormones are involved in blood sugar regulation, immune system function, and energy production. When hormone levels change as a result of aging or a physical disorder, however, other health issues tend to arise. Symptoms such as depression and mood swings, weight gain, muscle aches and joint stiffness, blood pressure changes, blood sugar imbalance, low sex drive, and cognitive decline may all be associated with hormonal shifts. And because many of these substances depend on each other to maintain balance, problems with one hormone can easily raise or lower another hormone. Thankfully, there are measures to bring the body back into equilibrium, as you will learn in this section.

32. DEHYDROEPIANDROSTERONE (DHEA)

Dehydroepiandrosterone (DHEA) is a building block of steroid hormones that is produced predominantly in the adrenal glands. It serves as a precursor to the sex hormones testosterone and estrogen in both men and women. DHEA is also a building block of the stress hormone cortisol (see page 256) and supports immune system function. DHEA may also increase insulin sensitivity, enhance fat metabolism, and act as an antioxidant.

There are two types of dehydroepiandrosterone: DHEA and its sulfate form, dehydroepiandrosterone sulfate (DHEAS). Because DHEAS remains in the bloodstream longer the DHEA, doctors generally test DHEAS numbers when they suspect a problem with this hormone. Typically, DHEAS levels are high in newborns and drop significantly after birth. They increase during puberty, peak soon after, and decline with age. Normal ranges are as follows.

REFERENCE RANGES FOR DHEA

Category	Age	DHEAS Normal Range (mcg/dL)
Men	18 to 19	108 to 441
	20 to 29	280 to 640
	30 to 39	120 to 520
	40 to 49	95 to 530
	50 to 59	70 to 310
	60 to 69	42 to 290
	69 and older	28 to 175
Women	18 to 19	145 to 395
	20 to 29	65 to 380
	30 to 39	45 to 270
	40 to 49	32 to 240
	50 to 59	26 to 200
	60 to 69	13 to 130
	69 and older	17 to 90

Keep in mind that reference ranges can differ slightly from lab to lab, so check the listing on your blood test for the range that applies to you.

WHAT CAUSES HIGH DHEA?

DHEA levels are naturally higher during youth, but there are a few conditions that can cause this hormone to become elevated beyond the normal range, including:

- Adrenal tumors
- Hyperplasia (adrenal swelling)
- Polycystic ovary syndrome (PCOS)

DHEA levels can vary widely from person to person. Your doctor will be able to verify whether or not the amount of this hormone in your blood is a problem.

WHAT ARE THE SYMPTOMS OF HIGH DHEA?

Because of its association with both male and female sex hormones, high DHEA levels can create a number of distressing symptoms. They can cause women to develop facial hair, male pattern baldness, and a deeper voice in a process known as masculinization. They can also lead to feminine traits in men, such as increased breast tissue and testicular wasting. Other possible symptoms include fatigue, sweating, and acne.

HOW CAN HIGH DHEA BE TREATED?

Because high DHEA is mainly associated with medical conditions such as adrenal tumors and PCOS, your doctor will have to treat these underlying issues in order to normalize this hormone.

WHAT CAUSES LOW DHEA?

Although DHEA levels decline naturally with age, they may also be lowered by conditions such as:

- Autoimmune diseases such Addison's disease, lupus, and rheumatoid arthritis
- Chronic stress

Unfortunately, some of the medications used to treat symptoms of these illnesses can also deplete DHEA in the body. These drugs include:

- Corticosteroids, including dexamethasone (Decadron), methylprednisolone (Medrol), and hydrocortisone
- Insulin

- Pain medications, including opiates and nonsteroidal anti-inflammatory drugs such as ibuprofen (Advil) and naproxen (Aleve)

Do not, however, attempt to adjust the dosage of your medication on your own. If your DHEA is low, your doctor will suggest the best way to remedy the problem.

WHAT ARE THE SYMPTOMS OF LOW DHEA?

Symptoms of low DHEA include extreme fatigue, muscle and joint pain, weight gain, trouble sleeping, lowered immunity, loss of sexual interest, decreased bone density, depression, and reduced muscle mass. Pay attention to these signs, as they can lead to conditions such as cardiovascular disease, type 2 diabetes, or osteoporosis. Interestingly, low DHEA—especially when combined with high cortisol levels—can also damage the hippocampus (memory center of the brain), in turn leading to short-term memory loss.

HOW CAN LOW DHEA BE TREATED?

To effectively treat low DHEA levels, adjustments to lifestyle and diet are crucial. Supplements can also prove beneficial.

SUPPLEMENTS

There are several natural products available that can help you cope with stress, as seen in the table below. Do not take any supplement to treat low levels of DHEA without speaking to your doctor first. You should also consult your doctor about exploring other treatment options, such as bioidentical hormone replacement therapy (see the inset on page 266), depending on the underlying cause of your imbalance.

SUPPLEMENTS FOR LOW DHEA

Supplement	Dosage	Considerations
Ashwagandha (standardized to 1.5-percent withanolides and 1-percent alkaloids)	450 to 900 mg once a day.	Use with caution when taking sedatives and hypnotics such as barbiturates, as their effects may be increased. May also alter thyroid hormone levels, so check with your doctor before using if you have a thyroid disorder. Consult your doctor before taking if you are on blood thinners or antiplatelet drugs. Substances similar to ashwagandha (adaptogens) that may also be beneficial include Rhodiola, American ginseng, and Manchurian ginseng.

Supplement	Dosage	Considerations
DHEA	25 to 50 mg once a day.	Regular blood tests are required when using this supplement. Do not use if you have a hormone-sensitive condition, such as breast cancer or uterine fibroids. Avoid use if you have a mood disorder or depression, liver problems, low HDL cholesterol, PCOS, or are pregnant or breastfeeding. If you are diabetic, monitor your blood sugar closely while taking DHEA.
Relora	250 mg two to three times a day.	This supplement helps alleviate stress by reducing the body's physiological response. Since it may cause drowsiness, do not take before driving an automobile or working with or around heavy machinery.
Whey protein	44 g once a day (added to a beverage).	Studies have shown that whey protein is a form of protein that is both easily digested and superior to other proteins for muscle building. It has also been reported to improve immunity and work as an antioxidant in the body. However, high doses can cause increased bowel movements, nausea, thirst, bloating, cramps, reduced appetite, fatigue, and headaches. Avoid use if you are pregnant or breastfeeding.

LIFESTYLE CHANGES

If chronic stress is behind decreased DHEA, do your best to eliminate the source of stress from your life. Getting at least eight hours of sleep every night can also help reduce stress, as can exercising aerobically for approximately thirty minutes a day, three to four times a week. As low DHEA levels may be associated with inflammation, it is wise to cut back on foods that can have an inflammatory reaction in your body, such as refined sugars and carbohydrates, fried food, baked goods, lunch meats, and fast food. Additionally, avoid eating items that may cause hormone imbalances, such as nonorganic meat and dairy, chemical additives and preservatives, and artificial sweeteners. Increase your consumption of antioxidant-rich foods, including yellow and red peppers, squashes, tomatoes, green leafy vegetables, garlic, onions, and cruciferous vegetables such as broccoli and Brussels sprouts. Also, be sure to quit smoking, as this habit negatively affects DHEA levels. In many cases, DHEA levels will return to normal by reducing stress, which decreases the demands of cortisol production in the body. Stress management through yoga, meditiation, or prayer have been shown to have a positive effect on stress response.

33. CORTISOL

Over the past decade, cortisol has been at the forefront of research on health and well-being. The rise of diabetes complications and short-term memory erosion has resulted in more studies highlighting the importance of cortisol management. Made in the adrenal glands, cortisol is a steroid hormone that increases blood sugar, suppresses the immune system, fights inflammation, decreases bone formation, and helps metabolize fat, protein, and carbohydrates when it is released in appropriate amounts. It is most commonly known as the "stress hormone," as it is released in response to both physical and psychological stress. While this reaction is normal and healthy in short bursts, chronic stress leads to the creation of too much cortisol, which results in a variety of imbalances in the body. Chronic elevation of cortisol can block the growth of nerve cells in the brain and damage the brain's memory center (hippocampus), which may begin to shrink when high cortisol and low DHEA occur together.

Normal cortisol levels rise and fall cyclically throughout the day. Generally, they will be highest in the early morning (between 6:00 and 8:00 AM) and lowest at midnight. They usually drop around noon or midday, and then again in the evening around 4:00 to 6:00 PM. The table below lists the traditionally accepted ranges for cortisol production in the blood for adults.

REFERENCE RANGES FOR CORTISOL

Time of Day	Cortisol Normal Range (mcg/dL)
AM	6.2 to 19.4*
PM	2.3 to 11.9
Target Range: AM: 10 to 14 mcg/dL; PM: Less than 7.0 mcg/dL	

*Some labs place the normal upper limit at 22.24 mcg/dL

Always check the reference ranges on your blood test, as they may vary slightly from the above. Cortisol may also be assessed using a four-point salivary cortisol test, which maps out cortisol output over the course of the day to determine if your body is releasing the appropriate amounts at specific times. These values are completely different from blood values and should not be confused with serum (blood) testing.

WHAT CAUSES HIGH CORTISOL?

Very high cortisol, also called *hypercortisolism,* has a number of potential causes, including:

- Adrenal tumors
- Anorexia or bulimia
- Chronic stress
- Cushing's syndrome
- Oral contraceptives
- Physical activity
- Pituitary tumors
- Pregnancy

While physical activity brings about an increase in cortisol, this condition is temporary. A more troublesome issue is chronic stress, which does not allow the body to recover from moments of raised cortisol, setting the stage for bigger problems.

WHAT ARE THE SYMPTOMS OF HIGH CORTISOL?

Symptoms of chronic high cortisol may include anxiety, cravings for sweets and carbohydrate-rich foods, mood swings, sleep pattern disturbances, memory impairment, increased susceptibility to colds and flu, joint aches and pain, blood sugar imbalances, increased belly fat, and gastrointestinal disturbances such as gas, bloating, diarrhea, and constipation.

HOW CAN HIGH CORTISOL BE TREATED?

While there are many lifestyle adjustments that can be made to lower chronically high cortisol levels, sometimes the problem is beyond these solutions and requires pharmaceutical treatment. Typically, extremely high levels related to a disease may require surgery or medication. When cortisol is slightly elevated, treatment will likely depend on alleviating symptoms of conditions like insomnia, anxiety, or other mood disorders, whether through drugs or other means. There are also plenty of natural ways to correct slight elevations in cortisol or levels that trend high, as explained in further detail below.

SUPPLEMENTS

Dietary supplements may be recommended to balance the production of cortisol. The following table lists these helpful substances.

SUPPLEMENTS FOR HIGH CORTISOL		
Supplement	**Dosage**	**Considerations**
Magnesium	400 mg one to two times a day.	Use magnesium aspartate, citrate, taurate, glycinate, or any amino acid chelate. Supports bone building and balances calcium intake. The ratio of calcium-to-magnesium intake should be between 1 to 1 and 2 to 1. This supplement is reported to improve blood vessel function and insulin resistance, in addition to decreasing LDL cholesterol, total cholesterol, and triglycerides. Also essential for phase-I liver detoxification. If you experience loose stools after taking magnesium, cut your dose in half and gradually increase over the course of a few months. Consult your health-care provider for dosage advice.
Melatonin	3 to 6 mg once a day, an hour before bedtime.	This is a natural hormone that improves sleep patterns and acts as an antioxidant in the body. It also resets the cortisol release pattern. Possible but rare side effects include dizziness and headache. People who are taking anticoagulants, immuno-suppressants, oral contraceptives, or diabetes medication must use with caution and only under the supervision of a health professional. Doses higher than the recommended amount can be taken only under the advice and guidance of a doctor.
Relora	250 mg two to three times a day.	This supplement helps alleviate stress by reducing the body's physiological response. Since it may cause drowsiness, do not take before driving an automobile or working with or around heavy machinery.
L-theanine	100 to 200 mg three times a day.	This supplement alleviates mental and physical stress, and decreases the level of phenethylamine (PEA) in the brain, a stimulatory neurotransmitter. Some medical sources say no side effects have been observed, but others warn that dizziness, headaches, and upset stomach are possible. Women who are pregnant or breastfeeding should avoid use.

LIFESTYLE CHANGES

Because cortisol is produced in reaction to inflammation, reducing inflammation is a good way to lower cortisol levels. Eliminate inflammatory foods from your diet, including products made with refined sugar and flour, fried food, sweets, processed snacks, soft drinks, and fast food in general. Choose organic free-range meat and steer clear of chemical flavoring agents, artificial sweetener, preservatives, and dyes. Eat at regular intervals and take time to enjoy the meal. Foster relaxation by going for long walks, doing yoga, or meditating. Additionally, moderate exercise of thirty to sixty minutes a day can help reduce stress hormones and balance your blood sugar. Finally, try to drink at least 2 to 3 liters of filtered water every day.

WHAT CAUSES LOW CORTISOL?

Although chronic stress causes cortisol levels to rise in the body, it may lead to cortisol deficiency if it persists long enough. When the adrenal glands constantly produce large amounts of cortisol, they can eventually begin to wear out and lose their ability to produce and regulate cortisol. This condition is commonly referred to as adrenal fatigue, but the term is not entirely accurate. Most of the time, the adrenal glands are not the problem, but rather the regulation of the adrenal glands by the brain's hypothalamus and pituitary glands. Stress alters the circuitry of brain signaling, and the net result is what is called *maladaptive stress syndrome*. In other words, the term "adrenal fatigue" is misleading and poorly chosen.

Although this scenario is the most common reason for altered patterns of cortisol production, the condition can also be caused by underlying medical disorders such as:

- Addison's disease
- Hypopituitarism
- Post-traumatic stress disorder (PTSD)

If you experience symptoms of low cortisol, make an appointment with your doctor for a blood test.

WHAT ARE THE SYMPTOMS OF LOW CORTISOL?

If low cortisol stems from chronic stress, you may experience many of the symptoms of high cortisol before you notice the effects of a drop in the hormone. Signs of low cortisol include chronic fatigue, muscle weakness, darkening of the skin, loss of appetite, unexplained weight loss, depression, irregular menstrual periods, low blood pressure, and low blood sugar. If traumatic stress or post-traumatic stress disorder (PTSD) is the cause of low levels, panic and anxiety may ensue when the brain begins to release cortisol again.

HOW CAN LOW CORTISOL BE TREATED?

Cortisol management is becoming increasingly important in treating chronic illness, as well as for maintaining good health in general. Although it is relatively rare to have a disease that causes a dramatic change in cortisol output, many people experience chronic health-related issues due to inappropriate cortisol release. It's critical for you to monitor your levels carefully. If Addison's disease or hypopituitarism is responsible for low cortisol levels, your doctor will treat these underlying conditions appropriately with medications such as corticosteroids. Otherwise, there are a few options for managing cortisol levels naturally.

SUPPLEMENTS

The following dietary supplements may help normalize cortisol levels.

SUPPLEMENTS FOR LOW CORTISOL

Supplement	Dosage	Considerations
Adrenal glandular supplement	100 to 200 mg one to three times a day.	Whole-gland extract may cause anxiety in individuals who have PTSD or artificially suppressed cortisol levels. To avoid health risks associated with Bovine Spongiform Encephalitis, buy supplements made from cattle in New Zealand, not Europe, where BSE infection rates are higher.
Ashwagandha (standardized to 1.5-percent withanolides and 1-percent alkaloids)	450 to 900 mg once a day.	Use with caution when taking sedatives and hypnotics such as barbiturates, as their effects may be increased. May also alter thyroid hormone levels, so check with your doctor before using if you have a thyroid disorder. Consult your doctor before taking if you are on blood thinners or anti-platelet drugs. Substances similar to ashwagandha (adaptogens) that may also be beneficial include Rhodiola, American ginseng, and Manchurian ginseng.
Licorice root (standardized to contain 20-percent glycyrrhizinic acid)	250 to 500 mg three times a day.	Do not take if you have heart disease, congestive heart failure, high blood pressure, fluid retention, diabetes, kidney disease, or liver disease. Women who are pregnant or breastfeeding should not take licorice. This supplement should not be used by anyone who is currently taking ACE inhibitors, diuretics, digoxin, or oral contraceptives, among other medications. Talk to your doctor before using.

LIFESTYLE CHANGES

If you suspect you are suffering from consistently elevated amounts of cortisol and wish to avoid the symptoms of adrenal burnout, follow the suggestions made earlier in connection with the treatment of high cortisol, such as cutting out refined carbohydrates and trying meditation. (See pages 257 to 258.) The goal is to bring your body back into balance before the circuitry between the hypothalamus, pituitary glands, and adrenal glands misfires and alters cortisol output.

Consider This

Cortisol levels fluctuate during the day. The best time to take a cortisol test is in the morning, between 7 and 9 a.m., when cortisol levels are lowest. Salivary tests can also be used to map out the pattern of your cortisol fluctuation over a 24-hour period, accounting for times of day when your stress response may be highest.

34. ESTROGEN

Although it has a number of functions, estrogen is a class of steroid hormones known primarily for its role in sexual development and reproduction. While this type of hormone is present in both sexes, adult women typically have significantly higher amounts than men, particularly during reproductive age. The three main forms of estrogen are estrone (E1), estradiol (E2), and estriol (E3). Estriol is normally the weakest estrogen and is produced in meaningful amounts only in pregnant women. Estradiol, the most potent form, is the main estrogen in women during their reproductive years. It is also present in males as a derivative of testosterone. Finally, estrone increases in females during menopause to become the predominant estrogen in postmenopausal women. As the ovaries lose the ability to make estradiol, the adrenal glands, liver, and fat cells compensate for the loss by producing estrone. The problem is that metabolized estrone can be harmful, and elevated levels can increase the risk of estrogen-related cancers like breast cancer. Because estrone may be secreted by fat cells, higher than normal amounts may be found in overweight individuals.

While they remain fairly constant in men, normal ranges for total estrogen levels in women vary considerably depending on stage of life. They also fluctuate during a woman's menstrual cycle. The table below gives the reasonable ranges for total estrogen, measured in picograms per milliliter (pg/mL), for both males and females.

REFERENCE RANGES FOR ESTROGEN

Category	Stage	Estrogen Normal Range (pg/mL)
Men	Prepubertal	12 to 55
	Adult	40 to 115
Women	Prepubertal	12 to 57
	Follicular Phase (Day 1 to 12 of menstrual cycle)	61 to 394
	Ovulation (Day 13 to 16 of menstrual cycle)	122 to 437
	Luteal Phase (Day 17 to 29 of menstrual cycle)	156 to 350
	Postmenopausal	20 to 40

Reference ranges can vary depending on the lab, so always rely on your doctor to determine whether or not your estrogen count is outside the norm for your age.

WHAT CAUSES HIGH ESTROGEN?

It goes without saying that pregnancy elevates estrogen levels, as do fertility treatments for those who are having trouble getting pregnant. There are, however, other unintended factors that may raise estrogen levels, including:

- Adrenal tumors
- Cirrhosis of the liver
- Environmental estrogens, such as those found in foods and cleaning products
- Increased consumption of phytoestrogen-containing foods such as soy, in combination with a low-fiber diet
- Ovarian tumors
- Stress

Certain medications also cause high estrogen readings, including:

- Anabolic steroids
- Antibiotics, including ampicillin (Omnipen) and tetracycline (Ala-Tet)
- Corticosteroids, including prednisone (Deltasone), cortisone, hydrocortisone, and methylprednisolone (Medrol)
- Hormone replacement therapy
- Oral contraceptives
- Phenothiazines, including chlorpromazine (Thorazine) and promethazine (Pentazine)

Elevated estrogen levels have been associated with such health conditions as breast cancer, hyperthyroidism, and liver damage. If you notice symptoms of this issue, see your doctor.

WHAT ARE THE SYMPTOMS OF HIGH ESTROGEN?

Symptoms of high estrogen include fatigue, insomnia, gas and bloating, abdominal swelling, irregular periods, weight gain, mood swings, gynecomastia, loss of concentration, and mental fogginess.

HOW CAN HIGH ESTROGEN BE TREATED?

When it comes to lowering estrogen levels, the best lifestyle choices you can make involve avoiding further ingestion of estrogenic compounds and boosting metabolism of this hormone. There are also supplements you can take to support hormone balance in general.

SUPPLEMENTS

To promote hormonal balance and a healthy system, you may wish to investigate the following supplements.

SUPPLEMENTS FOR HIGH ESTROGEN

Supplement	Dosage	Considerations
Calcium glucarate	500 mg one to two times a day.	Do not use if you are pregnant or breastfeeding.
DIM (diindolylmethane)	75 to 150 mg twice a day.	This supplement helps metabolize estrogen into a more beneficial form. Consult your health-care provider before using.
Probiotics	5 to 15 billion CFUs two to three times a day.	Probiotics help normalize beneficial flora in the gastrointestinal tract, and are reported to decrease triglyceride and cholesterol levels. They are also reported to improve BUN levels and quality of life in people with kidney disease. It's best to use heat-stable products that do not require refrigeration. If using an antibiotic, wait three hours before taking probiotics. If diarrhea occurs, decrease your dosage. If this side effect persists for longer than 48 hours, stop taking the supplement and contact your doctor. Live cultures should be guaranteed through the date of expiration on label. For optimal results, take probiotics with meals, as food improves the survivability of the cultures.

LIFESTYLE CHANGES

The first step should be to stop drinking out of plastic containers that contain chemicals such as phthalates and bisphenol A (BPA), which can leach into your beverage and disrupt hormone balance. Because it can contain high amounts of hormones, meat should not be eaten, unless you buy organic meat, which should be free of any chemical additives. As fat cells secrete estrogen, other foods to limit would be refined carbohydrates and sugars, and high-fat products, which encourage weight gain.

To help with estrogen metabolism, eat at least 30 g of fiber a day (with at least some from flax seed), and increase your consumption of cruciferous vegetables, including broccoli, cauliflower, and Brussels sprouts. Finally, reduce your alcohol consumption and get some exercise, particularly aerobic. Thirty minutes a day, three to four times a week is recommended.

WHAT CAUSES LOW ESTROGEN?

Low levels of estrogen are more common than high levels. They decrease naturally after giving birth, while breastfeeding, and at the onset of menopause. Because fat cells promote estrogen production, people who have extremely low amounts of body fat, such as athletes, may have low estrogen readings. There are, however, certain health factors that result in a reduction of this hormone, including:

- Anticonvulsant medication
- Eating disorders, including anorexia nervosa
- Hypogonadism
- Hypopituitarism
- Ovariohysterectomy
- Turner syndrome

Low levels of estrogen can lead to serious conditions such as osteoporosis, heart disease, and stroke, so it is important to recognize the symptoms of this issue.

WHAT ARE THE SYMPTOMS OF LOW ESTROGEN?

Low amounts of estrogen in the blood are associated with decreased libido, hot flashes and night sweats, depression, anxiety, memory problems, headaches, fatigue, joint pain, dry skin, and vaginal dryness. Do not ignore these symptoms; consult your doctor regularly.

HOW CAN LOW ESTROGEN BE TREATED?

As recently stated, the reduction of estrogen at menopause is a normal occurrence. Some women, however, may experience severe symptoms caused by low estrogen at this time and wish to alleviate them through the use of hormone replacement therapy (HRT), in which synthetic estrogen is administered to raise amounts of this hormone. In recent years, though, HRT has drawn considerable criticism. A number of large studies have linked synthetic estrogen replacement therapy to an increased risk of dementia, breast cancer, heart disease, stroke, and blood clots. For this reason, you may want to ask your doctor about bioidentical hormone replacement therapy (BHRT), which preliminary studies have shown to be safer (see the inset below). Supplements and lifestyle changes may also be recommended in place of or in addition to hormone therapy.

Bioidentical Hormone Replacement Therapy

Due to the safety concerns and side effects associated with traditional pharmaceutical hormone therapy, more and more doctors are turning to bioidentical hormones, or human-identical hormones. These hormones have the same chemical structure as hormones produced by the human body and, unlike nonbioidentical synthetic hormones, are generally thought to provide a safer and lower-risk side effect profile. Traditionally, hormone therapies took more of a "one-size-fits-all" approach. In contrast, bioidentical hormone replacement therapy (BHRT) can be individualized to meet the patient's unique needs and correct her hormonal imbalance.

Because a physician must prescribe bioidentical hormones, BHRT is considered a prescription drug therapy. The hormones can be compounded into creams for topical application, or manufactured in the form of a patch, like some traditional prescription drugs. The problem is that there have been few large-scale studies on BHRT, so some physicians are hesitant to prescribe or even recommend it to their patients. However, many smaller studies have concluded that bioidentical hormones are preferable to nonbioidentical synthetic hormone regimens, which are linked to numerous side effects and may increase the risk of several serious conditions, like blood clots, liver disease, and some cancers. Patients should be proactive and encourage their clinicians to call pharmacists and investigate bioidentical treatment options, risks, and starting dosages.

Bioidentical hormone therapy can be highly beneficial and improve your quality of life as you age. Still, it may not be right for everyone. If you have ever had breast cancer or liver disease, or if you are prone to blood clots, you should consider an alternative to hormone treatment. Find an experienced physician to help you incorporate BHRT into your long-term health plan. In most cases, your doctor will gradually increase your dosage to reduce your symptoms and achieve specific hormone levels.

SUPPLEMENTS

The supplements listed in the following table may be effective for increasing estrogen levels. Because elevated estrogen may contribute to a number of serious diseases, raising levels of this hormone should be attempted only under a doctor's supervision.

SUPPLEMENTS FOR LOW ESTROGEN

Supplement	Dosage	Considerations
Black cohosh (standardized to 1 mg triterpenes)	20 mg twice a day.	Do not use if you are pregnant or breastfeeding. Avoid use if you have a hormone-sensitive condition such as uterine fibroids or breast cancer. Do not use if you have liver disease, had a kidney transplant, or are suffering from protein-S deficiency.
Rhapontic rhubarb (2.2 mg rhaponticin and 1 mg desoxyrhaponticin)	4 mg once a day.	Do not take if you are pregnant or breastfeeding. Speak to your doctor before using if you have or have ever had a hormone-sensitive condition such as uterine fibroids or breast cancer.

LIFESTYLE CHANGES

When it comes to diet, the easiest step to take is to eat more phytoestrogen-rich foods. These include legumes such as chickpeas and lentils; fruits such as apples, cherries, and pomegranates; vegetables such as beets, carrots, and eggplant; grains such as barley, oats, and wheat; herbs and spices such as clover, garlic, and licorice; and seeds such as alfalfa, fennel, and sunflower seeds. As with any dietary supplementation, however, it is important that you consult with your doctor before making any major changes to your regime.

Consider This

Phytoestrogens are plant-derived chemicals that mimic the effect of estrogen on the body. They are abundant in beans, but can also be found in certain grains and seeds, including flaxseed, barley, and oats. While the effects of phytoestrogen are still being studied, there is some indication that increased consumption of phytoestrogen-rich food lowers the risk of osteoporosis, heart disease, breast cancer, and menopausal symptoms.

35. THYROID HORMONES

Located in the neck, the thyroid gland produces hormones that control metabolism and energy production. These hormones regulate how each cell converts food into calories and utilizes stored fat to create energy. They influence weight control, nerve and gastrointestinal health, nutrient absorption, and oxygen use. Initiated by thyroid-stimulating hormone (TSH) from the pituitary gland, thyroid hormone production includes two principal types: the active hormone triiodothyronine (T_3) and the inactive hormone thyroxine (T_4), which is converted to T_3.

In addition to a TSH count, thyroid hormone measurements can include levels of total T_3 and T_4, and free T_3 and T_4. Free levels refer to the amount of circulating hormone available for use by your cells, while total levels also include the amount of hormone bound to proteins. Typically, free T_3 and T_4 readings are considered more reliable indicators of thyroid disturbances than total readings. If your doctor suspects thyroid damage, which is commonly associated with autoimmune conditions such as Hashimoto's thyroiditis, the lab may test for thyroglobulin antibodies, thyroglobulin AB, or thyroid peroxidase (TPO), which helps convert T_4 to T_3. Another thyroid hormone called reverse T_3, which is typically produced in greater amounts when chronic stress is present, may also be measured. Reverse T_3 binds to T_3 receptors but does not have any effect. Normal ranges for the main thyroid hormones are listed below.

REFERENCE RANGES FOR THYROID HORMONES

Thyroid Hormone	Normal Range
Thyroid-stimulating hormone (TSH)	0.45 to 4.5 mcIU/mL (microinternational units per milliliter)
Free triiodothyronine (T_3)	200 to 440 pg/dL (picograms per deciliter)
Total triiodothyronine (T_3)	71 to 180 ng/dL (nanograms per deciliter)
Free thyroxine (T_4)	0.82 to 1.77 ng/dL (nanograms per deciliter)
Total thyroxine (T_4)	4.5 to 12 mcg/dL (micrograms per deciliter)
Thyroid peroxidase (TPO)	0 to 34 IU/mL (international units per milliliter)

Most doctors request only TSH and T_4 levels, following up with a T_3 reading if results fall outside out of the normal ranges. Some doctors place great importance on free T_3 levels right away, as it is the most active thyroid hormone. If T_3 levels are low compared to T_4 and TSH levels, it may signify low thyroid function even if the labs otherwise appear normal.

WHAT CAUSES HIGH THYROID HORMONES?

Normally, thyroid levels rise slightly during pregnancy. This is a good thing, as thyroid hormone is critical to the development of a baby's brain and nervous system. There are, however, unwanted reasons behind elevated thyroid hormones, also called *hyperthyroidism,* including:

- Environmental toxins, especially mercury, lead, and cadmium
- Estrogens
- Excess iodine in diet
- Graves' disease
- Oral contraceptives
- Pituitary gland disorder
- Stress
- Thyroid nodules
- Thyroiditis

In addition, certain medications may raise thryoid hormone levels. These substances include:

- Clofibrate (Atromid-S)
- Opiate pain relievers like morphine, demerol, and oxycodone

High thyroid hormone levels have been linked to heart disease, osteoporosis, eye problems, and skin conditions. If elevated thyroid hormones are a result of drugs, your doctor will determine how to address the problem. If your thyroid hormones are high, it is essential for you to be evaluated by an endocrinologist.

WHAT ARE THE SYMPTOMS OF HIGH THYROID HORMONES?

Symptoms of elevated thyroid hormones include bulging eyes, goiter, irregular heartbeat, anxiety, hand tremors, difficulty sleeping, weight loss, diarrhea, moist skin, muscle weakness, light or missed menstrual periods, and infertility.

HOW CAN HIGH THYROID HORMONES BE TREATED?

High thyroid hormones are a serious issue that will most likely be treated by pharmaceuticals prescribed by your physician. Although it is not often performed unless the situation is unmanageable, the surgical removal of the thyroid gland known as a thyroidectomy may be suggested. While there are lifestyle adjustments that may help alleviate the problem, these will likely be complementary to the treatment recommended by your doctor.

DRUGS

Beta blockers are typically prescribed to lessen the symptoms of high thyroid hormone levels, while antithyroid medications are used to decrease production of these hormones. One of the most common antithyroid drugs is listed in the table below. In addition, a nonradioactive iodide formula called Lugol's solution may be administered to inhibit thyroid hormone synthesis, while radioactive iodine may be used to kill active thyroid cells, possibly curing the condition.

DRUGS FOR HIGH THYROID HORMONES	
Drug	**Considerations**
Methimazole *Tapazole*	Side effects may include upset stomach, nausea, vomiting, mild rash, and itchiness.

SUPPLEMENTS

You may also wish to consider the following supplements to lower your thyroid hormone levels. Always talk to your physician about possible interactions between supplements and thyroid-reducing drugs. In addition, since bone loss is a common problem in hyperthyroidism, you should ask your doctor about taking a multiple mineral supplement containing calcium and magnesium, as well as vitamin D.

SUPPLEMENTS FOR HIGH THYROID HORMONES		
Supplement	**Dosage**	**Considerations**
L-carnitine	2 to 4 g once a day to start; for maintenance, 1 to 2 g once a day.	Can help lower triglycerides because it helps move fat into cells for the purpose of energy production. Also supports demineralization and has been reported to reverse and prevent symptoms related to hyperthyroidism. Food sources of the substance are meat, poultry, and dairy products.
Moducare	40 mg (2 capsules) twice a day.	Taken if thyroid antibodies are present.
Vitamin D (vitamin D_3, or cholecalciferol)	1,000 to 4,000 IU once a day.	Vitamin D is necessary for proper calcium absorption. Inform your doctor if you are taking any drug that can deplete vitamin D, such as

Supplement	Dosage	Considerations
Vitamin D *(continued)*		anticonvulsants, cholesterol-lowering medications, anti-ulcer drugs, or mineral oil. People with kidney disease or atherosclerosis should not take vitamin D. Excessive intake can increase the risk of hardened arteries and high blood calcium levels. People with sarcoidosis, tuberculosis, hyperparathyroidism, and lymphoma should use vitamin D only as directed by a physician. The tolerable upper limit for vitamin D intake is 4,000 IU per day. Higher dosages may be used to treat vitamin D deficiencies, but must be short term and medically supervised.

LIFESTYLE CHANGES

In the face of high thyroid production, you should stop eating foods that increase inflammation, including fried foods, refined sugar and carbohydrates, preserved or processed foods, artificial sweeteners, dyes or chemical additives, and saturated fats founds in fatty meats and dairy. Additionally, increase your intake of anti-inflammatory omega-3 fatty acids found in low-mercury fish like salmon (pregnant women have to be particularly vigilant when it comes to mercury levels in fish), walnuts, and wild game. Limit exposure to pesticides, antibiotics, and hormones by eating organic produce and free range organic meats. Fruits and vegetables should be favored in your diet. Also consider being tested for food intolerances or beginning an elimination diet to limit exposure to the foods to which your body may be sensitive. This might be a substantial step in taking a proactive approach to managing your thyroid condition, as Hashimoto's food antigen-induced thyroiditis, for example, is fairly common. You should also be tested for gluten intolerance and celiac disease, as gluten sensitivity is directly associated with an increased risk of both high and low thyroid function.

Because certain chemicals may leach out of products and into your body, do not microwave or drink out of plastic containers, which may have been made with bisphenol A, and do not use personal care products such as shampoos and face creams that contain phthalates. And while drinking two liters of filtered water a day is recommended, stay away from water supplies that contain fluoride or chlorine. Do not smoke, and drink only in moderation. Decrease stress by getting thirty to sixty minutes of exercise three to four times a week. Simply walking, doing yoga, or even gardening can be helpful. Finally, get six to eight hours or uninterrupted sleep per night.

WHAT CAUSES LOW THYROID HORMONES?

While chronic stress can lower thyroid hormone levels (particularly T_3 levels), also called *hypothyroidism*, often the problem is the result of a more serious factor such as:

- Environmental toxins, especially mercury
- Hashimoto's disease
- Hypothalamic disease
- Iodine deficiency in diet
- Pituitary disease

Pharmaceuticals that can prevent the thyroid gland from functioning properly include:

- Anabolic steroids (testosterone)
- Beta blockers
- Interferon alpha
- Lithium
- Phenytoin (Dilantin)
- Thalidomide

If you notice any symptoms of low thyroid, a blood test is needed to evaluate the reason behind the problem.

WHAT ARE THE SYMPTOMS OF LOW THYROID HORMONES?

A decreased amount of thyroid hormones can result in symptoms that include goiter, chills, cold hands and feet, muscle and joint pain, constipation, depression, weight gain, difficulty losing weight, decline in cognitive function and memory, fatigue, brittle hair and nails, and even hair loss.

HOW CAN LOW THYROID HORMONES BE TREATED?

In a traditional setting, hypothyroidism is most commonly treated with synthetic thyroid hormones. Low levels of selenium, iodine, tyrosine, and chromium can all play a role in reduced thyroid production, as can low iron and ferritin levels. If dietary changes, nutritional support, and lifestyle adjustments do not help, pharmaceutical options should be considered. Finding a doctor who is knowledgeable about managing thyroid balance can be tricky, so look around your community to locate a doctor with a strong reputation. A doctor worth consulting is one who considers all aspects of thyroid function, including food intolerance—particularly gluten intolerance and celiac disease—environmental burden, micronutrient status, and lifestyle factors such as stress and sleep.

DRUGS

The main drug used to treat low thyroid hormone levels is a synthetic form of thyroxine called levothyroxine (see the table below). Doctors who practice integrative medicine prefer the use of gland-based thyroid extracts because they provide all thyroid hormones in a single compound. However, if you have thyroid antibodies you will not be able to use natural thyroid. Another option is compounded T_4 and T_3 combined to personalize the thyroid prescription.

DRUGS FOR LOW THYROID HORMONES

Drug	Considerations
Armour Thyroid (prescription thyroid derived from glandular extracts)	Temporary hair loss may occur. See your doctor if you experience symptoms such as increased sweating, sensitivity to heat, tremors, shortness of breath, diarrhea, or mood changes.
Levothyroxine *Levoxyl, Synthyroid*	Must first be converted to T_3 in the body, which many doctors see as a shortcoming of the drug. Hair loss may occur at the beginning of treatment and last for a few months. If you experience increased perspiration, sensitivity to heat, tremors, mood swings, shortness of breath, or diarrhea, see your doctor right away.
Triiodothryonine (T_3) *Cytomel*	Temporary hair loss may occur. See your doctor if you experience symptoms such as increased sweating, sensitivity to heat, tremors, shortness of breath, diarrhea, or mood changes.

SUPPLEMENTS

The supplements in the table below may combat low thyroid production. If you have hypothyroidism, your doctor will likely prescribe some type of thyroid hormone. Do not take any supplement in combination with this pharmaceutical without first speaking to your physician.

SUPPLEMENTS FOR LOW THYROID HORMONES

Supplement	Dosage	Considerations
Fucus (seaweed)	300 to 600 mg once a day. Dosage should contain no more than 150 mcg of iodine a day.	Use high quality sea vegetables that have been tested for heavy metals and other contaminants. Do not use if you are pregnant or breastfeeding, or trying to become pregnant. Stop taking at least two weeks before any surgery. Avoid if you have an iodine allergy.

Supplement	Dosage	Considerations
GTF (Glucose Tolerance Factor) chromium	500 mcg twice a day.	Helps improve the conversion of T_4 to T_3. Chromium is also important for blood sugar and insulin regulation. Additionally, people who have a diet high in refined carbohydrates like sugar may also be low in chromium. Use under a doctor's supervision if you are diabetic, as it may affect medication dosage. Do not use if you have kidney or liver problems, chromate or leather contact allergy, or a behavioral psychiatric condition such as schizophrenia or depression.
Iodine	150 mcg once a day.	Clinicians may prescribe higher doses of iodine, but this should be done only under a doctor's supervision.
Moducare	40 mg (2 capsules) twice a day.	Taken if thyroid antibodies are present.
Selenium	100 to 200 mcg once a day.	Has been reported to help protect the kidneys. Selenium also helps protect the body against mercury toxicity, which can damage the liver and kidneys. Never take more than the recommended dose. Symptoms of selenium toxicity include vomiting, stomach pain, hair loss, brittle nails, and fatigue.
7-Keto-DHEA	75 to 100 mcg twice a day.	Helps improve the conversion of T_4 to T_3 in tissues.
Tyrosine	250 to 500 mg twice a day.	Do not use if you are pregnant or breastfeeding unless under a doctor's supervision.

LIFESTYLE CHANGES

Many of the dietary guidelines recommended to fight high thyroid hormone levels also apply to low thyroid hormone levels, such as avoiding foods that cause inflammation, increasing intake of anti-inflammatory foods, eating organic meats and produce, and drinking water that does not contain fluoride or chlorine. Because thyroid production depends on iodine, make sure you get enough iodized salt in your diet, and eat more seafood like shrimp and oysters. Don't overdo it, though, as too much salt can lead to high blood pressure and heart disease. Add more calcium-rich items to your meals, including leafy green vegetables and organic milk and cheese. Foods that contain selenium and iron may also help. Selenium can be found in whole grains, Brazil nuts, poultry, vegetables, beans, and shellfish. Foods high in iron include liver, beef, oysters, and turkey.

Do not use plastic containers or personal care items that contain bisphenol A or phthalates, as these chemicals disrupt hormone levels. Reduce stress by exercising for thirty minutes a day three to four times a week, and sleeping for six to eight hours a night.

Did You Know?

According to the American Thyroid Association, about 20 million Americans suffer from thyroid disease—and only about 40 percent of that twenty million are aware of their condition! More than twelve percent of all Americans will develop some form of thyroid disease over the course of their lifetime, with women five to eight times more susceptible than men; for these reasons, it is important to have your thyroid hormone levels evaluated by blood test.

36. PROGESTERONE

Although progesterone is found in both males and females, it is primarily known for its role in conception, pregnancy, and the regulation of a woman's menstrual cycle. Produced in the ovaries, adrenal glands, and the placenta of pregnant women, progesterone has several functions in addition to its role as a sex hormone. It supports bone density, protects against the proliferation of breast and uterine cells, and acts as a coating for the nerve fibers of the brain, reducing hyperexcitability. A female's progesterone levels rise and fall according to the stages of her life. While men also synthesize a small amount of this hormone, it is much less important than testosterone when it comes to sexual maturity. Synthetic forms of progesterone (progestins) are widely used in birth control pills and hormone replacement therapy.

Natural progesterone levels are suppressed in women who take synthetic forms, so blood tests are inaccurate in these cases. Otherwise, a blood test is usually administered twenty-one days after the start of a woman's period, if she is still menstruating. Because progesterone readings normally fluctuate in women, there are a number of normal adult ranges for this hormone, as shown in the table below.

REFERENCE RANGES FOR PROGESTERONE

Category	Progesterone Normal Range (ng/mL)
Men	0.2 to 1.4
Women (pre-ovulation)	Less than 1.0
Women (mid-menstrual cycle)	5 to 20
Women (pregnant, first trimester)	11.2 to 90
Women (pregnant, second trimester)	25.6 to 89.4
Women (pregnant, third trimester)	48.4 to 42.5
Women (postmenopausal)	Less than 1.0

While variations in progesterone levels may be perfectly normal, sometimes a high reading is cause for further testing.

WHAT CAUSES HIGH PROGESTERONE?

As stated earlier, ovulation, pregnancy, and bioidentical hormone replacement therapy (see the inset on page 266) can raise progesterone levels in the blood. Adrenal hyperplasia (abnormal functioning of the adrenal glands) can also raise levels, as can the use of drugs like hCG (human chorionic gonadotropin) and Clomid, which are most commonly used for ferility or stimulating testosterone synthesis in men. Oral contraceptives do not raise blood progesterone levels, as synthetic progestins have neither the same characteristics as natural progesterone nor the same risk profile.

WHAT ARE THE SYMPTOMS OF HIGH PROGESTERONE?

High progesterone levels can create symptoms such as breast tenderness, mood swings, irregular periods, incontinence, bloating, reduced sex drive, vaginal dryness, insulin resistance, weight gain, and depression.

HOW CAN HIGH PROGESTERONE BE TREATED?

Because estrogen and progesterone work to balance each other out, your doctor may recommend estrogen replacement therapy. Your first step, however, might be to try a variety of dietary and lifestyle changes to boost estrogen naturally. Because progesterone fluctuates, treating a high level of this hormone may not be necessary. Follow your doctor's advice when it comes to analyzing this reading.

SUPPLEMENTS

If you are interested in supplements that might help balance your level, consider the following products.

SUPPLEMENTS FOR HIGH PROGESTERONE

Supplement	Dosage	Considerations
Black cohosh (standardized to 1 mg triterpenes)	20 mg twice a day.	Do not use if you are pregnant or breastfeeding. Avoid use if you have a hormone-sensitive condition such as uterine fibroids or breast cancer. Do not use if you have liver disease, had a kidney transplant, or are suffering from protein-S deficiency.
Calcium glucarate	500 mg one to two times a day.	Do not use if you are pregnant or breastfeeding.
DIM (diindolyl-methane)	75 to 150 mg twice a day.	This supplement helps metabolize estrogen into a more beneficial form. Consult your health-care provider before using.

Supplement	Dosage	Considerations
Maca	500 to 1,000 mg three times a day.	Do not use if you are pregnant or breastfeeding.
Omega-3 essential fatty acids DHA and EPA (fish oil)	1,000 mg twice a day.	Fish oil acts as an antioxidant and decreases inflammation in the body, in addition to supporting heart and blood vessel health. Speak to your doctor before taking if you are on blood-thinning medication, as fish oil may increase the risk of bleeding. Be sure to use only high-quality oils that have been tested for contaminants.
Probiotics	5 to 15 billion CFUs one to three times a day.	Probiotics help normalize beneficial flora in the gastrointestinal tract, and are reported to decrease triglyceride and cholesterol levels. They are also reported to improve BUN levels and quality of life in people with kidney disease. It's best to use heat-stable products that do not require refrigeration. If using an antibiotic, wait three hours before taking probiotics. If diarrhea occurs, decrease your dosage. If this side effect persists for longer than 48 hours, stop taking the supplement and contact your doctor. Live cultures should be guaranteed through the date of expiration on label. For optimal results, take probiotics with meals, as food improves the survivability of the cultures.

LIFESTYLE CHANGES

Adding phytoestrogen-containing foods like pomegranates and snap peas, eating more cruciferous vegetables such as broccoli and cabbage, and increasing your fiber intake with flaxseeds, bran, and beans can help raise beneficial forms of estrogen in the body. Remove refined sugars and carbohydrates from your diet, decrease calories from fat, and increase lean protein consumption. Diets that are high in saturated fat and refined sugars but low in fiber have been reported to alter estrogen metabolism, in turn affecting progesterone levels. You should also avoid soft drinks, as the phosphorous and caffeine they contain foster bone loss, and opt for filtered water instead. Try not to drink from plastic containers, though, which may leach hormone-disrupting chemicals such as bisphenol A and phthalates. In addition, limit your use of personal care products that have these substances.

As stated earlier, stress can lead to hormonal imbalances. You may cut your stress levels by walking, meditating, doing yoga, gardening, or engaging in thirty minutes of moderate exercise five times a week. Finally, make sure to get seven to eight hours of sleep a night.

WHAT CAUSES LOW PROGESTERONE?

Progesterone levels can decrease naturally or as the result of illness or lifestyle. The main factors behind low progesterone include:

- Chronic stress
- Environmental pollutants
- High estrogen
- Lack of exercise
- Menopause
- Oral contraceptives
- Polycystic ovarian syndrome (PCOS)
- Poor diet

If left untreated, this issue can lead to serious conditions such as infertility, miscarriage, heart disease, ovarian or uterine cysts, breast or ovarian cancer, and osteoporosis.

WHAT ARE THE SYMPTOMS OF LOW PROGESTERONE?

Low progesterone levels can cause symptoms that include anxiety, depression, trouble sleeping, fatigue, memory loss, fibrocystic breasts, headaches, hot flashes, night sweats, breast tenderness, loss of libido, mood swings, irregular or heavy periods, lowered immunity, high blood pressure, and bone loss.

HOW CAN LOW PROGESTERONE BE TREATED?

Your doctor may suggest treatment with synthetic progesterone or naturally derived bioidentitcal hormone replacement therapy (see the inset on page 266). Follow the directions of your doctor when taking bioidentical hormones and have your hormones tested regularly. Although low progesterone levels may simply be attributable to a normal phase of life, they can be the result of something more serious. Discuss all treatment options with your doctor.

SUPPLEMENTS

Depending on the cause of your low progesterone level, chasteberry may be beneficial. Do not take this substance before discussing its use with a doctor.

SUPPLEMENTS FOR LOW PROGESTERONE		
Supplement	**Dosage**	**Considerations**
Chasteberry (standardized to contain at least 0.5-percent agnuside and 0.6-percent aucubin)	100 to 200 mg every morning, preferably on an empty stomach, one hour before or two hours after breakfast.	Do not use if you are pregnant or breastfeeding. Avoid use if you have a hormone-sensitive condition such as uterine fibroids or breast cancer. Use with caution if taking dopamine agonist drugs, including metoclopramide and levodopa.

LIFESTYLE CHANGES

In some cases, lifestyle change may have enough impact on progesterone production to bring about a normal reading. Cutting out processed foods and refined sugars, getting more exercise, and reducing stress are ways to bring balance to hormone levels.

Did You Know?

Although progesterone is normally associated with reproductive health, recent studies have indicated that it plays a role in protecting the neurological system, too. Noting that in every age group, women were significantly less likely than men to die from a traumatic brain injury (brain injury caused by sudden impact, as in a fall, a car collision, or a blow to the head), scientists have hypothesized that progesterone--found in higher levels in women--reduces swelling around the brain and perhaps eliminates free radicals that cause cell death.

37. TESTOSTERONE

Although both males and females produce testosterone, this hormone is ten times more abundant in men. It is primarily associated with male sexual development, but also plays a role in the brain function, muscle mass, fat distribution, and energy levels of both sexes. Testosterone is typically attached to a protein in the bloodstream known as bound testosterone. When this hormone is unattached, it is known as free testosterone, which is the form that is most available for use by the body. Generally, a blood test will measure the combination of both types of testosterone, called total testosterone. If the reading appears problematic, your doctor will likely follow up with a free testosterone count, which typically gives more accurate clues for diagnosis. Total testosterone ranges are listed in the table below.

REFERENCE RANGES FOR TOTAL TESTOSTERONE	
Category	**Total Testosterone Normal Range (ng/mL)**
Men (13 to 17 years old)	28 to 1110
Men (over 18 years old)	280 to 800
Women (under 18 years old)	6 to 82

If your doctor requests a reading of free testosterone levels, you can match your results to the ranges below.

REFERENCE RANGES FOR FREE TESTOSTERONE	
Category	**Free Testosterone Normal Range (pg/mL)**
Men (20 to 29 years old)	9.3 to 26.5
Men (30 to 39 years old)	8.7 to 25.1
Men (40 to 49 years old)	7.2 to 24
Men (50 to 59 years old)	6.8 to 21.5
Men (older than 59 years old)	6.6 to 18.1
Women (20 to 59 years old)	0 to 2.2
Women (older than 59 years old)	0 to 1.8

While testosterone levels can vary, a consistently low or high reading will need to be addressed by your physician.

WHAT CAUSES HIGH TESTOSTERONE?

Testosterone levels may be elevated for a number of reasons, some of which are more serious conditions than others. The list below details the causes behind this issue.

- Environmental contaminants like lead, mercury, plastics, and pesticides
- Excessive exercise
- High DHEA levels
- Medications, including anabolic steroids, androgen replacement therapy; anticonvulsants, including phenytoin (Dilantin), and barbiturates

In addition to these factors, women have their own causes of high testosterone, including:

- Acromegaly
- Adrenal neoplasm disorders
- Androgen-producing adrenal or ovarian tumor
- Certain oral contraceptives
- Congenital adrenal hyperplasia
- Cushing's syndrome
- Diabetes
- Dwarfism
- Hormone replacement therapy (HRT)
- Multiple endocrine neoplasm 1 and 2
- Polycystic ovary syndrome (PCOS)
- Thyroid disorders

While women can have elevated amounts of testosterone in the blood, most of the conditions that lead to this result are still quite rare.

WHAT ARE THE SYMPTOMS OF HIGH TESTOSTERONE?

Symptoms of high testosterone levels in men include acne, testicular shrinkage, reduced fertility, receding hair line, anger, aggressiveness, and enlarged prostate gland. These signs are particularly important to acknowledge, since elevated testosterone has been associated with prostate cancer. Symptoms of high testosterone in women include hirsutism (excessive body and facial hair), male pattern baldness, deepening of the voice, redistribution of body fat, increased perspiration, raised libido, and cessation of menstruation.

HOW IS HIGH TESTOSTERONE TREATED?

Depending on the severity of high testosterone levels in the blood, medical intervention may be recommended. In extremely serious cases such as advanced prostate cancer, an orchiectomy, or removal of the testicles, may be suggested. This procedure stops most testosterone production and increases the chance of survival. However, both drugs and lifestyle change can promote healthy testosterone levels.

DRUGS

Elevated amounts of testosterone may be treated with pharmaceuticals, including the following medications.

DRUGS FOR HIGH TESTOSTERONE

Drug	Considerations
Antiandrogens (bicalutamide, flutamide, and cyproterone acetate) *Casodex, Cyprostat, Eulixin*	Side effects are possible when taking this drug. Use only under a doctor's supervision.
5-alpha reductase inhibitors (finasteride) *Proscar*	Use only under the guidance and supervision of your doctor. Seek medical attention if you experience any side effects.
Ketoconazole *Nizoral*	Follow your doctor's instructions for taking this drug.
LHRH analogs (goserelin and leuprolide) *Zoladex, Lupron*	Use only under your physician's guidance.

LIFESTYLE CHANGES

There are also a few lifestyle adjustments that may help alleviate high testosterone. Because inflammatory foods can lead to imbalances in testosterone levels, try to decrease the consumption of these troublesome edibles, which include high-carbohydate or high-sugar items, products made with high-fructose corn syrup, fried foods, lunch meats, and fast food in general. Avoid chemical additives, preservatives, dyes, and artificial sweeteners, and buy organic meats, which are raised without antibiotics or hormones. Instead, eat more antioxidant-rich foods, such as yellow and red peppers, squash, tomatoes, leafy greens, garlic, onions, and cruciferous vegetables like broccoli and Brussels sprouts. In addition to dietary changes, make sure to get between seven and eight hours of sleep every night, stop smoking, and engage in physical activities like yoga or pilates.

WHAT CAUSES LOW TESTOSTERONE?

While a descrease in testosterone levels is a normal part of aging, it can also be caused by other factors, including:

- Chemotherapy and radiation therapy
- Chronic stress
- Drugs such as Minoxidil (Rogaine), opiate pain medications, including meperidine (Demerol), oxycodone (Oxycontin), and morphine; and steroids, including prednisone (Deltasone) and dexamethasone (Decadron)
- Environmental contaminants like lead, mercury, plastics, and pesticides
- Head trauma
- Obesity
- Ovary problems in women
- Scrotal injury

Low testosterone levels have been linked to type 2 diabetes, heart disease, and a higher death rate in men, so listen to your body and pay attention to any symptoms you might experience.

WHAT ARE THE SYMPTOMS OF LOW TESTOSTERONE?

Decreased amounts of testosterone may result in symptoms such as erectile dysfunction, changes in mood, fatigue, sleep disturbances, high blood pressure, low libido, muscle atrophy, joint aches and pains, increased body fat (particularly belly fat), loss of body hair, poor concentration, and blood sugar imbalances.

HOW CAN LOW TESTOSTERONE BE TREATED?

Testosterone replacement therapy—administered as injections, patches, or a gel—may be recommended for men with low testosterone counts, although it is not approved for women at this time. Both men and women, however, can support balanced testosterone with supplements, dietary measures, and general lifestyle changes. While all of these methods may be helpful, the treatment you use will depend upon your particular situation and the advice of your doctor.

SUPPLEMENTS

Supplements that may benefit people with low testosterone levels are listed below. Be sure to speak to your doctor before beginning a regimen, as some supplements are contraindicated by certain medications.

SUPPLEMENTS FOR LOW TESTOSTERONE		
Supplement	**Dosage**	**Considerations**
Saw palmetto (standardized to at least 85-percent fatty acids and astaxanthin)	400 mg three times a day.	May be used by men to treat low testosterone and improve overall prostate health. Consult your physician before using.
Tongkat ali	300 mg twice a day.	May be used by men to treat low testosterone. Avoid if you have a prostate condition such as BPH or prostate cancer.
Zinc	50 mg once a day.	Zinc is important in immunity and acts as an antioxidant. It is also reported to help regulate blood sugar. May also be used by men to treat low testosterone and support prostate health. Take zinc in the form of an amino acid chelate or citrate. Check with your doctor before using.

LIFESTYLE CHANGES

Diet and lifestyle are key factors in raising low testosterone. First, increase your intake of quality protein, including organic turkey, beef, or bison. Add coldwater fish like wild salmon and wild halibut to your meals, and eat more antioxidant-rich produce, including yellow and red peppers, squash, tomatoes, leafy greens, broccoli, Brussels sprouts, garlic, and onions. Because zinc and selenium benefit reproductive health, opt for lean meats, liver, eggs, high-quality seafood (especially oysters), garlic, cabbage, cucumbers, and radishes.

Aside from dietary adjustments, get at least seven hours of sleep every night, as lack of sleep and sleep distruptions have been shown to lower tesosterone. Drink two to three liters of filtered water every day and restrict alcohol use as well. Additionally, exercise for thirty minutes a day three to four times a week. Try yoga, pilates, or simply walking.

38. PROSTATE-SPECIFIC ANTIGEN (PSA)

The prostate is a small gland—about the size and shape of a walnut—located below the bladder in men. It produces and releases the liquid component of semen and helps discharge sperm during ejaculation. Prostate-specific antigen, or PSA, is one of the proteins synthesized by prostate cells. Although it is not a hormone, it was once used as a screening marker for prostate cancer, but this practice has become controversial because it leads to many unnecessary procedures. Still, many doctors rely on this test as a screening for at-risk males. Ordinarily, there is a small amount of PSA in a man's blood. However, aging can bring about prostate problems, such as enlarged prostate and prostate cancer. This causes PSA levels to rise as it attempts to suppress the growth of prostate cells.

While PSA levels increase naturally over time, there are reference ranges for this hormone, as shown in the table below. Clinicians look at the rate of change in PSA between two readings for evidence of early signs of prostate problems. If the number suddenly jumps within six months to a year, your doctor may require further testing or an examination. The night before a PSA test, do not engage in sexual activity, particularly if it results in ejaculation. This can create false-positive lab values.

REFERENCE RANGES FOR PROSTATE-SPECIFIC ANTIGEN

Total PSA (ng/mL)	Category
4.0 to 10.0	High
0.0 to 4.0	Normal

As evidenced by the normal range for this protein, low PSA levels are not a factor.

WHAT CAUSES HIGH PSA?

Although the process of aging is responsible for slight increases in PSA, there are a number of other reasons for an elevated PSA reading, including:

- Anabolic steroid use
- Benign prostatic hyperplasia (BPH)
- Bicycle riding
- Digital rectal exam (DRE)
- Frequent ejaculation
- Pituitary disease
- Prostate biopsy
- Testicular disease
- Prostate cancer

A high PSA reading may be cause for concern, but does not mean that you have cancer. Your doctor will discuss it with you, perhaps recommending further testing or simply deciding to keep an eye on it.

WHAT ARE THE SYMPTOMS OF HIGH PSA?

Symptoms of elevated PSA may include painful or frequent urination, trouble urinating, a feeling of fullness in the bladder, decreased libido, fertility problems, erectile dysfunction, or pain in the groin area.

HOW CAN HIGH PSA BE TREATED?

If PSA is raised due to a specific medical condition, your doctor will attempt to treat the underlying cause. If the reason is prostate cancer, there are several options available, including surgery, proton radiation, and drug therapy. Prostate cancer can be slow to progress, so depending on your age and severity of the condition, surgery may not be necessary. The supplements and lifestyle modifications discussed in the following sections may help reduce PSA, as well as promote a healthy level.

SUPPLEMENTS

The substances listed in the table below can help lower PSA levels. Consult your physician before using any supplement to make sure it is appropriate for your health needs.

SUPPLEMENTS FOR HIGH PSA

Supplement	Dosage	Considerations
Omega-3 essential fatty acids DHA and EPA (fish oil)	1,000 mg twice a day.	Fish oil acts as an antioxidant and decreases inflammation in the body, in addition to supporting heart and blood vessel health. Speak to your doctor before taking if you are on blood-thinning medication, as fish oil may increase the risk of bleeding. Be sure to use only high-quality oils that have been tested for contaminants.
Saw palmetto (standardized to at least 85-percent fatty acids and astaxanthin)	160 mg three times a day.	May be used by men to treat low testosterone and improve overall prostate health. Consult your physician before using.

Supplement	Dosage	Considerations
Zinc	15 to 30 mg once a day.	Zinc is important in immunity and acts as an antioxidant. It is also reported to help regulate blood sugar. May also be used by men to treat low testosterone and support prostate health. Take zinc in the form of an amino acid chelate or citrate. Check with your doctor before using.

LIFESTYLE CHANGES

There are also lifestyle modifications you can make to help lower PSA levels. The first step is to lose weight. The second step is to avoid inflammatory foods, which include foods that are high in carbohydrates and sugar. Additionally, items that may contain trans fats—such as many fried foods and baked goods—should be avoided. In general, stay away from processed foods, lunch meats, and fast food. Because zinc and selenium may have a protective effect on prostate health, increase your intake of foods that contain these minerals, such as pumpkin seeds, liver, eggs, oysters, cabbage, celery, and radishes.

As is the case in the treatment of many of imbalances, sleep and exercise are important. Get at least seven to eight hours of uninterrupted sleep nightly, and engage in moderate physcial activity for thirty minutes a day, three to four days a week. Stop smoking and drink alcohol only in moderation. Finally, drink 2 to 3 liters of filtered water each day.

CONCLUSION

Now that you know more about hormones, you can see how important they are to numerous vital functions in the body. From sexual development and energy production to blood sugar regulation and the health of your immune system, hormones play a role in your well-being every second of every day. When one hormone is thrown out of balance by age, illness, nutritional deficiency, or environmental toxins, symptoms begin to occur, and other hormones may become elevated or suppressed. Maintaining hormonal equilibrium is key when it comes to feeling healthy, especially as you age, and there are a variety of ways to manage hormone levels throughout your lifetime. Lifestyle measures and nutritional supplements can be very helpful, and when they are not enough, medications—particularly bioidentical hormones—may lend a hand. So listen to your body, pay attention to symptoms of possible hormone imbalance, and consult your doctor as needed.

PART 6

Optional Tests

In addition to the traditional blood test panels discussed in this book, there are a number of labs that, though optional, are equally vital to your well-being. Among them are *homocysteine*, an amino acid byproduct; *C-reactive protein* (CRP), a marker of inflammation; and essential nutrients like *vitamin D* and *magnesium*.

Homocysteine, which is part of a comprehensive lipid profile, may be measured to evaluate an individual's total cardiovascular risk. This lab value can also be measured to determine whether or not the body has a sufficient supply of B vitamins. CRP is another lab included in a complete heart risk assessment, as high levels are usually a sign of inflammation in the body. People who have a history or higher risk of conditions like heart disease, stroke, and peripheral artery disease.

Two nutrients in particular are also worth testing. The first is vitamin D, which has been a subject of attention in recent years due to the growing amount of research on its health benefits. Vitamin D is crucial to heart health, immunity, calcium absorption, and insulin regulation, and may lower the risk of medical conditions like hypertension, osteoporosis, some autoimmune disorders, and even certain types of cancer. Although more and more doctors recommend the test to their patients, vitamin D is still usually measured only when calcium levels are high, or when a person has a condition that may lead to low vitamin D. This is also the case for magnesium, an essential nutrient that, like vitamin D, performs a wide range of functions in the body. Unfortunately, most Americans do not take in sufficient amounts of the mineral, as the standard diet in the United States is filled with refined sugars and saturated fats—substances tht actually increase the body's magnesium requirement. Therefore, keeping an eye on magnesium levels with regular blood tests can help ensure proper metabolism, bone formation, blood sugar regulation, and other basic physiological processes.

Although this section focuses on four labs—homocysteine, CRP, vitamin D, and magnesium—there are many others that are just as valuable when it comes to achieving and maintaining good health. By reviewing the information in the following pages, you will be in a better position to have a meaningful conversation with your physician about the present and future state of your health.

Consider This:

The average adult has 5 liters, or 10 pints, of blood, accounting for about 7 percent of total body weight. A person can lose about 10 to 15 percent of his total blood volume with no ill effect; the standard unit for blood donation is 450 milliliters, or about a pint.

39. HOMOCYSTEINE

Homocysteine is not included in the traditional lipid profile but may be measured as part of a complete heart risk assessment. A byproduct of amino acids, homocysteine is generated when *methionine*—an amino acid found primarily in meats, fish, and dairy products—is metabolized, and used by the body to make protein and maintain tissues. When adequate levels of vitamins B_2, B_6, B_{12}, and folic acid are present in the body, leftover homocysteine is normally recycled and used to make methionine. Elevated homocysteine, therefore, usually indicates that the body is deficient in B-complex vitamins or unable to metabolize methionine properly. Studies have found that an excess of homocysteine in the blood can damage the arteries, cause blood-clotting problems, and increase the risk of coronary artery disease, peripheral artery disease, and stroke. Heightened risk of Alzheimer's disease, dementia, and kidney disease is also associated with high levels of homocysteine.

The following reference ranges are used to categorize homocysteine levels, which are measured in micromoles per liter (μmol/L).

REFERENCE RANGES FOR HOMOCYSTEINE

Homocysteine (μmol/L)	Category
Greater than 29	Very high risk
15 to 29	High risk
11 to 15	Intermediate risk
Less than 11	Normal
Target Range: 6 to 8 μmol/L	

A homocysteine test is requested by a doctor when comprehensive blood work is needed to evaluate total cardiovascular risk. Most often, doctors order a homocysteine blood test when an individual has heart problems without the usual risk factors, such as smoking and obesity. The test may also be recommended if one or more of the individual's immediate family members have high homocysteine levels or developed heart conditions at a young age. In addition, people who take medications like metformin, a diabetes drug, should ask for a homocysteine test, as many pharmaceuticals can increase the amount in the blood. If you take any of the medications listed on pages 292 to 293, speak to your physician about having your level tested. Usually, a simple supplement regimen of vitamin B_6, vitamin B_{12}, or folic acid can restore blood homocysteine to normal levels.

It's equally important that your blood is not too low on homocysteine, since the substance is essential for a number of physiological functions. More specifically, cysteine is needed to produce *glutathione,* which is one of the most important antioxidants and a vital molecule for intracellular function. Reduced availability of glutathione can result in a number of health conditions, ranging from cataracts and accelerated aging to cancer, AIDS, and even schizophrenia. Studies have shown that insufficient cysteine can also affect levels of taurine and sulfate, which are essential for liver function, among other physiological processes. If your blood test shows that your homocysteine level is abnormal, you should work with your health practitioner to determine and then eliminate the cause. This section focuses on high levels of homocysteine, which is a more common condition.

WHAT CAUSES HIGH HOMOCYSTEINE?

Elevated homocysteine levels are usually related to a deficiency in B vitamins, which are found in a variety of foods, especially meat, poultry, and dairy products. (See the table on page 296.) The list below contains common reasons for a high level of homocysteine.

- Being overweight or obese (BMI of 25 or above)
- Binge drinking or excessive alcohol consumption
- B-vitamin deficiency
- Chronic stress
- Excessive caffeine intake
- Genetics (See the inset on page 293)
- Insufficient exercise or lack of exercise
- Insulin resistance
- Kidney disease
- Menopause
- Smoking

The following medications can also cause an increase:

- Antacids containing magnesium and aluminum
- Anticonvulsants
- Antiepileptic drugs
- Anti-ulcer drugs
- Biguanides, such as metformin
- Cholestyramine
- Corticosteroids
- Cyclosporine
- Diuretics

- Fenofibrate
- Levodopa
- Methotrexate
- Niacin
- Nonsteroidal anti-inflammatory drugs (NSAIDs)
- Oral contraceptives
- Theophylline

The amount of homocysteine in the blood increases with aging, so levels tend to be higher in middle-aged and elderly adults. Elevated homocysteine is strongly correlated with coronary heart disease, since it can contribute to atherosclerosis. Although researchers do not yet fully understand the relationship between high homocysteine levels and chronic disease, they have identified it as a potential factor in the development of Alzheimer's disease and dementia, blood clots, chronic inflammation, depression, erectile dysfunction, glaucoma, insulin resistance and type 2 diabetes, intestinal disorders, kidney disease, and liver disease. High homocysteine is also associated with thyroid hormone imbalance, sleep problems, and pregnancy complications, including miscarriage.

WHAT ARE THE SYMPTOMS OF HIGH HOMOCYSTEINE?

Elevated homocysteine does not produce symptoms on its own. However, when heart disease is present, people may experience chest pain, shortness of breath, leg cramps, and similar warning signs. Such symptoms require prompt

MTHFR Gene Test

When vitamin-B deficiency is the suspected cause of an elevated homocysteine level, the methylenetetrahydrofolate reductase (MTHFR) gene test may be recommended by your health practitioner. This test analyzes a sample of DNA, checking for small genetic variations called *single nucleotide polymorphisms*, or SNPs, which act as biological markers of disease. Testing positive for a MTHFR gene SNP (pronounced "snip") means that the body cannot effectively process folic acid and convert it into its bioactive form, methyltetrahydrofolate. In addition to elevated homocysteine levels, this genetic abnormality is associated with breast cancer, colon cancer, and depression. The most common MTHFR variant is the C677T mutation, which is correlated with high homocysteine levels as well as heart disease, kidney disease, and Alzheimer's disease. The MTHFR gene test is performed at almost every major lab in the United States, so your doctor can easily order the test if necessary.

medical attention, especially if they persist. A vitamin-B deficiency may be indicated by hair thinning or hair loss, headaches, depression, irritability, and subtle cognitive deficits. Speak to your doctor if one or more of these symptoms apply to you.

HOW CAN HIGH LEVELS OF HOMOCYSTEINE BE TREATED?

In contrast to other lipid panel biomarkers, medications are not a mainstay of treatment for elevated homocysteine levels. Dietary modification and nutritional supplements are often sufficient for keeping levels within a normal range.

SUPPLEMENTS

If your homocysteine level is abnormally high, you need a healthcare professional to prescribe higher doses of key nutrients. Specifically, B-complex vitamins, betaine (also called trimethylglycine, or TMG), and omega-3 fatty acids are known to help lower homocysteine. Moreover, you can decrease inflammation by taking fiber, probiotics, or aged garlic extract, which is also cardioprotective. Keep in mind that supplements are meant to enhance your nutrition; they do not and cannot replace a healthy diet.

SUPPLEMENTS FOR HIGH HOMOCYSTEINE

Supplement	Dosage	Considerations
Aged garlic extract	600 mg one to three times a day.	Aged garlic extract is used to protect the heart and blood vessels, and is reported to help decrease oxidative stress markers, including those related to blood sugar regulation problems. Aged garlic has also been reported to reduce liver enzymes and fatty liver, as well as decrease the formation of advanced glycation end-products (AGEs), which are implicated in various health problems, such as heart disease, kidney problems, and cancer. Aged garlic is not reported to interfere with blood thinners.
B-complex vitamins (containing at least 50 mg B_6)	1 tablet or capsule once a day, or as directed on the product label.	Typically listed as a B-25, B-50, or 5-100 supplement. Quality B-complex vitamins generally contain vitamins B_1 (thamin), B_2 (riboflavin), B_3 (niacin), B_5 (pantothenic acid), B_6 (pyridoxine), folic acid, and B_{12} (cyanocobalamin). Betaine (TMG) should also be added for increased protection. B vitamins can be found in quality multivitamins and mineral supplements as well. Speak to your health-care provider before taking if you have a medical condition, including anemia, diabetes, and liver problems.

Supplement	Dosage	Considerations
Fiber	Check the product label for dosage guidelines. The recommendation for women is 25 g per day, and for men, 30 g per day.	Guar gum (Sunfiber) is an excellent source of soluble dietary fiber. Potential side effects include abdominal discomfort and bloating. Excess fiber may also interfere with the absorption of certain nutrients like iron and calcium.
Omega-3 essential fatty acids DHA and EPA (fish oil)	1,000 mg two to three times a day.	Fish oil is one of the first supplements recommended by doctors for lowering triglycerides. In addition to its anti-inflammatory properties, fish oil is reported to lower total cholesterol levels and decrease oxidative stress, which is associated with LDL, or "bad" cholesterol. Speak to your doctor before taking if you are on blood-thinning medication, as fish oil may increase the risk of bleeding. Be sure to use only high-quality oils that have been tested for contaminants.
Probiotics	5 to 10 billion CFUs two to three times a day.	Probiotics help normalize beneficial flora in the gastrointestinal tract, and are reported to decrease triglyceride and cholesterol levels. They are also reported to improve BUN levels and quality of life in people with kidney disease. It's best to use heat-stable products that do not require refrigeration. If using an antibiotic, wait three hours before taking probiotics. If diarrhea occurs, decrease your dosage. If this side effect persists for longer than 48 hours, stop taking the supplement and contact your doctor. Live cultures should be guaranteed through the date of expiration on label. For optimal results, take probiotics with meals, as food improves the survivability of the cultures.

LIFESTYLE CHANGES

The set of nutrients that is most important for balancing homocysteine includes four water-soluble B vitamins: B_2 (riboflavin), B_6 (pyridoxine), vitamin B_9 (more commonly referred to as folic acid or folate), and B_{12} (cyanocobalamin). In addition to improving energy production, enhancing immunity, and supporting detoxification, these vitamins are needed to recycle homocysteine into methionine. Fortunately, B vitamins are abundant in a variety of foods, making it easier to reverse a nutritional deficiency. Some of these foods are listed in the table below. Keep in mind that dietary sources of B vitamins cannot alone lower homocysteine and, therefore, should not be considered a replacement for B-vitamin supplements.

FOOD SOURCES OF B VITAMINS

Vitamin B_2 (Riboflavin)	Vitamin B_6 (Pyridoxine)	Folic Acid (Folate, Vitamin B_9)	Vitamin B_{12} (Cyanocobalamin)
Almonds	Bananas	Asparagus	Cheese, particularly Swiss, Gjetost, mozzarella, and parmesan
Asparagus	Bell peppers (red)	Beets	Crab
Broccoli	Brown rice	Black beans	Eggs
Chard	Buckwheat flour	Broccoli	Fish, especially mackerel, herring, salmon, tuna, sardines, and cod
Collard greens	Cabbage	Brewer's yeast	Fortified cereals
Eggs	Celery	Brussels sprouts	Lamb (mutton)
Fish, especially mackerel, wild-caught Atlantic salmon, and trout	Chestnuts	Cantaloupe	Liver
Liver	Chick peas (garbanzo beans)	Cauliflower	Lobster
Milk (cow and goat)	Fish, particularly cod, halibut, and yellowfin tuna	Chick peas (garbanzo beans)	Meat and poultry (beef, bison, chicken, turkey)
Mushrooms	Fortified cereals	Collard greens	Shellfish (clams, oysters, mussels)
Mustard greens	Meat and poultry (beef, chicken, pork, turkey)	Eggs	
Romaine lettuce	Potatoes	Fortified cereals	
Soybeans	Shiitake mushrooms	Grapefruit	
Spinach	Spinach	Lentils	
Tomatoes		Liver	
Turnip greens		Mustard greens	
Venison		Oranges	
Yogurt		Papaya	
		Pinto, kidney, and lima beans	
		Romaine lettuce	
		Spinach	
		Sprouts	
		Squash	
		String beans	
		Sunflower seeds	
		Turnip greens	
		Wheat germ	
		Whole grain breads and cereals	

In addition to foods rich in B vitamins, you should include the following foods and nutrients in your daily dietary intake.

• **Antioxidants.** Citrus fruits like grapefruit, lemons, oranges, and tangerines will strengthen your body's defenses against harmful free radicals, which cause inflammation and chronic health problems, including arterial plaque buildup and heart disease. Additionally, eat vegetables such as bell peppers, kale, and romaine lettuce, which contain fiber and antioxidants in addition to their anti-inflammatory properties.

• **Cold-water fish.** Halibut, salmon, tuna, and haddock are excellent sources of omega-3 fatty acids and anti-inflammatory compounds, which support cardiovascular health.

• **Lean meats.** Choose leaner—and when possible, organic—beef, bison, chicken, and turkey that is grass-fed or free-range, which is lower in saturated fats and cholesterol. Organic free-range poultry and grass-fed meats are also higher in omega-3 fatty acids, making them beneficial for your heart.

• **Limited amounts of alcohol.** Although excessive alcohol consumption can deplete B vitamins and raise homocysteine levels, drinking alcohol in moderation has been known to lower some health risks. Moderate alcohol intake is generally defined as no more than one to two drinks per day—the equivalent of 1 to 2 ounces of hard liquor, 12 ounces of beer, or 4 to 8 ounces of wine. Still, if your homocysteine level is high, it is best to avoid alcohol completely.

• **Magnesium.** High levels of homocysteine may reduce the amount of magnesium in your body. Compensate for this loss by eating magnesium-rich foods such as nuts and seeds, which also help to control blood pressure and prevent blood vessel spasms. Other foods high in magnesium include spinach, Swiss chard, soybeans, mustard greens, broccoli, summer squash, and halibut. (See page 312 to read more about magnesium.)

You should also avoid foods that accelerate the loss of B vitamins, particularly foods containing refined sugar. Cut out candy, commercial baked goods, jams, jellies, and condiments like barbecue sauce and ketchup from your diet. Also, stay away from soda, energy drinks, and sweetened beverages, which are loaded with added sugars. The following guidelines are helpful when it comes to reducing homocysteine and other sources of inflammation:

• Cut back on coffee. Caffeine consumption is associated with high homocysteine levels, so you should stick to one or two cups of coffee per day if you're a coffee drinker. Use a French press to extract more of the coffee's essential health-promoting properties, like antioxidants, or drink espresso, which contains less caffeine. You may also want to consider switching to low-caffeine coffee.

- Exercise. Thirty- to sixty-minute sessions of physical activity about four days a week is all it takes to give your health a boost. Swimming, jogging, and even walking can be hugely beneficial.

- Lose weight. Very often, weight loss can be achieved through simple diet and exercise. Shedding even a few extra pounds can go a long way in improving cardiovascular health.

- Manage stress. Studies have shown that mental health and physical wellness are closely connected. To reduce your anxiety and improve your overall well-being, try stress management techniques such as biofeedback, meditation, yoga, imagery exercises, or regular physical activity, such as swimming, dancing, or walking.

- Sleep. When it comes to sleeping, quality is as important as quantity. Poor sleep patterns—including inadequate sleep and interrupted sleep—can lead to oxidative stress and inflammation. Aim for seven to eight hours of restful sleep each night.

- Reduce exposure to toxins. Whether you realize it or not, every day you are exposed to a host of toxic substances, including paint, pesticides, plastics, and household cleaning products. Avoid overexposure to these harmful toxins by storing food in glass rather than plastic containers, using all-natural cleaners and hygiene products, and buying organic food whenever possible.

- Throw away the cigarettes. This bad habit greatly increases oxidative stress and inflammation and puts harmful toxins such as cadmium, an extremely poisonous heavy metal, into your system. Smoking is also a major contributor to heart disease, so if you smoke, quit.

40. C-REACTIVE PROTEIN (CRP)

It was initially believed that *C-reactive protein*, or CRP, was produced by the liver. However, recent research has shown that vascular tissues and epithelial cells, which line the respiratory tract and kidneys, make CRP, as do fat cells called adipocytes. CRP, a component of the immune system, becomes elevated when inflammation is present in the body, whether due to infection, diabetes, cancer, obesity, overexercising, poor diet, or heart-related conditions like atherosclerosis. CRP is not included in a standard lipid panel blood test, but it is an important lab value to measure, especially you are at risk for certain medical conditions based on your age, weight, family history, or other factors. The CRP blood test is called the *high-sensitivity CRP* (hs-CRP) *test*, and it is also used to determine your cardiovascular risk. Many studies have shown that there is a correlation between inflammation and the development of cardiovascular problems, as well as stroke and peripheral artery disease. As such, CRP lab values—which are measured in milligrams per liter (mg/L)—are categorized according to heart disease risk:

REFERENCE RANGES FOR C-REACTIVE PROTEIN (CRP)	
CRP (mg/L)	**Category**
Greater than 2.9	High risk
1.0 to 2.9	Intermediate risk
Less than 1.0	Low risk
Target Range: Less than 1.0	

Since elevated CRP does not produce physical symptoms, a blood test is the only way to know if your level is high. A level above 2.4 mg/L has been shown to double the risk of a cardiovascular event as compared with levels below 1.0 mg/L. If a lipid blood test shows that you have a high level of the protein, further testing may be needed to determine the cause and location of the inflammation.

WHAT CAUSES HIGH C-REACTIVE PROTEIN?

The most common and direct cause of elevated CRP is inflammation, which may be acute or chronic. Acute inflammation occurs as a normal reaction to burns, injuries, or other physical traumas. Bacterial infections—which may be caused by an illness such as pneumonia, rheumatic fever, or tuberculosis—also trigger acute inflammation. This inflammatory state is temporary, and CRP levels should return to normal once the injury or infection has healed. Chronic inflammation, however, develops over a long period of time, perhaps years. This condition is linked to many types of cancer, atherosclerotic heart disease, insulin resistance and diabetes, and inflammatory bowel disease (IBD). Autoimmune disorders, including connective tissue diseases like arthritis, are also examples of chronic inflammatory conditions that raise CRP levels. Other factors that can influence CRP are:

- Aging
- Depression
- Diet high in inflammatory foods
- Environmental toxicity due to heavy metals, pesticides, or other contaminants
- Genetic factors (See the inset below)
- Hormone replacement therapy (estrogen and progesterone)
- Oral contraceptives
- Pregnancy

Keep in mind that high CRP may simply indicate a minor infection. However, if no other signs of infection (such as elevated white blood cells) are present, it might signal a current or future medical issue.

Genetics and CRP Levels

Although the primary cause of elevated CRP is inflammation, scientists have identified a few genes that may also cause levels to be higher than normal. There are four gene polymorphisms, or variations, that can influence CRP, and studies have shown that any combination of these four gene snips can increase the risk of *ischemic heart disease*—which is caused by reduced blood flow to the heart—by 32 percent. Certain gene combinations can also raise the risk of *cerebrovascular disease,* or reduced blood flow to the brain, resulting in a stroke. Like other genes, these can lie dormant or be "turned on" by factors such as diet, environment, and hormone imbalance, in turn causing CRP to be produced. Since lifestyle choices can have a significant impact on gene expression, you should follow the guidelines provided on pages 304 to 306. Adopting healthy behaviors will also help to prevent other causes of high CRP and boost your general well-being.

WHAT ARE THE SYMPTOMS OF HIGH C-REACTIVE PROTEIN?

Elevated CRP does not produce physical symptoms by itself; a blood test is the only way to be certain that your level is too high. But there are several factors that may put you at a greater risk for a higher-than-normal level, including high cholesterol, high blood pressure, and a diet high in inflammation-causing foods. Being overweight or obese also increases your risk of heightened CRP, as well as insufficient exercise, poorly controlled diabetes, and bad habits like smoking. If any of these risk factors apply to you, or if you have had a heart attack or stroke, you should have your CRP level tested.

HOW CAN HIGH LEVELS OF C-REACTIVE PROTEIN BE TREATED?

When a hs-CRP blood test indicates an intermediate or high risk of heart disease, it is absolutely necessary to correct the problem. Fortunately, there are long-term solutions for restoring healthy levels, as well as medications that can be used when circumstances call for them. Both categories of treatment are described below.

DRUGS

There are essentially two types of drugs that can effectively lower your CRP level—statins and anti-inflammatory drugs. Anti-inflammatory medication can be further broken down into three separate categories: Aspirin, corticosteroids, and nonsteroidal anti-inflammatory drugs (NSAIDs). The table below covers these drug classes in more detail. Keep in mind that all of these agents—even those available over the counter, like aspirin—should be taken under the direction and guidance of a healthcare professional. However, you may not need medication. If taking a drug is appropriate, your prescription will be based on the cause of your elevated CRP level. Before taking any substance, make sure you discuss interactions, side effects, and proper dosing with your physician.

DRUGS FOR HIGH CRP

Drug	Considerations
Aspirin *Anacin, Bayer, Bufferin, Sloprin*	Tell your healthcare provider if you are on other medications before using aspirin. If you experience persistent or recurring symptoms such as nausea, stomach pain, or heartburn, consult your health-care provider. This drug should not be taken by anyone who is eighteen years old or younger.

Drug	Considerations
Corticosteroids (dexamethasone, methylprednisolone) *Decadron, Medrol*	Side effects can include bone loss, cataracts, constipation, diarrhea, dizziness, depression, fluid retention, immune imbalances, liver and/or kidney problems, mental confusion, nausea and/or vomiting, sleep problems, and weight gain. Corticosteroids can also deplete the body of essential nutrients, including calcium, DHEA, folic acid, magnesium, potassium, selenium, vitamin C, vitamin D, and zinc. Taking a quality daily multivitamin or mineral supplement is recommended when using corticosteroids.
Nonsteroidal anti-inflammatory drugs (NSAIDs) *Advil, Aleve, Motrin, Naprosyn*	Side effects vary among different NSAIDs, but can include constipation, diarrhea, gastrointestinal bleeding, headache, liver and/or kidney problems, and upset stomach. These drugs can also deplete the body of essential nutrients, such as DHEA, folic acid, melatonin, and zinc. You should take a quality daily multivitamin or mineral supplement while using NSAIDs. If you have trouble sleeping, taking 1 to 5 mg of melatonin one hour before bedtime may help. Start at the lowest possible dose and increase as necessary if your sleep cycle does not improve.
Statins (rosuvastatin, atorvastatin, lovastatin, pravastatin) *Crestor, Lipitor, Mevacor, Pravachol*	Statin drugs can deplete essential nutrients from the body, including CoQ_{10}, vitamin D, and vitamin E. Take 100 mg of CoQ_{10} daily along with a multivitamin or mineral supplement to prevent nutritional deficiencies. Side effects may include headache, muscle pain, nausea, weakness, elevated liver enzymes, memory loss, and kidney problems. Inform your doctor or pharmacist if you are currently on cholesterol-lowering drugs to avoid adverse drug interactions. Do not take with grapefruit juice.

SUPPLEMENTS

Nutritional supplements are also helpful, but should not take the place of a wholesome diet and healthy lifestyle (see pages 304 to 306). Some supplements that can be used for reducing inflammation and lowering CRP are presented in the table below. Supplements do not require a prescription, but you should check with your doctor before taking any substance due to potential side effects and interactions. You should also work with your doctor or other health-care professional to determine a dose that is appropriate for your needs.

SUPPLEMENTS FOR HIGH CRP		
Supplement	**Dosage**	**Considerations**
Aged garlic extract	600 mg one to three times a day.	Aged garlic extract is used to protect the heart and blood vessels, and is reported to help decrease oxidative stress markers, including those related to blood sugar regulation problems. Aged garlic has also been reported to reduce liver enzymes and fatty liver, as well as decrease the formation of advanced glycation end-products (AGEs), which are implicated in various health problems, such as heart disease, kidney problems, and cancer. Aged garlic is not reported to interfere with blood thinners.
Curcumin	250 mg twice a day.	Curcumin, an antioxidant, has anti-inflammatory activity and is reported to help decrease CRP levels. If stomach discomfort occurs, take with food.
Grape seed extract	100 to 150 mg twice a day.	Grape seed has anti-inflammatory and antioxidant activity, and is reported to help decrease the oxidation of LDL cholesterol, as well as the risk of heart disease. Side effects, though uncommon, may include dizziness, headache, itchy scalp, and nausea. It may also increase the risk of blood thinning, especially if you are taking aspirin or anticoagulant drugs. If you are taking blood thinners, NSAIDS, or heart medication, take only under a doctor's supervision. Do not use if you are allergic to grapes. Use an extract that is standardized to 90-percent proanthocyanidins.
Green tea or green tea extract	3 to 6 cups (tea) or 250 mg one to two times a day (extract).	Helps improve antioxidant and lipid levels. When taken with other supplements and diet/lifestyle chances, green tea extract is reported to assist in weight loss. It can also help regulate glucose levels, lower triglycerides, and prevent kidney stones, which may result from high calcium. If taking an extract, use a form standardized to 90-percent polyphenols (specifically EGCG). Tell your doctor if you are currently taking aspirin or anti-coagulant drugs like warfarin (Coumadin), as green tea extract may increase the risk of bleeding.
Magnesium	250 to 500 mg twice a day.	Use magnesium aspartate, citrate, taurate, glycinate, or any amino acid chelate. Supports bone building and balances calcium intake. The ratio of calcium-to-magnesium intake should be between 1 to 1 and 2 to 1. This supplement is reported to improve blood vessel function and insulin resistance, in addition to decreasing LDL cholesterol, total cholesterol, and triglycerides. Also essential for phase-I liver detoxification. If you

Supplement	Dosage	Considerations
Magnesium *(continued)*		experience loose stools after taking magnesium, cut your dose in half and gradually increase over the course of a few months. Consult your health-care provider for dosage advice.
Omega-3 essential fatty acids DHA and EPA (fish oil)	1,000 mg two to three times a day.	Fish oil is one of the first supplements recommended by doctors for lowering triglycerides. In addition to its anti-inflammatory properties, fish oil is reported to lower total cholesterol levels and decrease oxidative stress, which is associated with LDL, or "bad" cholesterol. Speak to your doctor before taking if you are on blood-thinning medication, as fish oil may increase the risk of bleeding. Be sure to use only high-quality oils that have been tested for contaminants.
Vitamin C (ascorbic acid/ ascorbate)	1,000 mg once a day.	Vitamin C has been found to lower CRP by about 25 percent when levels are elevated. Doses higher than 5,000 mg per day may cause diarrhea. Mineral ascorbates and Ester-C are buffered forms of vitamin C that decrease the likelihood of diarrhea. Do not take in large doses if you are prone to gout or kidney stones.
Vitamin D (vitamin D_3, or chole-calciferol)	1,000 to 4,000 IU once a day.	Low vitamin D levels are associated with increased CRP. Vitamin D is also necessary for proper calcium absorption. Inform your doctor if you are taking any drug that can deplete vitamin D, such as anti-convulsants, cholesterol-lowering medications, anti-ulcer drugs, or mineral oil. People with kidney disease or atherosclerosis should not take vitamin D. Excessive intake can increase the risk of hardened arteries and high blood calcium levels. People with sarcoidosis, tuberculosis, hyperparathyroidism, and lymphoma should use vitamin D only as directed by a physician. The tolerable upper limit for vitamin D intake is 4,000 IU per day. Higher dosages may be used to treat vitamin D deficiencies, but must be short term and medically supervised.

LIFESTYLE CHANGES

If your CRP level falls into the "intermediate risk" range, cautionary action is necessary even if you are currently in presumably good health. An anti-inflammatory diet can have a huge impact on CRP, as can the use of certain nutritional supplements. I have seen a number of cases in which a concerted effort to improve overall lifestyle has singlehandedly lowered CRP to the "low risk" category. Effective CRP management is possible with only a handful of lifestyle adjustments, such as:

- Avoid inflammation-causing foods. Ingredients that promote inflammation include trans fats and refined and added sugars like high-fructose corn syrup. Stay away from foods that contain these ingredients, like commercial baked goods, condiments, soft drinks, and any food fried in partially hydrogenated oils. Their inflammatory properties can lead to chronic medical conditions such as heart disease, digestive imbalance, liver problems, and even cancer.

- Consider following a Mediterranean-type diet. This kind of diet qualifies as an anti-inflammatory diet and facilitates weight loss. Several studies have shown that any diet that helps you lose weight tends to lower CRP as well. The Mediterranean diet cuts out refined carbohydrates and replaces "bad" fats with "good" fats like olive oil. It also includes fish and lean meats, as well as plenty of plant-based foods like fruits, vegetables, and legumes.

- Get tested for food allergies. Food allergies are a common source of inflammation because the immune cells involved produce various inflammatory substances that increase CRP. Managing food allergies is necessary to lower internal inflammation and, therefore, CRP levels.

- Increase intake of omega-3s. Omega-3 fatty acids have anti-inflammatory properties that can help keep your CRP level in check, in turn protecting your heart and offering other health benefits, such as mood enhancement, improved insulin sensitivity, and weight management. Cold-water fish, walnuts, flax seeds, and vegetables such as cabbage and cauliflower are top sources of omega-3s.

- Load up on fruits and vegetables. In particular, you should eat fruits and vegetables containing flavonoids and carotenoids, naturally occurring plant compounds that boost the amount of antioxidants in your body, bolster your immune system, and fight inflammation. Enjoy fruits such as apples, blueberries, blackberries, and peaches, as well as vegetables like broccoli, cabbage, spinach, and green beans. Aim for at least seven servings (combined) of fruits and vegetables every day, eating no more than one fruit serving per every three vegetable servings, as fruit is high in natural sugars.

- Make magnesium a dietary priority. Studies show that low intake of magnesium is correlated with elevated CRP levels. Therefore, you should eat magnesium-rich foods like nuts and seeds, which also help to control blood pressure and reduce blood vessel spasms. Other foods high in magnesium include broccoli, halibut, soybeans, and spinach. (See page 312 for more information on magnesium.)

Other healthy habits, like regular exercise, are helpful as well. Engaging in some form of physical activity, from biking to Pilates and/or strength training, in thirty- to sixty-minute sessions about four times a week will enhance your cardiovascular health and help you lose weight. You should also moderate your alcohol intake and quit smoking, as tobacco smoke increases inflammation and, therefore, CRP levels. Your doctor should be able to recommend an effective smoking cessation program.

Did You Know?

Many people get the results of their cholesterol tests and assume that because their levels are normal, they are not at risk for heart disease. This is not always the case. The high-sensitivity C-reactive protein test accounts for error by testing for inflammation, a separate indicator of coronary artery disease and heart damage. The American Heart Association recommends the test for anyone who is thought to have an intermediate risk of heart disease because of age, weight, or family history. If you are forward thinking about your health, consider getting a hs-CRP.

41. VITAMIN D

Vitamin D has garnered a tremendous amount of attention over the past decade because of the extensive health-related research that has been published on it. Also called the sunshine vitamin, vitamin D is a fat-soluble vitamin that is produced mainly when the skin comes into contact with the sun's UV radiation. Small amounts of vitamin D may also be found in foods such as fish and dairy products. There are approximately 2,700 binding sites for vitamin D in the human genome (DNA), which suggests that vitamin D exerts influence on various nearby genes associated with autoimmune diseases.

There are two main forms of vitamin D that are taken in from food or supplements—*ergocalciferol,* also known as D_2, and *cholecalciferol,* or D_3. Vitamin D_3 is converted into 25-hydroxycholecalciferol in the body, and then 1,25-dihydroxyvitamin D (calcitrol) in the kidneys. Calcitrol is the most potent and active steroid form of vitamin D_3, but is generally not measured unless an individual has kidney disease or if there is reason to believe the body is not converting the vitamin into its active form.

Vitamin D plays a key role in the absorption of calcium from the intestines and is vital to bone strength. In addition, an adequate level of this nutrient is important for immune function, health of the heart and blood vessels, insulin regulation, and mood. Measured in nanograms per milliliter (ng/mL), adult ranges of vitamin D may be found in the table below. Reference ranges for high and low values may vary according to the lab, so be sure to look at the ranges provided on your blood test form.

REFERENCE RANGES FOR TOTAL VITAMIN D

Total Vitamin D (ng/mL)	Category
Greater than 85	High
25 to 85	Normal
Less than 25	Low

Target Range: Ranges vary for individuals, so consult your physician.

Although getting a vitamin D count on a routine blood test is becoming more common, not all doctors request it. Ask your physician to include the reading when you get blood drawn.

WHAT CAUSES HIGH VITAMIN D?

Although exposure to sunlight initiates the synthesis of vitamin D, it cannot cause excessive levels of this nutrient, also known as *hypervitaminosis D*. The body regulates the amount of vitamin D created by UV light. In addition, due to the relatively small degree of vitamin D in food, it is quite difficult to get too much of this substance from your diet. Typically, too much vitamin D is the result of excessive supplement intake, which can be fixed by lowering your dosage. If your high vitamin D level is left untreated, it could easily lead to dehydration and an excess of calcium in the bloodstream known as *hypercalcemia* (see page 81), as well as contribute to kidney problems.

WHAT ARE THE SYMPTOMS OF HIGH VITAMIN D?

Symptoms of excessive vitamin D are all related to a toxic buildup of calcium in the blood and include nausea, vomiting, constipation, weakness, increased frequency of urination, loss of appetite, kidney stones, and heart rhythm abnormalities.

HOW CAN HIGH VITAMIN D BE TREATED?

If your vitamin D reading is severely raised, your doctor may recommend IV hydration, as well as therapy with drugs that reduce blood calcium. Additional lifestyle-related measures are also necessary. Always follow your doctor's advice when it comes to treatment of high vitamin D levels.

LIFESTYLE CHANGES

The first step to take in the treatment of hypervitaminosis D is to stop vitamin D supplementation until levels return to normal. It is also advisable to restrict calcium intake in order to avoid the serious health conditions associated with hypercalcemia. This means cutting back on dairy products and calcium-fortified foods and beverages. Additionally, you should aim to drink approximately 2 to 3 liters of filtered water on a daily basis.

WHAT CAUSES LOW VITAMIN D?

Low amounts of vitamin D in the blood may be the result of a number of factors, including:

- Aging
- Dark skin
- Fat malabsorption syndromes
- Genetics

- Hypocalcemia (low calcium levels)
- Inflammatory bowel disease
- Kidney disease
- Lack of sun exposure, which includes wearing clothing that covers the skin
- Obesity
- Poor diet

Additionally, infants may have low vitamin D levels if they are exclusively breastfed. The following medications can also cause a depletion of vitamin D:

- Anticonvulsants, including carbamazepine (Carbatrol), fosphenytoin (Cerebyx), phenytoin (Dilantin), and barbiturates
- Bile acid sequestrants, including cholestyramine (Questran) and colestipol (Colestid)
- Corticosteroids
- H2-receptor antagonists, including such as cimetidine (Tagamet), famotidine (Pepcid), nizatidine (Axid), and ranitidine (Zantac)
- Isoniazid (Tubizid)
- Mineral oil
- Rifampin (Rifadin)
- Statin drugs

Although it may not seem like a serious issue, never ignore low levels of vitamin D. If the problem becomes severe enough, it could lead to health conditions such as rickets, hyperparathyroidism, a softening of the bones known as *osteomalacia,* a loss of bone density known as osteoporosis, or kidney disease. Low vitamin D is also associated with autoimmunity, blood glucose control problems, gastrointestinal tract issues, increased risk of cardiovascular disease and hypertension, and certain cancer risks.

WHAT ARE THE SYMPTOMS OF LOW VITAMIN D?

Symptoms of low vitamin D include brittle bones that increase your risk of fractures, raised susceptibility to infections such as colds and flu, muscle and joint pain, thyroid hormone imbalances, fatigue, weight gain, and mood swings.

HOW CAN LOW VITAMIN D BE TREATED?

The following lifestyle guidelines are generally recommended for low vitamin D, but check with your physician before adopting any of these modifications.

SUPPLEMENTS

Most of the time, vitamin D deficiency will need to be treated with dietary supplements. In addition to a regular vitamin D supplement, your doctor may suggest calcium and magnesium to deal with possible low levels of calcium in association with decreased vitamin D production. Another option is 1,25-dihydroxyvitamin D, which requires a prescription from your doctor. If you have celiac disease, make sure that the supplement you take is gluten-free, as gluten-containing agents are sometimes used in the manufacturing process. Your dosage of vitamin D_3 will depend upon the result of your blood test. If the lab value is 25 ng/mL or less, you should consider taking 5,000 IU daily. If your level is between 25 and 40 ng/mL, 1,000 to 2,000 IU plus a regular multivitamin every day may be the solution. Your doctor will recommend the correct amount for your situation and likely retest your blood in a few months.

SUPPLEMENTS FOR LOW VITAMIN D

Supplement	Dosage	Considerations
Calcium	500 mg one to three times a day.	Take a highly absorbable form of calcium, such as calcium aspartate, citrate, or hydroxyapatite. If using calcium to help sleep problems, take one 500-mg dose at bedtime.
Magnesium	200 to 400 mg twice a day.	Use magnesium aspartate, citrate, taurate, glycinate, or any amino acid chelate. Supports bone building and balances calcium intake. The ratio of calcium-to-magnesium intake should be between 1 to 1 and 2 to 1. This supplement is reported to improve blood vessel function and insulin resistance, in addition to decreasing LDL cholesterol, total cholesterol, and triglycerides. Also essential for phase-I liver detoxification. If you experience loose stools after taking magnesium, cut your dose in half and gradually increase over the course of a few months. Consult your health-care provider for dosage advice.

Supplement	Dosage	Considerations
Vitamin D (vitamin D_3, or cholecalciferol)	1,000 to 5,000 IU once a day.	Low vitamin D levels are associated with increased CRP. Vitamin D is also necessary for proper calcium absorption. Inform your doctor if you are taking any drug that can deplete vitamin D, such as anticonvulsants, cholesterol-lowering medications, anti-ulcer drugs, or mineral oil. People with kidney disease or atherosclerosis should not take vitamin D. Excessive intake can increase the risk of hardened arteries and high blood calcium levels. People with sarcoidosis, tuberculosis, hyperparathyroidism, and lymphoma should use vitamin D only as directed by a physician. The tolerable upper limit for vitamin D intake is 4,000 IU per day. Higher dosages may be used to treat vitamin D deficiencies, but must be short term and medically supervised.

LIFESTYLE CHANGES

The easiest way to raise vitamin D levels is to increase your sun exposure. Ten to twenty minutes of sunlight three times a week is recommended. Wait at least one hour before bathing after being in the sun, so that the vitamin D produced has time to be fully absorbed. However, this does not guarantee adequate vitamin D levels. It is strongly recommended that you monitor your level, especially if you live in a cold climate that requires you to be indoors a majority of the time or in a region where it isn't often sunny. It's best to get tested at the peak of the season in which it's sunniest, and then again at the time when you have the least exposure to sunshine. This will allow you to more accurately gauge your vitamin D needs.

Helpful dietary measures include eating more foods that contain vitamin D, such as fortified dairy products, egg yolks, and coldwater fish like salmon, herring, or halibut. Because diminished vitamin D will likely lower calcium levels, you should also increase your intake of calcium-containing foods such as green leafy vegetables and nuts. Similarly, you should avoid soft drinks, as the phosphoric acid in these beverages robs the body of calcium.

42. MAGNESIUM

Along with calcium, phosphorus, sodium, potassium, and chloride, magnesium is one of the six essential minerals required by the human body in significant quantities. Involved in more than 300 enzyme reactions in the body, magnesium is necessary for bone formation, muscle activity, nerve transmission, energy production, and blood pressure regulation. It also plays an important role in blood sugar balance, as well as the metabolism of carbohydrates, fats, and proteins. Low magnesium status is directly associated with increased risk of metabolic syndrome, type 2 diabetes, and cardiovascular disease.

The functions of magnesium are so diverse that nearly every body system depends on it to operate properly, and yet, it is not monitored as frequently as other minerals. Blood levels of magnesium are typically measured only when an individual displays symptoms of magnesium deficiency (hypomagnesemia) or excess (hypermagnesemia), or when a malabsorptive disorder is suspected. However, many people experience functional deficiencies that go unrecognized. The fact is, most Americans do not consume enough magnesium from the foods they commonly eat. The American diet tends to be high in refined sugar and saturated fats, which yield very little magnesium. Therefore, a magnesium test is recommended for a comprehensive metabolic assessment. Normal ranges for serum (blood) magnesium, which is measured in milliequivalents per liter (mEq/L), are listed in the table below, but keep in mind that these values may vary slightly by the testing laboratory.

REFERENCE RANGES FOR SERUM MAGNESIUM

Category	Normal Range
Adult	1.8 to 2.6 mEq/L
Child (2 to 18 years old)	1.7 to 2.1 mEq/L
Infant	1.5 to 2.2 mEq/L

Although these are the ranges that are generally accepted as normal, serum magnesium is not reflective of total body stores. Therefore, you may test in the normal range for serum magnesium but still exhibit signs of functional magnesium deficiency. According to some experts, by the time your serum magnesium hits the low or mid-low range, your body already has a significant cellular magnesium deficiency. The reason for this is that your bloodstream needs magnesium in order to buffer its pH. If the magnesium supply in the blood is low, the body must "steal" magnesium from the bones and tissues in order to keep the blood's buffer system intact. While some doctors may perform a red blood cell test if deficiency is suspected, the reality is that there is no accurate test for measuring total magnesium stores. Your physician will evaluate your blood test results and any symptoms you experience to determine whether or not your lab is actually abnormal.

WHAT CAUSES HIGH MAGNESIUM?

In most cases, high magnesium levels in the blood (hypermagnesemia) are caused by underlying kidney problems or excessive consumption of the mineral through supplements or magnesium-containing laxatives. More specifically, high magnesium may be due to one of the following conditions:

- Adrenal disorders, such as Addison's disease
- Dehydration
- Electrolyte imbalance caused by chemotherapy
- Hyperparathyroidism
- Hypothyroidism
- Kidney failure
- Overuse of medications containing magnesium, including antacids, thyroid medication, lithium, and certain antibiotics

High levels may also result from factors not listed above. If a blood test shows that your blood magnesium is abnormally high, your doctor will work with you to identify the root of the problem and begin an appropriate course of treatment.

WHAT ARE THE SYMPTOMS OF HIGH MAGNESIUM?

The most common symptom associated with high magnesium levels is diarrhea, especially when the cause is excessive intake through supplements. Other signs of hypermagnesemia include confusion, muscle weakness, and reduced reflex response. Severe elevations in magnesium levels in the blood may lead to complications such as kidney dysfunction.

HOW CAN HIGH MAGNESIUM BE TREATED?

In general, correcting a high level depends upon proper treatment of the underlying condition. However, the following dietary and lifestyle modifications may be recommended to support your treatment and to maintain balanced levels in the long term. Never attempt to treat yourself without your doctor's supervision. Labs that are out of range should always be assessed by a health-care professional.

LIFESTYLE CHANGES

The guidelines below are recommended for maintaining proper magnesium levels.

- Cut out simple carbohydrates like refined sugars and grains to balance your blood sugar and insulin levels.
- Drink approximately 2 to 3 liters of filtered water daily.
- Eat foods that promote kidney detoxification, such as artichokes, asparagus, melons, and parsley.
- Increase your intake of foods that contain calcium, which is the main mineral that interacts with magnesium and blocks its absorption in the body.

WHAT CAUSES LOW MAGNESIUM?

Reasons for low levels of magnesium in the blood (hypomagnesemia) include:

- Chronic stress, especially when it is due to surgery or a physical injury such as severe burns
- Diabetes or insulin resistance
- Diet high in refined sugar and saturated fats
- Excessive alcohol consumption
- Excessive sweating or urination
- Gastrointestinal disorders, such as Crohn's disease, celiac disease, and inflammatory bowel disease
- High calcium levels (hypercalcemia)
- High intake of coffee, tea, or carbonated beverages
- Hypoparathyroidism
- Kidney disease
- Low dietary intake
- Prolonged diarrhea
- Uncontrolled diabetes
- Use of medications like corticosteroids, loop and thiazide diuretics, estrogen replacement therapy, oral contraceptives, and tetracycline antibiotics
- Weight gain

Additionally, aging, illness, and alcohol addiction raise your risk of magnesium depletion. Lower levels are also frequently seen in pregnant women and people who exercise regularly. In fact, people who exercise all or most days need about 20 percent more magnesium than those who are sedentary. If these factors or any of the conditions above apply to you, it's advised that you request detailed magnesium testing from your physician, as low levels can lead to chronic inflammation, blood sugar elevation, insulin resistance, and mood disturbances.

WHAT ARE THE SYMPTOMS OF LOW MAGNESIUM?

Because magnesium is essential to the body, even a marginal deficiency can result in a number of symptoms that range in severity. This list includes muscular and neurological symptoms, such as migraines, twitching, muscle spasms, restless limbs, cramps, and weakness of the muscles. Fatigue, irregular heartbeat, loss of appetite, nausea, and vomiting may also be signs of magnesium deficiency. In addition, people with low levels may experience anxiety, depression, decreased cognitive abilities, bone loss, insomnia, constipation, blood sugar disorders, high blood pressure, and kidney stones.

HOW CAN LOW MAGNESIUM BE TREATED?

As already mentioned, most Americans do not get enough magnesium in their diet. It's estimated that the standard American diet—which is high in refined sugar and saturated fats—supplies less than two-thirds of the magnesium required for proper functioning of the body. While medical attention is necessary for very low magnesium, as well as deficiencies caused by underlying conditions, in general, the best plan of action is to raise dietary intake through food sources and supplements.

SUPPLEMENTS

General recommendations for taking magnesium are provided in the table below. Magnesium is available in various supplement forms, including capsules, tablets, powders, liquids, and even topical creams. Not all magnesium supplements are created equal, of course, so be sure to seek the advice of your doctor. It's important that you choose a supplement that is highly bioavailable, has the greatest solubility and absorption, and will be well tolerated by your body. If you experience any unusual side effect while taking magnesium, it's crucial that you speak to your physician.

SUPPLEMENTS FOR LOW MAGNESIUM		
Supplement	**Dosage**	**Considerations**
Magnesium	250 to 500 mg twice a day.	Use magnesium aspartate, citrate, taurate, glycinate, or amino acid chelate. Supports bone building and balances calcium intake. The ratio of calcium-to-magnesium intake should be between 1 to 1 and 2 to 1. This supplement is reported to improve blood vessel function and insulin resistance, in addition to decreasing LDL cholesterol, total cholesterol, and triglycerides. Also essential for phase-I liver detoxification. If you experience loose stools after taking magnesium, cut your dose in half and gradually increase over the course of a few months. Consult your health-care provider for dosage advice.

LIFESTYLE CHANGES

Some guidelines for correcting a magnesium imbalance through changes to diet and lifestyle are below.

- Eat foods low in calcium, which can interfere with proper magnesium absorption. This list includes asparagus, beets, cantaloupe, chicken, cottage cheese, eggplant, grapes, pineapple, and strawberries.

- Consume green vegetables rich in magnesium, especially chard, kale, spinach, and collard and mustard greens. Pumpkin seeds are the single richest source of magnesium. Other good food sources of magnesium include halibut, salmon, celery, and bell peppers.

- Increase your intake of high-quality lean proteins, particularly fish, turkey, bison, and ostrich. Organic, free-range meats are ideal, as they lack chemical additives, hormones, and antibiotics. Legumes like beans are also good sources of quality protein.

- Limit or cut out soft drinks, especially dark-colored sodas. These beverages contain high levels of phosphates (phosphoric acid), which inhibit the absorption of essential minerals. It's also a good idea to reduce your consumption of caffeinated drinks like coffee and tea, which increase the amount of magnesium that is released from the kidneys and removed from the body.

- Lower your intake of refined sugar and carbohydrates, which tend to create fluctuations in blood sugar and, in turn, affect magnesium levels.

- Reduce stress. Cortisol, the stress hormone, increases the excretion of magnesium from the body, in turn causing low levels.

- Start an exercise program, which should consist of thirty to sixty minutes of physical activity at least three or four times per week. A combination of aerobic exercise and strength training is ideal, but your main priority should be to make physical activity a part of your lifestyle. Exercise prevents bone loss, thereby decreasing your need for calcium supplements, which are often recommended for women at risk for osteoporosis. Remember, though, that exercising regularly increases your body's magnesium requirement by about 20 percent.

In addition, if you are taking one or more of the drugs listed on page 314, find out if your doctor can change your prescription. If you must take a magnesium-lowering medication, eat more foods rich in magnesium and consider taking an additional magnesium supplement.

CONCLUSION

This section presents sufficient evidence that an optional test is far from being a less important one. While homocysteine, CRP, vitamin D, and magnesium are not typically included in traditional blood panels, they are of equal value when it comes to assessing total health. Homocysteine and CRP can provide a more accurate picture of cardiovascular risk, as well as indicate the presence of more generalized conditions like vitamin deficiency and inflammation. Moreover, vitamin D and magnesium blood tests can play a key role in the prevention and proper diagnosis of common conditions ranging from blood sugar imbalance to osteoporosis. Discussing this information with your physician and requesting these tests, especially if you are at risk for certain diseases, is the first step towards better health and a better future.

Conclusion

The body changes with age—that's a fact of life. But if you are proactive and do what is necessary to reduce health risks, you can enjoy the same state of health at seventy years of age as you did at age twenty. The future of your health is within your control. Chronic disease and medical problems are not inevitable. You *can* avoid symptoms like weakness, fatigue, cognitive impairment, and bone loss, and even serious conditions such as diabetes, heart disease, and kidney disorders. The key is detecting the problem as early as possible—or ideally, before it develops into a full-blown condition—and taking the steps necessary to get your health back on the right track. And a blood test can show you the way.

As you now know, the main purpose of a blood test is to help you and your doctor determine the current state of your health. Lab values are a reflection of the internal workings of your body—its cardiovascular system, metabolism, liver function, immune health, ability to efficiently transport oxygen, hormone production and regulation, and many other vital processes. Lab values can tell you if you are at risk of developing a condition or disease, or if a particular disease has already taken hold. Blood test results give you the information you need to make critical changes to your lifestyle or begin an appropriate course of treatment, which can add years, even decades, to your life.

At the same time, blood tests have benefits that go beyond disease prevention and detection; they can also help you significantly improve your quality of life. Results of a hormone test, for example, can push you to take necessary measures to correct a mood disorder, restore energy, or alleviate negative symptoms associated with aging. In other words, regular blood testing can lead to good physical health, as well as enhance your overall well-being as you advance through each stage of life.

But it's up to you to take the first step. I encourage you to consult your physician and schedule a comprehensive blood test as soon as possible, especially if you already know that you are at risk for one or more of the conditions mentioned in this book. Now that you have read this book, I hope that filing your lab reports away with other miscellaneous paperwork, or worse, throwing them away, will be a thing of the past. With *Your Blood Never Lies* serving as your manual and guide, you will be able to have a meaningful conversation with your doctor about your test results and, moreover, understand their implications for your health. I hope that you will no longer dismiss "normal" results as healthy, but instead study them more closely and determine whether or not they are trending towards the upper- or lower-normal range. And most important, I hope that you will strive towards not just better health but *optimal* health by adopting lifestyle practices that promote wellness, energy, and vitality.

This book is meant to serve as a starting point on the road to health and longevity. By understanding, using, and sharing the information it contains, you will become not only a better patient, but also the proactive, self-advocating individual that your body deserves. When you take control of your health, you take control of your life—and it all begins with remembering that your blood never lies.

Testing Laboratories

When planning to have a blood test, your best resource is your physician. Still, it's helpful to be familiar with laboratories that offer comprehensive blood testing and have locations in most states. The labs listed below are accredited testing service providers that meet a variety of patient needs. Remember to research each laboratory and speak to your doctor before scheduling an appointment.

American Metabolic Laboratories

1818 Sheridan Street, Suite 102
Hollywood, FL 33020
Phone: 954-929-4814 • 954-929-4895
Website: www.americanmetabolic laboratories.net

American Metabolic Laboratories is the only laboratory in the United States that offers specialty panels like the Cancer Profile and Longevity Profile, tests developed by the company's founder, Dr. Emil K. Schandl. In addition, they provide conventional lab tests to assess cardiovascular health, metabolism, hormone balance, liver function, and blood components. Tests can be ordered by both patients and physicians. Phone consultations to discuss results are also available. Visit the company's website for more information or contact them directly to speak to a representative.

HealthCheckUSA

8700 Crownhill Road, Suite 110
San Antonio, TX 78209
Phone: 800-929-2044
Website: www.healthcheckusa.com

HealthCheckUSA allows patients to order blood tests directly rather than through a healthcare provider. The company's website allows you to select from an array of blood tests and schedule an appointment at a nearby testing center. Test results are sent to an accredited website for analysis and can be viewed online upon receiving an email notification. For more information, visit the HealthCheckUSA website.

LabCorp

358 South Main Street
Burlington, NC 27215
Phone: 336-584-5171
Website: www.LabCorp.com

With an extensive network of labs located across the country, LabCorp's laboratory services range from routine testing, including basic blood counts and cholesterol tests, to more complex blood work that can assist in diagnosing genetic conditions, cancers, and other diseases. In addition, LabCorp offers a wide range of other services, including drug testing, DNA and paternity testing, bone marrow engraftment monitoring, and clinical trials for pharmaceutical and drug development companies. Visit LabCorp's website to find a location in your area or schedule an appointment.

Private MD Labs

445 Highway 46 South, Suite 29-214
Dickson, TN 37055
Phone: 877-283-7882 • 615-560-2180
Website: www.privatemdlabs.com

Private MD Lab Services provides confidential clinical laboratory testing directly to patients in a variety of areas, including heart health, diabetes and cancer screenings, immune function, allergies, hormones and metabolism, and liver and kidney disease. Tests can be ordered online and administered at one of the company's testing centers, which are located in most states. Results are available to patients through the website.

Quest Diagnostics

3 Giralda Farms
Madison, NJ 07940
Phone: 800-222-0446
Website: www.questdiagnostics.com

A leader in diagnostic testing worldwide, Quest services cover a broad spectrum of areas, ranging from conventional blood testing—such as lipid profiles and complete blood counts—to genetic and molecular tests. They have expertise in tests to detect and help diagnose cancer, cardiovascular disease, infectious disease, and neurological problems. The Quest website allows patients to search for specific tests by name, medical condition, or medical specialty, as well as find a Quest location, schedule an appointment, and use a variety of additional patient services.

A Guide to Reference Ranges

To save you the time and trouble of flipping pages trying to find a specific lab value, the table below includes a list of normal ranges for every lab value discussed in this book. This guide should serve as an easy reference tool when reading the results of your blood test. Keep in mind, though, that not every lab uses the same set of reference ranges. Moreover, normal values are not necessarily *optimal,* so be sure to refer to the appropriate section of this book to find out the specific target range for a given lab. Analyze your lab report carefully and direct any questions to your physician so that you can work towards optimum health and well-being.

REFERENCE RANGES FOR BASIC LABS

Lab	Normal Range
Lipid Panel	
Triglycerides	Less than 150 mg/dL
Total Cholesterol	Less than 200 mg/dL
LDL Cholesterol	Less than 100 mg/dL
HDL Cholesterol	**Men:** 40 to 50 mg/dL **Women:** 50 to 60 mg/dL
Basic Metabolic Panel	
Glucose	65 to 99 mg/dL
Calcium	8.6 to 10.2 mg/dL
Potassium	3.5 to 5.4 mEq/L
Sodium	134 to 143 mmol/L
Chloride	97 to 108 mmol/L

Lab	Normal Range
Carbon Dioxide	21 to 33 mmol/L
Blood Urea Nitrogen (BUN)	6 to 20 mg/dL
Creatinine	0.5 to 1.1 mg/dL
BUN/Creatinine Ratio	10:1 to 20:1
Glomerular Filtration Rate (GFR)	90 to 120 mL/min
Hepatic Function Panel	
Total Protein	6.5 to 8.0 g/dL
Albumin	3.7 to 5.0 g/dL
Globulin	2.0 to 3.5 g/dL
Albumin/Globulin (A/G) Ratio	1.1 to 2.4
Bilirubin	Total: 0.2 to 1.4 mg/dL Direct: 0.0 to 0.4 mg/dL
Alanine Aminotransferase (ALT)	0 to 40 IU/L
Alkaline Phosphatase (ALP)	25 to 150 IU/L
Aspartate Aminotransferase (AST)	5 to 40 IU/L
Gamma-Glutamyl Transferase (GGT)	0 to 45 IU/L
Complete Blood Count (CBC)	
Red Blood Cells (RBCs)	**Men:** 4.7 to 6.1 million cells/mcL **Women:** 4.2 million to 5.4 million cells/mcL **Children** (under 18 years old): 4.0 to 5.5 million cells/mcL **Infants:** 4.8 to 7.1 million cells/mcL
Hemoglobin	**Men:** 14 to 18 g/dL **Women:** 12 to16 g/dL **Children** (under 18 years old): 11 to 13 g/dL
Hematocrit	**Men:** 36 to 50 percent **Women:** 34 to 44 percent **Children** (under 18 years old): 29 to 40 percent
Mean Corpuscular Hemoglobin (MCH)	80 to 100 fL
Mean Corpuscular Volume (MCV)	26 to 43 pg/cell
Mean Corpuscular Hemoglobin Concentration (MCHC)	31 to 37 g/dL
Platelets	150,000 to 400,000 mm^3

Lab				
	Normal Range			
White Blood Cells (WBCs)				
Total	4,500 to 11,000 mcg/L			
Neutrophils	1,800 to 7,800 mcg/L			
Lymphocytes	1,000 to 4,800 mcg/L			
Monocytes	0 to 800 mcg/L			
Eosinophils	0 to 450 mcg/L			
Basophils	0 to 200 mcg/L			
	Hormones			
Dehydroepiandrosterone (DHEA)	**Men (by age)**		**Women (by age)**	
	18 to 19	108 to 441 mcg/dL	18 to 19	145 to 395 mcg/dL
	20 to 29	280 to 640 mcg/dL	20 to 29	65 to 380 mcg/dL
	30 to 39	120 to 150 mcg/dL	30 to 39	45 to 270 mcg/dL
	40 to 49	95 to 530 mcg/dL	40 to 49	32 to 240 mcg/dL
	50 to 59	70 to 310 mcg/dL	50 to 59	26 to 200 mcg/dL
	60 to 69	42 to 290 mcg/dL	60 to 69	13 to 130 mcg/dL
	69 and over	28 to 175 mcg/dL	69 and over	17 to 90 mcg/dL
Cortisol	**AM:** 6.2 to 19.4 mcg/dL **PM:** 2.3 to 11.9 mcg/dL			
Estrogen (Total)	**Men**		**Women**	
	Prepubertal	12 to 55 pg/mL	Prepubertal	12 to 57 pg/mL
	Adult	40 to 115 pg/mL	Follicular	61 to 394 pg/mL
			Ovulation	122 to 437 pg/mL
			Luteal	156 to 350 pg/mL
			Postmenopausal	20 to 40 pg/mL
Thyroid Hormones				
TSH	0.45 to 4.5 mcIU/mL			
T_3, Free	200 to 440 pg/dL			
T_3, Total	71 to 180 ng/dL			
T_4, Free	0.82 to 1.77 ng/dL			
T_4, Total	4.5 to 12.0 mcg/dL			
TPO	0 to 34 IU/mL			
Progesterone	**Men**		**Women**	
	0.2 to 1.4 ng/mL		Pre-ovulation	Less than 1.0 ng/mL

Lab	Normal Range			
Progesterone (continued)			Mid-menstrual cycle	5.0 to 20.0 ng/mL
			Pregnant, 1st trimester	11.2 to 90.0 ng/mL
			Pregnant, 2nd trimester	25.6 to 89.4 ng/mL
			Pregnant, 3rd trimester	42.5 to 48.4 ng/mL
			Post-menopausal	Less than 1.0 ng/mL
Testosterone	**Total**		**Free**	
	Men, 13 to 17 years old	28 to 1,110 pg/mL	Men, 20 to 29 years old	9.3 to 26.5 pg/mL
	Men, 18 years and over	280 to 800 pg/mL	Men, 30 to 39 years old	8.7 to 25.1 pg/mL
	Women over 18 years old	6 to 82 pg/mL	Men, 40 to 49 years old	7.2 to 24.0 pg/mL
			Men, 50 to 59 years old	6.8 to 21.5 pg/mL
			Men over 59 years old	6.6 to 18.1 pg/mL
			Women, 20 to 59 years old	0 to 2.2 pg/mL
			Women over 59 years old	0 to 1.8 pg/mL
Prostate-Specific Antigen (PSA)	0 to 4.0 ng/mL			
Optional Tests				
Homocysteine	Less than 11µmol/L			
C-Reactive Protein (CRP)	Less than 1.0 mg/L (Low risk)			
Vitamin D	25 to 85 ng/mL			
Magnesium (Serum)	**Adult:** 1.8 to 2.6 mEq/L **Child** (2 to 18 years old): 1.7 to 2.1 mEq/L **Infant:** 1.5 to 2.2 mEq/L			

Key to Measurement Abbreviations

cells/mcL = cells per microliter

fL = femtoliters

g/dL = grams per deciliter

IU/dL = international units per deciliter

IU/mL = international units per milliliter

IU/L = international units per liter

mcg/dL = micrograms per deciliter

mcg/L = micrograms per liter

mcIU/mL = microinternational units per milliliter

mEq/L = milliequivalents per liter

mg/dL = milligrams per deciliter

mg/L = milligrams per liter

mL/min = milliliters per minute

mm^3 = millimeters cubed

mmol/L = millimoles per liter

ng/dL = nanograms per deciliter

ng/mL = nanograms per milliliter

pg/cell = picograms per cell

pg/dL = picograms per deciliter

pg/mL = picograms per milliliter

µmol/L = micromoles per liter

Tracking Your Blood Test Results

It's important that you not only keep a copy of your lab report, but also keep track of any changes or improvements in your results. The chart below is designed to help you compare the results of your blood tests and, therefore, monitor the progress of medical treatments, supplement regimens, dietary modifications, or any other lifestyle changes that may have an effect on your lab values. Record the results of your blood test in the first empty column, and make arrangements with your doctor to have follow-up blood work. Document the results of each blood test in the appropriate columns, and continue to strive for optimal values.

YOUR BLOOD TEST RESULTS

Lab	Results of 1st Test	Results of 2nd Test	Results of 3rd Test
Lipid Panel			
Triglycerides			
Total Cholesterol			
LDL Cholesterol			
HDL Cholesterol			
Basic Metabolic Panel			
Glucose			
Calcium			
Potassium			
Sodium			

Lab	Results of 1st Test	Results of 2nd Test	Results of 3rd Test
Chloride			
Carbon Dioxide			
Blood Urea Nitrogen (BUN)			
Creatinine			
BUN/Creatinine Ratio			
Glomerular Filtration Rate (GFR)			
Hepatic Function Panel			
Total Protein			
Albumin			
Globulin			
Albumin/Globulin (A/G) Ratio			
Bilirubin			
Alanine Aminotransferase (ALT)			
Alkaline Phosphatase (ALP)			
Aspartate Aminotransferase (AST)			
Gamma-Glutamyl Transferase (GGT)			
Complete Blood Count (CBC)			
Red Blood Cells (RBCs)			
Hemoglobin			
Hematocrit			
Mean Corpuscular Volume (MCV)			
Mean Corpuscular Hemoglobin (MCH)			
Mean Corpuscular Hemoglobin Concentration (MCHC)			

Lab	Results of 1st Test	Results of 2nd Test	Results of 3rd Test
Platelets			
White Blood Cells			
Total			
Neutrophils			
Lymphocytes			
Monocytes			
Eosinophils			
Basophils			
Hormones			
Dehydroepiandrosterone (DHEA)			
Cortisol			
Estrogen (Total)			
Thyroid Hormones			
TSH			
T_3, Free			
T_3, Total			
T_4, Free			
T_4, Total			
TPO			
Progesterone			
Testosterone			
Prostate-Specific Antigen (PSA)			
Optional Tests			
Homocysteine			
C-Reactive Protein (CRP)			
Vitamin D			
Magnesium (Serum)			

References

PART 1—THE LIPID PANEL

Abeywardena, M, and Patten, G. "Role of *w*3 longchain polyunsaturated fatty acids in reducing cardio-metabolic risk factors." *Endoc Metab Immune Disord Drug Targets* 2011: [Epub ahead of print].

Anderson, R. "Effects of chromium on body composition and weight loss." *Nutr Rev* 1998; 56(9):266–270.

Anton, SD, et al. "Effects of chromium picolinate on food intake and satiety." *Diabetes Technol Ther* 2008; 10(5):405–412.

Assmann, G, Cullen, P, and Schulte, H. "Non-LDL-related dyslipidaemia and coronary risk: a case-control study." *Diab Vasc Dis Res* 2010; 7(3):204–212.

Bertolini, S, et al. "Lipoprotein changes induced by pantethine in hyperlipoproteinemic patients: adults and children." *Int J Clin Pharmacol Ther Toxicol* 1986; 24(11):630–637.

Budoff, M. "Aged garlic extract retards progression of coronary artery calcification." *J Nutr* 2006; 136 (3 Suppl):741S–744S.

Bundy, R, et al. "Artichoke leaf extract (Cynara scolymus) reduces plasma cholesterol in otherwise healthy hypercholesterolemic adults: a randomized, double blind placebo controlled trial." *Phytomedicine* 2008; 15(9):668–675.

Chan, DC, et al. "Plasma markers of cholesterol homeostasis and apolipoprotein B-100 kinetics in the metabolic syndrome." *Obes Res* 2003; 11(4):591–596.

Cheng, T. "Green tea may inhibit warfarin." *Int J Cardiol* 2007; 115(2):236.

Cronin, J. "Green tea extract stokes thermogenesis: Will it replace ephedra?" *Alternative and Complementary Therapies* 2000; 296–300.

Devine, A, et al. "Tea drinking is associated with benefits on bone density in older women." *Am J Clin Nutr* 2007; 86(4):1243–1247.

Eslick, GD, et al. "Benefits of fish oil supplementation in hyperlipidemia: a systematic review and meta-analysis." *Int J Cardiol* 2009; 136(1):4–16.

Englisch, W, et al. "Efficacy of artichoke dry extract in patients with hyperlipoproteinemia." *Arzneimittelforschung* 2000; 50(3):260–265.

Folkers, K, et al. "Lovastatin decreases coenzyme Q10 levels in humans." *Proc Natl Acad Sci USA* 1990; 87(22):8931–8934.

Fujita, H, et al. "Human volunteers study on antihypertensive effect of 'Katsuobushi Oligopeptide' (II)." *Jpn Pharmacol Ther* 1997; 25(8):2161–2165.

Gaziano, J, et al. "Cholesterol reduction: weighing the benefits and risks." *Ann Intern Med* 1996; 124(10):914–918.

Gil, M, et al. "Antioxidant activity of pomegranate juice and its relationship with phenolic composition and processing." *J Agric Food Chem* 2000; 48(10):4581–4589.

Hadjistavri, LS, et al. "Beneficial effects of oral magnesium supplementation on insulin sensitivity and serum lipid profile." *Med Sci Monitor* 2010; 16(6):CR307–312.

Harris, WS, et al. "Omega-3 fatty acids and coronary heart disease risk: clinical and mechanistic perspectives." *Atherosclerosis* 2008;197(1):12–24.

Hollman, P, and Katan, M. "Dietary flavonoids: intake, health effects and bioavailability." *Food Chem Toxicol* 1999;37(9–10):937–942.

Holvoet, P, et al. "Oxidized LDL and the metabolic syndrome." *Future Lipidol* 2008; 3(6):637–649.

Hu, Y, et al. "Relations of glycemic index and glycemic load with plasma oxidative stress markers." *Am J Clin Nutr* 2006; 84(1):70–76.

Hsu, CH, et al. "Effect of green tea extract on obese women: a randomized, double-blind, placebo-controlled trial." *Clin Nutr* 2008; 27(3):363–370.

Jenkins, DJ, et al. "Effect of a dietary portfolio of cholesterol-lowering foods given at 2 levels of intensity of dietary advice on serum lipids in hyperlipidemia: a controlled trial." *JAMA* 2011; 306(8):831–839.

Leifert, WR, Abeywardena, M. "Cardioprotective actions of grape polyphenols." *Nutr Res* 2008; 28(11):729–737.

Libby, P. "Inflammation and cardiovascular disease mechanisms." *Am J Clin Nutr* 2006; 83(2):456S–460S.

Liu, J, et al. "Chinese red yeast rice (Monascus purpureus) for primary hyperlipidemia: a meta-analysis of randomized, controlled trials." *Chin Med* 2006; 1:4.

Lorenzo, C, et al. "Relation of low glomerular filtration rate to metabolic disorders in individuals without diabetes and with normoalbuminuria." *CJASN* 2008; 3(3):783–789.

Lukaczer, D. "Case study: A case study evaluating the effects of bonito peptides and coenzyme Q10 in a patient with hypertension." *Metagenics Inc*; 051HTN804.

Mattar M, and Obeid, O. "Fish oil and the management of hypertriglyceridemia." *Nutr Health* 2009; 20(1):41–49.

McCarty, M. "Inhibition of acetyl-CoA carboxylase by cystamine may mediate the hypotriglyceridemic activity of pantethine." *Med Hypotheses* 2001; 56(3):314–317.

McCormick, S. "Lipoprotein(a): biology and clinical importance." *Clin Biochem Rev* 2004; 25(1):69–80.

Natella, F, et al. "Grape seed proanthocyanidins prevent plasma postprandial oxidative stress in humans." *J Agric Food Chem* 2002; 50(26):7720–7725.

O'Byrne, D, et al. "Studies of LDL oxidation following alpha-, gamma-, or delta-tocotrienyl acetate supplementation of hypercholesterolemic humans." *Free Radic Biol Med* 2000; 29(9): 834–845.

Ooi, L, and Liong, M. "Cholesterol-lowering effects of probiotics and prebiotics: a review of in vivo and in vitro findings." *Int J Mol Sci* 2010; 11(6):2499–2522.

Plat, J, et al. "Plant stanol and sterol esters in the control of blood cholesterol levels: mechanism and safety aspects." *Am J Cardiol* 2005; 96(1A):15D–22D.

Quinzii, C, et al. "Human coenzyme Q10 deficiency." *Neurochem Res* 2007; 32:723–727.

Ranganathan, S, et al. "Effect of pantethine on the biosynthesis of cholesterol in human skin fibroblasts." *Atherosclerosis* 1982; 44(3):261–273.

Steptoe, A, et al. "The effects of chronic tea intake on platelet activation and inflammation: a double blind placebo controlled trial." *Atherosclerosis* 2007; 193(2):277–282.

Terra, X, et al. "Grape-seed procyandins prevent low-grade inflammation by modulating cytokine expression in rats fed a high-fat diet." *J Nutri Biochem* 2009; 20(3):210–218.

Tokede, O, et al. "Effects of cocoa products/dark chocolate on serum lipids: a meta-analysis." *Eur J Clin Nutr* 2011; 65(8):879–886.

Vakkilainen, J, et al. "Relationships between low-density lipoprotein particle size, plasma lipoproteins, and progression of coronary artery disease: the Diabetes Atherosclerosis Intervention Study (DAIS)." *Circulation* 2003; 107(13):1733–1737.

Whelton, SP, et al. "Effect of dietary fiber on blood pressure: a meta-analysis of randomized controlled clinical trials." *J Hypertens* 2005; 23(3):475–481.

Williams MJ, et al. "Aged garlic extract improves endothelial function in men with coronary artery disease." *Phytother Res* 2005; 19(4):314–319.

Zhang, WZ, et al. "Detrimental effect of oxidized LDL on endothelial arginine metabolism and transportation." *Int J Biochem Cell Biol* 2008; 40(5):920–928.

PART 2—THE BASIC METABOLIC PANEL

Al-Maroof, RA, et al. "Serum zinc levels in diabetic patients and the effect of zinc supplementation on glycemic control of type 2 diabetics." *Saudi Med J* 2006; 27(3):344–350.

Bardini, G, et al. "Inflammation markers and metabolic characteristics of subjects with 1-h plasma glucose levels." *Diabetes Care* 2010; 33(2):411–413.

Basch, E, et al. "Bitter melon (Momordica charantia): a review of efficacy and safety." *Am J Health Syst Pharm* 2003; 60(4):356–359.

Beletate, V, et al. "Zinc supplementation for the prevention of type 2 diabetes mellitus." *Cochrane Database Syst Rev* 2007 Jan 24;(1):CD005525.

Belin, RJ, and He, K. "Magnesium physiology and pathogenic mechanisms that contribute to the development of the metabolic syndrome." *Magnes Res* 2007; 20(2):107–129.

Bourdel-Marchasson, I, et al. "Insulin resistance, diabetes and cognitive function: consequences for preventative strategies." *Diabetes Metab* 2010; 36(3):173–181.

Branch, JD. "Effect of creatine supplementation on body composition and performance: a meta-analysis." *Int J Sport Nutr Exerc Metab* 2003; 13(2):198–226.

Bulló, M, et al. "Inflammation, obesity and comorbidities: the role of diet." *Public Health Nutr* 2007; 10(10A):1164–1172.

Chen, Q, et al. "Bitter melon (Momordica charantia) reduces adiposity, lowers serum insulin and normalizes glucose tolerance in rats fed a high fat diet." *J Nutr* 2003; 133(4):1088–1093.

Christina, AJ, et al. "Antilithiatic effect of Asparagus racemosus Willd on ethylene glycol-induced lithiasis in male albino Wistar rats." *Methods Find Exp Clin Pharmacol* 2005; 27(9):633–638.

de Luca, C, and Olefsky, JM. "Inflammation and insulin resistance." *FEBS Lett* 2008; 582(1):97–105.

De Mattia G, et al. "Influence of reduced glutathione infusion on glucose metabolism in patients with non-insulin-dependent diabetes mellitus." *Metabolism* 1998; 47(8):993–997.

—. "Reduction of oxidative stress by oral N-acetyl-L-cysteine treatment decreases plasma soluble vascular cell adhesion molecule-1 concentrations in non-obese, non-dyslipidaemic, normotensive patients with non-insulin-dependent diabetes." *Diabetologia* 1998; 41(11):1392–1396.

De Vries, N, and De Flora, S. "N-Acetyl-l-cysteine." *J Cell Biochem* 1993; 17F:S270–S277.

Facchini, FS, et al. "Hyperinsulinemia: the missing link among oxidative stress and age-related diseases?" *Free Radic Biol Med* 2000 Dec; 29(12):1302–1306.

Feldman, L, et al. "N-acetylcysteine may improve residual renal function in hemodialysis patients: A pilot study." *Hemodial Int* 2012; 16(4):512–516.

Fletcher, RH, and Fairfield, KM. "Vitamins for chronic disease prevention in adults: clinical applications." *JAMA* 2002; 287(23):3127–3129.

Florez, JC, et al. "The inherited basis of diabetes mellitus: implications for the genetic analysis of complex traits." *Annu Rev Genomics Hum Genet* 2003; 4:257–291.

Fried, SK, and Rao, SP. "Sugars, hypertriglyceridemia, and cardiovascular disease." *Am J Clin Nutr* 2003; 78(4):873S–880S.

Gautam, M, et al. "Immunomodulatory activity of Asparagus racemosus on systemic Th1/Th2 immunity: implications for immunoadjuvant potential." *J Ethnopharmacol* 2009; 121(2):241–247.

Gibson, K, et al. "Therapeutic potential of N-acetylcysteine as an antiplatelet agent in patients with type-2 diabetes." *Cardiovasc Diabetol* 2011; 10:43.

Goldfine, AB, et al. "Metabolic effects of vanadyl sulfate in humans with non-insulin-dependent diabetes mellitus: in vivo and in vitro studies." *Metabolism* 2000; 49(3):400–410.

Guruprasad, R, et al. "Chromium picolinate positively influences the glucose transporter system via affecting cholesterol homeostasis in adipocytes cultured under hyperglycemic diabetic conditions." *Mutat Res* 2006; 610(1–2):93–100.

Henriksen, EJ. "Exercise training and the antioxidant alpha-lipoic acid in the treatment of insulin resistance and type 2 diabetes." *Free Radic BiolMed* 2006; 40(1):3–12.

Institute of Medicine, Food, and Nutrition Board. "Dietary reference intakes for calcium and vitamin D." Washington, DC: National Academy Press, 2010.

Isbir, T, et al. "Zinc, copper and magnesium status in insulin dependent diabetes." *Diabetes Res* 1994; 26(1):41–45.

Itoh, Y, et al. "Preventative effects of green tea on renal stone formation and the role of oxidative stress in nephrolithiasis." *J Urol* 2005; 173(1):271–275.

Joffe, D, and Yanagisawa, RT. "Metabolic syndrome and type 2 diabetes: can we stop the weight gain with diabetes?" *Med Clin North Am* 2007; 91(6):1107–23, ix.

Kallio, P, et al. "Dietary carbohydrate modification induces alterations in gene expression in abdominal subcutaneous adipose tissue in persons with the metabolic syndrome: the FUNGENUT Study." *Am J Clin Nutr* 2007; 85(5):1417–1427.

Kanoni, S, et al. "Total zinc intake may modify the glucose-raising effect of a zinc transporter (SLC30A8) variant: a 14-cohort meta-analysis." *Diabetes* 2011; 60(9):2407–2416.

Keltikangas-Järvinen, L, et al. "Relationships between the pituitary-adrenal hormones, insulin, and glucose in middle-aged men: moderating influence of psychosocial stress." *Metabolism* 1998; 47(12):1440–1449.

Kuo, YC, et al. "Cordyceps sinensis as an immunomodulatory agent." *Am J Chin Med.* 1996; 24(2):111–125.

Lewis, JL. "Disorders of calcium concentration." *The Merck Manual* 2009. http://www.merckmanuals.com/professional/endocrine_and_metabolic_disorders/electrolyte_disorders/disorders_of_calcium_concentration.html.

Lima, V, et al. "Parameters of glycemic control and their relationship with zinc concentrations in blood and with superoxide dismutase enzyme activity in type 2 diabetes patients." *Arq Bras Endocrinol Metabol* 2011; 55(9):701–707.

Mang, B, et al. "Effects of a cinnamon extract on plasma glucose, HbA, and serum lipids in diabetes mellitus type 2." *Eur J Clin Invest* 2006; 36(5):340–344.

Matsunaga, N, et al. "Bilberry and its main constituents have neuroprotective effects against retinal neuronal damage in vitro and in vivo." *Mol Nutr Food Res* 2009; 53(7):869–877.

Menik, HL, et al. "Genetic association between insulin resistance and total cholesterol in type 2 diabetes mellitus—A preliminary observation." *Online J Health Allied Scs* 2005; 1:4.

Muth, ER, et al. "The effect of bilberry nutritional supplementation on night visual acuity and contrast sensitivity." *Altern Med Rev* 2000; 5(2):164–173.

Nutall, FQ, et al. "The metabolic response to a high-protein, low carbohydrate diet in men with type 2 diabetes mellitus." *Metabolism* 2006; 55(2):243–251.

Palacios, C. "The role of nutrients in bone health, from A to Z." *Crit Rev Food Sci Nutr* 2006; 46(8):621–628.

Parihar, MS, Hemnani, T. "Experimental excitotoxicity provokes oxidative damage in mice brain and attenuation of extract by Asparagus racemosus." *J Neural Transm* 2004; 111(1):1–12.

Park, SK, et al. "Low-level lead exposure, metabolic syndrome, and heart rate variability: the VA Normative Aging Study." *Environ Health Perspect* 2006; 114(11):1718–1724.

Pham, A, et al. "Cinnamon supplementation in patients with type 2 diabetes mellitus." *Pharmacotherapy* 2007; 27(4):595–599.

Poh, ZX, and Goh, KP. "A current update on the use of alpha lipoic acid in the management of type 2 diabetes mellitus." *Endocr Metab Immune Disord Drug Targets* 2009; 9(4):392–398.

Resende, NM, et al. "Metabolic changes during a field experiment in a world-class windsurfing athlete: a trial with multivariate analyses." *OMICS* 2011; 15(10):695–704.

Ribeiro, G, et al. "N-acetylcysteine on oxidative damage in diabetic rats." *Drug Chem Toxicol* 2011; 34(4):467–474.

Rozen, P, et al. "Calcium supplements interact significantly with long-term diet while suppressing rectal epithelial proliferation of adenoma patients." *Cancer* 2001; 91(4):833–840.

Roussel, A, et al. "Antioxidant effects of a cinnamon extract in people with impaired fasting glucose that are overweight or obese." *J Am Coll Nutr* 2009; 28(1):16–21.

Saha, SA, and Tuttle, KR. "Influence of glycemic control on the development of diabetic cardiovascular and kidney disease." *Cardiol Clin* 2010; 28(3):497–516.

Savoca, MR, et al. "Food habits are related to glycemic control among people with type 2 diabetes mellitus." *J Am Diet Assoc* 2004; 104(4):560–566.

Sharma, S, et al. "Beneficial effect of chromium supplementation on glucose HbA1C and lipid variables in individuals with newly onset type-2 diabetes." *J Trace Elem Med Biol* 2011; 25(3):149–153.

Slama, G, et al. "Low glycemic index foods should play a role in improving overall glycemic control in type-1 and type-2 diabetic patients and, more specifically, in correcting excessive postprandial hyperglycemia." *Nestle Nutr Workshop Ser Clin Perform Programme* 2006; 11:73–81.

Takahashi, T, et al. "Hydrolyzed guar gum decreases postprandial blood glucose and glucose absorption in the rat small intestine." *Nutr Res* 2009; 29(6):419–425.

Tucker, KL. "Osteoporosis prevention and nutrition." *Curr Osteoporos Rep* 2009;7(4):111–117.

Virdi, J, et al. "Antihyperglycemic effects of three extracts from Mormordica charantia." *J Ethnopharmacol* 2003; 88(1):107–111.

Wang, Y, et al. "Protection of chronic renal failure by a polysaccharide from Cordyceps sinensis." *Fitoterapia* 2010; 81(5): 397–402.

Wolf, RL, et al. "Factors associated with calcium absorption efficiency in pre- and perimenopausal women." *AJCN* 2000; 72(2):466–471.

Zhou, X, et al. "Cordyceps fungi: natural products, pharmacological functions and developmental products." *J Pharm Pharmacol* 2009; 61(3): 279–291.

PART 3—THE HEPATIC FUNCTION PANEL

Castell, LM, et al. "Glutamine and the effects of exhaustive exercise upon the immune response." *Can J Physiol Pharmacol* 1998; 76(5):524–532.

Murphy, CG, et al. "Glutamine preconditioning protects against local and systemic injury induced by orthopaedic surgery." *J Nutr Health Aging* 2012; 16(4):365–369.

Nseir, W, et al. "Soft drink consumption and nonalcoholic fatty liver disease." *World J Gastroenterol* 2010; 16(21):2579–2588.

Tetri, LH, et al. "Severe NAFLD with hepatic necroinflammatory changes in mice fed trans fat and a high-fructose corn syrup equivalent." *Am J Physiol Gastrointest Liver Physiol* 2008; 295(5):G987–995.

York, LW, et al. "Nonalcoholic fatty liver disease and low-carbohydrate diets." *Annu Rev Nutr* 2009; 29:365–379.

PART 4—COMPLETE BLOOD COUNT

Cakir-Atabek, H, et al. "Effects of resistance training intensity on deformability and aggregation of red blood cells." *Clin Hemorheol Microcirc* 2009; 41(4):251–261.

Killip, S, et al. "Iron deficiency anemia." *Am Fam Physician* 2007; 75(5):671–678.

Sotelo A, et al. "Role of oxate, phytate, tannins and cooking on iron bioavailability from foods commonly consumed in Mexico." *Int J Food Sci Nutr* 2010; 61(1):29–39.

Tang, WH, and Yeo, PS. "Epidemiology of anemia in heart failure." *Heart Fail Clin* 2010; 6(3):271–278.

PART 5—HORMONES

Adly, L, et al. "Serum concentrations of estrogens, sex hormone-binding globulin, and androgens and risk of breast cancer in postmenopausal women." *Int J Cancer* 2006; 119(10):2402–2407.

Alsantali, A, and Shapiro, J. "Androgens and Hair Loss." *Curr Opin Endocrinol Diabetes Obes* 2009; 16(3): 246–253. Review.

Andriole, G, et al. "Dihydrotestosterone and the prostate: the scientific rationale for 5alpha-reductase inhibitors in the treatment of benign prostatic hyperplasia." *J Urol* 2004;172 (4 Pt 1):1399–1403.

Bednarek-Tupikowska, G, et al. "The correlations between endogenous dehydroepiandrosterone sulfate and some atherosclerosis risk factors in premenopausal women." *Med Sci Monit* 2008;14(1):CR37–41.

Biondi, B, et al. "Effects of subclinical thyroid dysfunction on the heart." *Ann Intern Med* 2002;137(11):904–14.

Brown, LM, and Clegg, DJ. "Central effects of estradiol in the regulation of food intake, body weight, and adiposity." *J Steroid Biochem Mol Biol* 2010; 122(1–3):65–73.

Buford, TW and Willoughby, DS. "Impact of DHEA(S) and cortisol on immune function in aging: a brief review." *Appl Physiol Nutr Metab* 2008; 33(3):429–433.

Cao, J, et al. "Sex hormones and androgen receptors: risk factors of coronary heart disease in elderly men." *Chin Med Sci J* 2010; 25(1):44–49.

Cauley, JA, et al; for the Osteoporotic Fractures in Men Study (MrOS) Research Group. "Sex steroid hormones in older men: longitudinal associations with 4.5 year change in hip bone mineral density—the Osteoporotic Fractures in Men Study." *J Clin Endocrinol Metab* 2010; 95(9):4314–4323.

Childs, E, et al. "Effects of acute progesterone administration upon responses to acute psychosocial stress in men." *Exp Clin Psychopharmacol* 2010; 18(1):78–86.

Clarke, BL, and Khosla, S. "Physiology of bone loss." *Radiol Clin North Am* 2010; 48(3):483–495.

Crewther, BT, et al. "Validating the salivary testosterone and cortisol concentration measures in response to short high-intensity exercise." *J Sports Med Phys Fitness* 2010; 50(1):85–92.

Deandrea, S, et al. "Alcohol and breast cancer risk defined by estrogen and progesterone receptor status: a case-control study." *Cancer Epidemiol Biomarkers Prev* 2008; 17(8):2025–2028.

Domingues, TS, et al. "Tests for ovarian reserve: reliability and utility." *Curr Opin Obstet Gynecol* 2010; 22(4): 271–276.

Etminan, M, et al. "Intake of selenium in the prevention of prostate cancer: a systematic review and meta-analysis." *Cancer Causes Control* 2005; 16(9):1125–1131.

Fernández, MF, et al. "Assessment of total effective xenoestrogen burden in adipose tissue and identification of chemicals responsible for the combined estrogenic effect." *Anal Bioanal Chem* 2004; 379(1):163–170.

Gelenberg AJ, and Gibson, CJ. "Tyrosine for the treatment of depression." *Nutr Health* 1984; 3(3):163–173.

Grosman, H, et al. "Lipoproteins, sex hormones and inflammatory markers in association with prostate cancer." *Aging Male* 2010; 13(2):87–92.

Grossmann, M, et al. "Low testosterone levels are common and associated with insulin resistance in men with diabetes." *J Clin Endocrinol Metab* 2008; 93(5):1834–1840.

Halden, RU. "Plastics and health risks." *Annu Rev Public Health* 2010; 31:179–194. Review.

Ho, E, and Song, Y. "Zinc and prostatic cancer." *Curr Opin Clin Nutr Metab Care* 2009; 12(6):640–645. Review.

Jeon, GH, et al. "Association between serum estradiol level and coronary artery calcification in postmenopausal women." *Menopause* 2010; 17(5):902–907.

Khaw, KT and Barrett-Connor, E. "Lower endogenous androgens predict central adiposity in men." *Ann Epidemiol* 1992; 2(5):675–682.

Leonetti, HB, et al. "Transdermal progesterone cream for vasomotor symptoms and postmenopausal bone loss." *Obstet Gynecol* 1999; 94:225–228.

Longcope, C, et al. "Diet and sex hormone-binding globulin." *J Clin Endocrinol Metab* 2000; 85(1):293–296.

Lunenfeld, B. "Replacement therapy in the aging male." *J Endocrinol Invest* 2002; 25(10 Suppl):2–9.

Maarin, P, et al. "Cortisol secretion in relation to body fat distribution in obese premenopausal women." *Metabolism* 1992; 41(8):882–886.

Mathur, R, and Braunstein, GD. "Androgen deficiency and therapy in women." *Curr Opin Endocrinol Diabetes Obes* 2010; 17(4):342–349.

Möller, MC, et al. "Effects of testosterone and estrogen replacement therapy on memory function." *Menopause* 2010; 17(5):983–989.

Muller, M, et al. "Endogenous sex hormones and progression of carotid atherosclerosis in elderly men." *Circulation* 2004; 109(17):2074–2079.

Mulligan, T, et al. "Prevalence of hypogonadism in males aged at least 45 years: the HIM study." *Int J Clin Pract* 2006; 60(7):762–769.

Munarriz, R, et al. "Androgen replacement therapy with dehydroepiandrosterone for androgen insufficiency and female sexual dysfunction: androgen and questionnaire results." *J Sex Marital Ther* 2002; 28 Suppl 1:165–173.

Nawata, H, et al. "Sex hormone and neuroendocrine aspects of the metabolic syndrome." *Prog Brain Res* 2010; 182:175–187.

Oettel, M, et al. "Selected aspects of endocrine pharmacology of the aging male." *Exper Gerontol* 2003; 38(1–2):189–198.

Panjari, M, and Davis, SR. "DHEA therapy for women: effect on sexual function and wellbeing." *Hum Reprod Update* 2007; 13(3):239–248.

Rasmusson, AM, et al. "A decrease in the plasma DHEA to cortisol ratio during smoking abstinence may predict relapse: a preliminary study." *Psychopharmacology* (Berl) 2006; 186(3):473–480.

Riesco, E, et al. "Synergic effect of phytoestrogens and exercise training on cardiovascular risk profile in exercise-responder postmenopausal women: a pilot study." *Menopause* 2010; 17(5):1035–1039.

Rosano, GM, et al. "Effects of androgens on the cardiovascular system." *J Endocrinol Invest* 2005; 28(3 Suppl):32–38. Review.

Rossouw, JE, et al. "Risks and benefits of estrogen plus progestin in healthy postmenopausal women: principal results from the Women's Health Initiative randomized controlled trial." *JAMA* 2002; 288(3):321–333.

Sallinen, J, et al. "Dietary intake, serum hormones, muscle mass and strength during strength training in 49–73-year-old men." *Int J Sports Med* 2007; 28(12):1070–1076.

Shumaker, SA, et al. "Estrogen plus progestin and the incidence of dementia and mild cognitive impairment in postmenopausal women: the Women's Health Initiative Memory Study: a randomized controlled trial." *JAMA* 2003; 289(20):2651–2662.

Stener-Victorin, E, et al. "Are there any sensitive and specific sex steroid markers for polycystic ovary syndrome?" *J Clin Endocrinol Metab* 2010 Feb; 95(2):810–819. [Epub 2009 Dec 16]

Tang, YJ, et al. "Serum testosterone level and related metabolic factors in men over 70 years old." *J Endocrinol Invest* 2007; 30(6):451–458.

Tannenbaum, C, et al. "A longitudinal study of dehydroepiandrosterone sulphate (DHEAS) change in older men and women: the Rancho Bernardo Study." *Eur J Endocrinol* 2004; 151(6):717–725.

Tivisten, A, et al. "Low serum testosterone and high serum estradiol associate with lower extremity peripheral arterial disease in elderly men." *J Am Coll Cardiol* 2007; 50(11):1070–1076.

Tsai, EC, et al. "Association of bioavailable, free, and total testosterone with insulin resistance." *Diabetes Care* 2004; 27(4):861–868.

Vandenput, L, et al. "Androgens and glucuronidated androgen metabolites are associated with metabolic risk factors in men." *J Clin Endocrinol Metab* 2007; 92(11):4130–4137.

Villareal, DT. "Effects of dehydroepiandrosterone on bone mineral density: what implications for therapy?" *Treat Endocrinol* 2002; 1(6):349–357.

Williams, NI, et al. "Estrogen and progesterone exposure is reduced in response to energy deficiency in women aged 25-40 years." *Hum Reprod* 2010; 25(9):2328–2339.

Woods, MN, et al. "Low-fat, high fiber diet and serum estrone sulfate in premenopausal women." *Am J Clin Nutr* 1989; 49(6):1179–1183.

Woods, NF, et al. "Cortisol levels during the menopausal transition and early postmenopause; observations from the Seattle Midlife Women's Health Study." *Menopause* 2009; 16(4):708–718.

PART 6—OPTIONAL TESTS

Annweiler, C, et al. "Vitamin D and aging: neurological issues." *Neuropsychobiology* 2010; 62(3):139–150.

Ahmad, M, et al. "Aged garlic extract and S-allyl cysteine prevent formation of advanced glycation end products." *Eur J Pharmacol* 2007; 561(1–3):32–38.

Amer, M, and Qayyum, R. "Relation between serum 25-hydroxyvitamin D and C-reactive protein in asymptomatic adults (from the Continuous Health and Nutrition Examination Survey 2001 to 2006)." *Am J Cardiol* 2011; 109(2):226–230.

Barnes, PJ. "Pathiophysiology of allergic inflammation." *Immunol Rev* 2011; 242(1):31–50.

Bartoszewska, M, et al. "Vitamin D, muscle function, and exercise performance." *Pediatr Clin North Am* 2010; 57(3):849–861. Review.

Beydoun, MA, et al. "Associations among 25-hydroxyvitamin D, diet quality, and metabolic disturbance differ by adiposity in United States adults." *J Clin Endocrinol Metab* 2010; 95(8):3814–3827.

Bischoff-Ferrari, HA, et al. "Prevention of nonvertebral fractures with oral vitamin D and dose dependency: a meta-analysis of randomized controlled trials." *Arch Intern Med* 2009; 169(6):551–561.

Block, G, et al. "Vitamin C treatment reduces C-reactive protein." *Free Radic Biol Med* 2009; 46(1):70–77.

Chellappa, P, and Ramaraj, R. "Depression, homocysteine concentration, and cardiovascular events." *JAMA*. 2009; 301(15):154–1542.

Chen, K, et al. "Induction of leptin resistance through direct interaction of C-reactive protein with leptin." *Nat Med* 2006; 12(4):425–432.

He, K, et al. "Magnesium intake and the metabolic syndrome: epidemiologic evidence to date." *J Cardiometab Syndr* 2006; 1(5):351–355.

Danescu, LG. "Vitamin D and diabetes mellitus." *Endocrine* 2009; 35(1):11–17.

Dobnig, H, et al. "Independent association of low serum 25-hydroxyvitamin D and 1,25-dihydroxyvitamin D levels with all-cause and cardiovascular mortality." *Arch Intern Med* 2008; 168(12):1340–1349.

Hollis, BW. "Circulating 25-hydroxyvitamin D levels indicative of vitamin D sufficiency: implications for establishing a new effective dietary intake recommendation for vitamin D." *J Nutr* 2005; 135(2):317–322.

Holmøy, T, and Moen, SM. "Assessing vitamin D in the central nervous system." *Acta Neurol Scand* 2010 (Suppl); 190:88–92.

Laverny, G, et al. "Efficacy of a potent and safe vitamin D receptor agonist for the treatment of inflammatory bowel disease." *Immunol Lett* 2010; 131(1):49–58.

Llewellyn, DJ, et al. "Vitamin D and risk of cognitive decline in elderly persons." *Arch Intern Med* 2010; 170(13):1135–1141.

May, HT, et al. "Association of vitamin D levels with incident depression among a general cardiovascular population." *Am Heart J* 2010; 159(6):1037–1043.

McBeth J, et al; "Musculoskeletal pain is associated with very low levels of vitamin D in men: results from the European Male Aging Study." *Ann Rheum Dis* 2010; 69(8):1448–1452.

McCully, KS. "Homocysteine, vitamins, and vascular disease prevention." *Am J Clin Nutr* 2007; 86(5):1563S–1568S.

Pearson, TA, et al. "Markers of inflammation and cardiovascular disease: application to clinical and public health practice. A statement for healthcare professionals from the Centers for Disease Control and Prevention and the American Heart Association." *Circulation* 2003; 17: 499–511.

Pilz, S, et al. "Association of vitamin D deficiency with heart failure and sudden cardiac death in a large cross-sectional study referred for coronary angiography." *J Clin Endocrinol Metab* 2008; 93(10):3927–3935

Reinders, I, et al. "Association of serum n-3 polyunsaturated fatty acids with C-reactive protein in men." *Eur J Clin Nutr* 2012; 66(6):736–741.

Ridker, PM. "Clinical application of C-reactive protein for cardiovascular. disease detection and prevention." *Circulation* 2003; 107(3): 363–369.

—. "C-reactive protein." *Circulation* 2003; 108:e81–e85.

Shoji, T, et al. "Lower risk for cardiovascular mortality in oral 1alpha-hydroxy vitamin D3 users in a haemodialysis population." *Nephrol Dial Transplant* 2004; 19:179–184.

Sugden, JA, et al. "Vitamin D improves endothelial function in patients with type 2 diabetes mellitus and low vitamin D levels." *Diabet Med* 2008; 25(3):320–325.

Tucker, KL, et al. "Potassium, magnesium, and fruit and vegetable intakes are associated with greater bone mineral density in elderly men and women." *Am J Clin Nutr* 1999; 69(4):727–736.

Verstuyf, A, et al. "Vitamin D: a pleiotropic hormone." *Kidney Int* 2010; 78(2):140–145.

Vieth, R. "Vitamin D supplementation, 25-hydroxyvitamin D concentrations, and safety." *Am J Clin Nutr* 1999; 69(5):842–856.

Wasserman, RH. "Vitamin D and the dual processes of intestinal calcium absorption." *J Nutr* 2004; 134(11):3137–3139.

Yeh, E, and Willerson, J. "Coming of age of C-reactive protein: using inflammation markers in cardiology." *Circulation* 2003; 107(3):370–372.

About the Author

James LaValle, RPh, CCN, is a nationally recognized clinical pharmacist, author, and board-certified clinical nutritionist. He is the founder of LaValle Metabolic Institute, an interdisciplinary clinic in Cincinnati, and Integrative Health Resources, an industry consulting company. He was awarded the Natural Products Association's Clinician Award in 2011 for excellence in integrative medicine modalities. In 2010, LaValle started a venture with Life Time Fitness, the largest publicly traded fitness company in the United States. As their lead nutrition and metabolism expert, he develops Life Time's national nutrition education, protocol design, and product development initiatives. LaValle was also named one of the "50 Most Influential Pharmacists" by *American Druggist* magazine, and was one of only nine Americans selected to participate in the inaugural Dietary Supplement Education Alliance and Dietary Supplement Information Bureau.

In addition to serving as the nutrition correspondent for *Body Shaping,* the top fitness show on ESPN II, LaValle is the author of over eighteen books, including *Cracking the Metabolic Code, Smart Medicine for Healthier Living, The Nutritional Cost of Prescription Drugs,* and comprehensive reference charts on drug-induced nutrient depletion, herbs, and vitamins. He served as an adjunct associate professor at Cincinnati College of Pharmacy for over fourteen years and currently serves as adjunct professor of metabolic medicine at the University of South Florida Medical School. He has written hundreds of articles and developed and organized education seminars on natural therapeutics across various healthcare professions, as well as for consumer audiences globally.

Index

OTHER SQUAREONE TITLES OF INTEREST

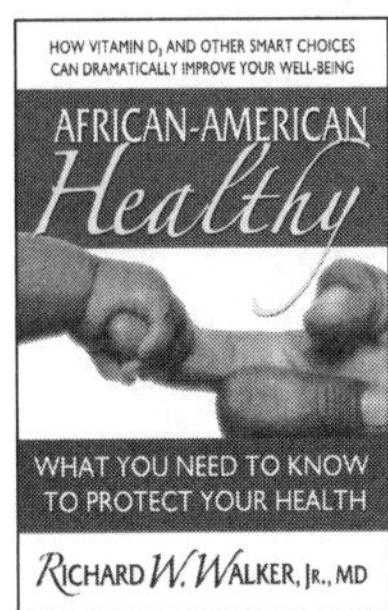

AFRICAN-AMERICAN HEALTHY

What You Need to Know to Protect Your Health

Richard W. Walker, Jr., MD

It's no secret that African Americans top the list of groups afflicted by hypertension, stroke, diabetes, heart disease, kidney failure, and cancer. As an African-American physician, Dr. Richard Walker has studied these conditions among his patients for many years. Now, for the first time, the author offers a commonsense way to prevent, reduce, and possibly eliminate these killers, turning the tide of black health.

Dr. Walker begins by looking at the black community's lifestyle. He then focuses on each major illness affecting this community and explores what it is, what its symptoms are, and how the reader can avoid or treat the problem through diet, exercise, and essential supplements such as vitamin D_3. A concise yet critical guide, *African-American Healthy* is an important first step towards achieving a healthier, longer life for millions of people.

$15.95 US • 160 pages • 6 x 9-inch quality paperback • ISBN 978-0-7570-0361-5

WHY YOU CAN'T LOSE WEIGHT

Why It's So Hard to Shed Pounds and What You Can Do About It

Pamela Wartian Smith, MD, MPH

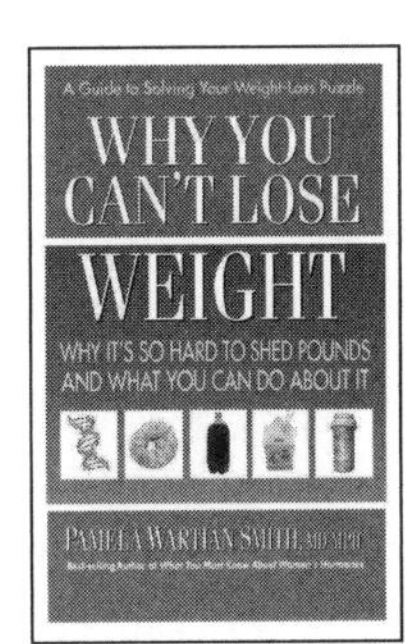

If you have tried diet after diet without shedding pounds, it may not be your fault. In this revolutionary book, Dr. Pamela Smith discusses the eighteen most common reasons why you can't lose weight, and guides you in overcoming the obstacles that stand between you and a trimmer body.

Why You Can't Lose Weight is divided into four parts. Part I looks at lifestyle practices, such as insufficient exercise and sleep. Part II examines health disorders, such as food allergies and thyroid hormone dysfunction. And Part III discusses biochemical problems, such as insulin resistance and depression. For each difficulty discussed, the author explains how the problem can be recognized, how it contributes to weight gain, and how you can take steps towards a slimmer body. The last part guides you in putting together a customized, easy-to-follow weight-loss program.

If you've been frustrated by one-size-fits-all diet plans, it's time to learn what's really keeping you from reaching your goal. With *Why You Can't Lose Weight,* you'll discover how to lose weight and enjoy radiant health.

$16.95 US • 256 pages • 6 x 9-inch quality paperback • ISBN 978-0-7570-0312-7

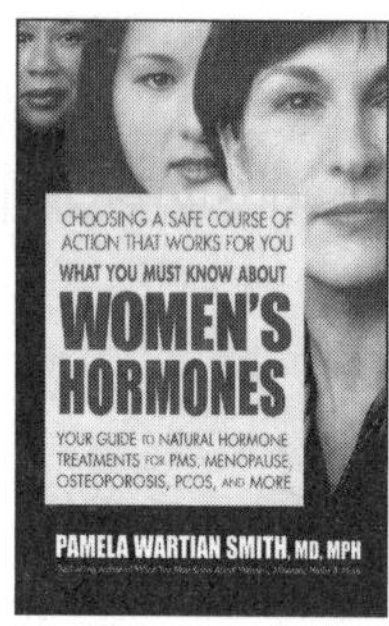

WHAT YOU MUST KNOW ABOUT WOMEN'S HORMONES

Your Guide to Natural Hormone Treatments for PMS, Menopause, Osteoporosis, PCOS, and More

Pamela Wartian Smith, MD, MPH

Hormonal imbalances can occur at any age and for a variety of reasons. While most related problems are associated with menopause, fluctuating hormonal levels can also cause a variety of other conditions. *What You Must Know About Women's Hormones* is a guide to the treatment of hormonal irregularities without the health risks associated with standard hormone replacement therapy.

Part I of this book describes the body's own hormones, looking at their functions and the problems that can occur if they are not at optimal levels. Part II focuses on the most common problems that arise from hormonal imbalances, such as PMS and endometriosis. Part III details hormone replacement therapy, focusing on the difference between natural and synthetic treatments. *What You Must Know About Women's Hormones* can make a profound difference in your life.

$17.95 US • 256 pages • 6 x 9-inch quality paperback • ISBN 978-0-7570-0307-3

WHAT YOU MUST KNOW ABOUT BIOIDENTICAL HORMONE REPLACEMENT THERAPY

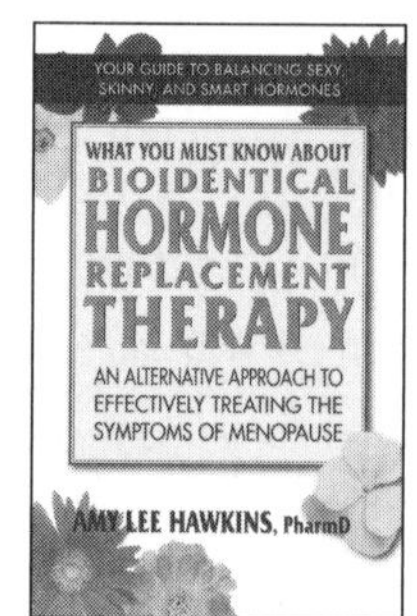

An Alternative Approach to Effectively Treating the Symptoms of Menopause

Amy Lee Hawkins, PharmD

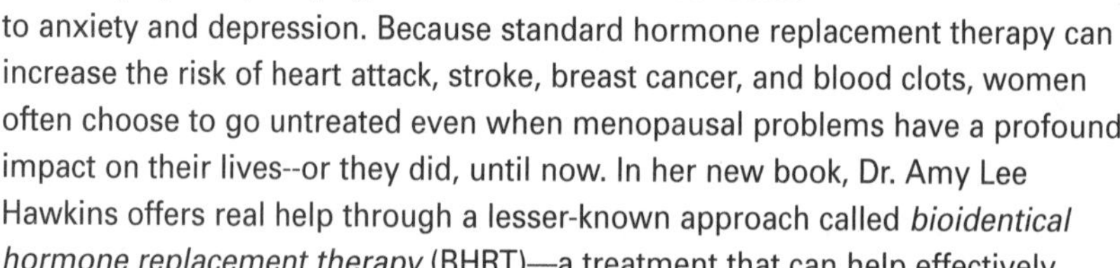

Although normal and natural, menopause can cause severe symptoms, ranging from insomnia and hot flashes to anxiety and depression. Because standard hormone replacement therapy can increase the risk of heart attack, stroke, breast cancer, and blood clots, women often choose to go untreated even when menopausal problems have a profound impact on their lives--or they did, until now. In her new book, Dr. Amy Lee Hawkins offers real help through a lesser-known approach called *bioidentical hormone replacement therapy* (BHRT)—a treatment that can help effectively diminish menopausal symptoms without the dangers of synthetic drugs.

If you are struggling with menopause-related problems, you want the safest, most effective route to feeling better. *What You Must Know About Bioidentical Hormone Replacement Therapy* provides the information you need to make the best possible decisions about your health.

$17.95 US • 240 pages • 6 x 9-inch quality paperback • ISBN 978-0-7570-0380-6

What You Must Know About Vitamins, Minerals, Herbs & More

Choosing the Nutrients That Are Right for You

Pamela Wartian Smith, MD, MPH

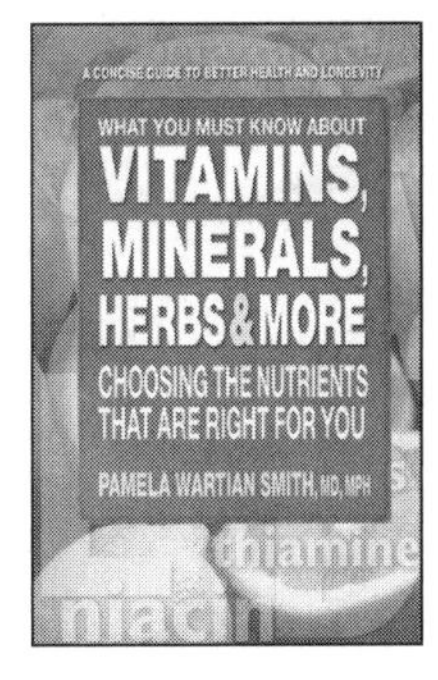

Almost 75 percent of health and longevity is based on lifestyle, environment, and nutrition. Yet even if you follow a healthful diet, you probably don't get all the nutrients you need to prevent disease. In this book, Dr. Pamela Smith explains how you can maintain health through the use of nutrients.

Part One of this easy-to-use guide discusses the individual nutrients necessary for good health. Part Two offers personalized nutritional programs for people with a wide variety of health concerns. People without prior medical problems can look to Part Three for their supplementation plans. Whether you want to maintain good health or you are trying to overcome a medical condition, *What You Must Know About Vitamins, Minerals, Herbs & More* can help you make the best choices for the health and well-being of you and your family.

$15.95 US • 448 pages • 6 x 9-inch quality paperback • ISBN 978-0-7570-0233-5

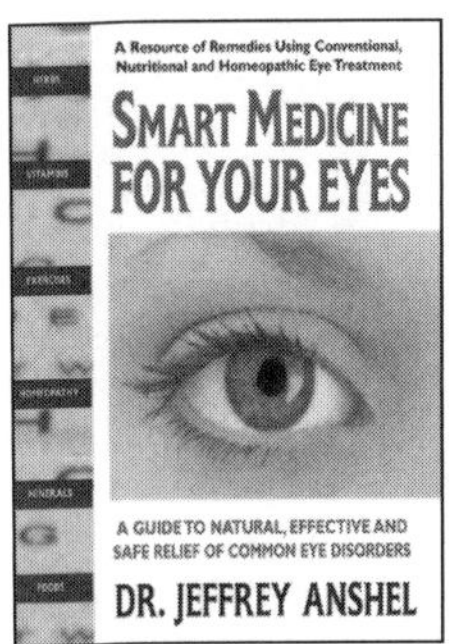

Smart Medicine for Your Eyes

A Guide to Natural, Effective, and Safe Relief of Common Eye Disorders

Jeffrey Anshel, OD

Trouble can start with headaches and blurred vision, or simply with redness and tearing. Certainly going to an eye-care professional is essential, but to be part of the solution, you must be informed. Designed for everyone who wants to take an active part in their own eye care, *Smart Medicine for Your Eyes* is an A-to-Z guide to the most common eye disorders and their treatments, using both conventional and alternative treatments.

This easy-to-understand book is divided into three parts. Part One provides an overview of eye function and introduces treatment methods, Part Two is a comprehensive directory to eye disorders and their therapy options, and Part Three guides you in using the recommended procedures. Here is a reliable source of information that you will turn to time and again to protect the greatest of your possessions--your eyes.

$19.95 US • 424 pages • 7.5 x 9-inch quality paperback • ISBN 978-0-7570-0301-1

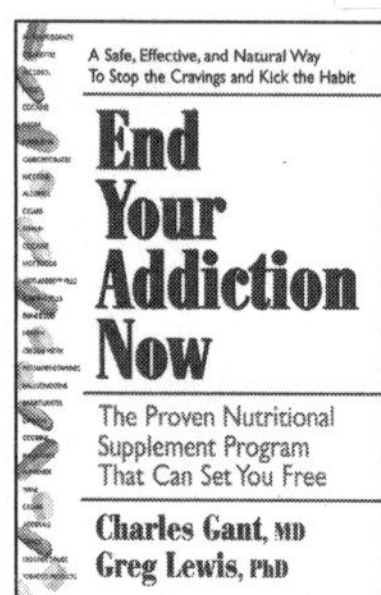

End Your Addiction Now

The Proven Nutritional Supplement Program That Can Set You Free

Charles Gant, MD, and Greg Lewis, PhD

While a number of rehabilitation programs are available, too many people with addictions return to their old habits. *End Your Addiction Now* explores the biochemical factors that are the real cause of this problem and offers proven advice on how to break addictions once and for all. A distinctive program of nutritional supplements is designed to jump-start recovery, which begins with a natural process of detoxification. Biochemical testing pinpoints the specific deficiencies that must be addressed to achieve complete recovery.

$16.95 US • 304 pages • 6 x 9-inch quality paperback • ISBN 978-0-7570-0313-4

15 Natural Remedies for Migraine Headaches

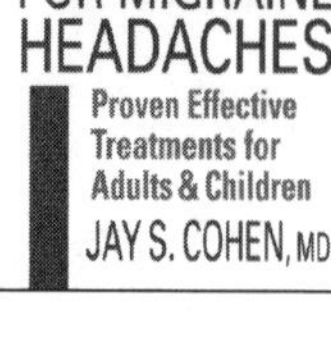

Proven Effective Treatments for Adults and Children

Jay S. Cohen, MD

Over the last few years, several powerful prescription migraine drugs have become available. Although many work, most have side effects that can cause individuals to stop treatment. For anyone who has yet to find relief from migraines, best-selling author Jay Cohen offers a concise and practical guide to natural remedies that are just as effective as their conventional counterparts, but much safer.

The book begins by explaining what migraines are and examining their causes, symptoms, and triggers. It then provides a comprehensive list of the most valuable natural migraine therapies available. Each entry includes an easy-to-understand explanation of the remedy, how it works, and its recommended dosage. The author also details which of these remedies can prevent migraines in children and adolescents. Finally, he reveals which treatments may be used to stop an acute migraine attack.

$7.95 US • 160 pages • 4 x 7-inch mass paperback • ISBN 978-0-7570-0358-5